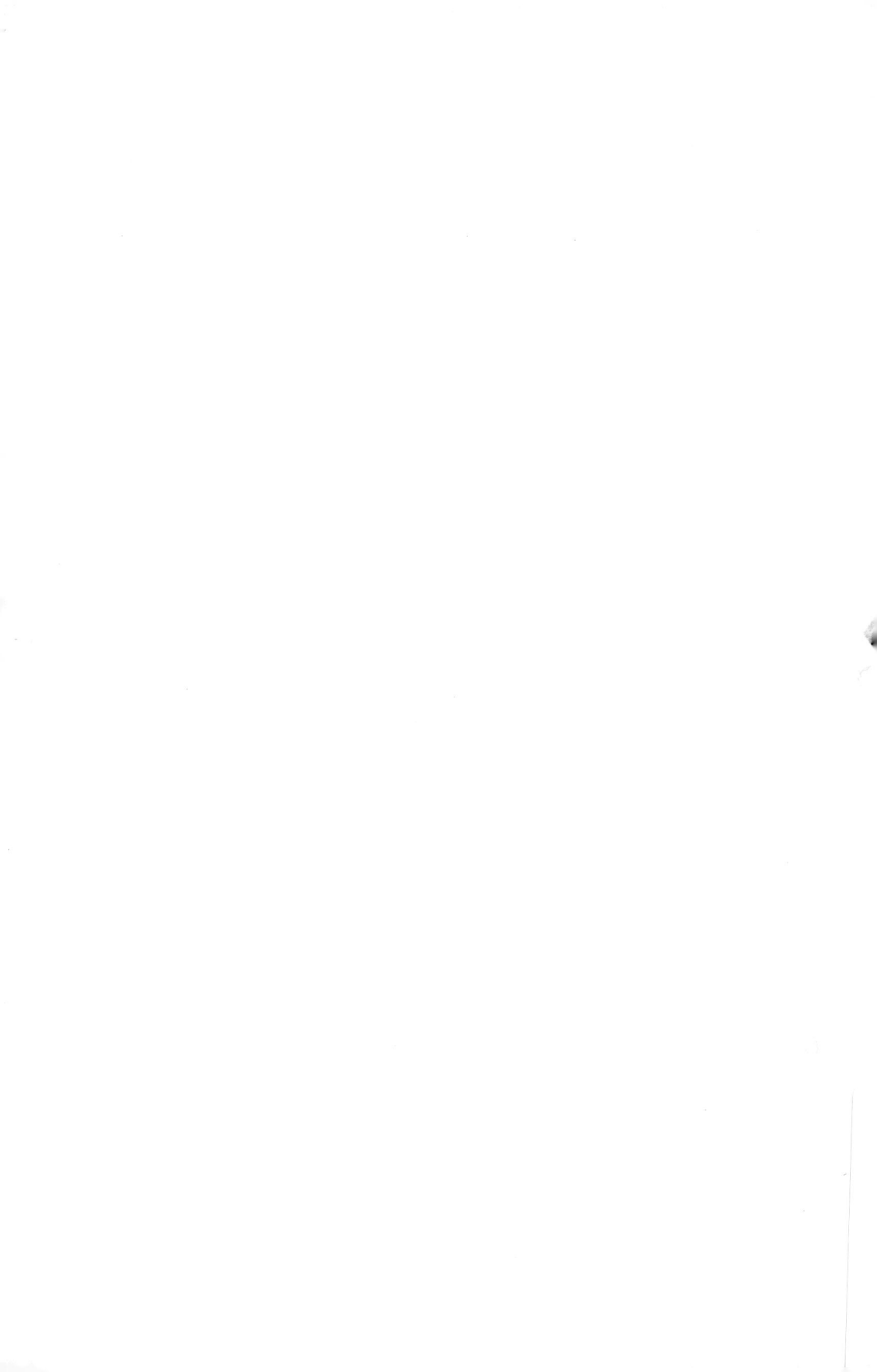

Self-Help in Mental Health

T. Mark Harwood · Luciano L'Abate

Self-Help in Mental Health

A Critical Review

Springer

T. Mark Harwood
Director of Clinical Training
Associate Professor of Clinical Psychology
Wheaton College
Psychology Department
Wheaton, IL 60185
USA

Luciano L'Abate
Georgia State University
Department of Psychology
33 Gilmer Street
Atlanta, GA 30303-3082
USA

ISBN 978-1-4419-1098-1   e-ISBN 978-1-4419-1099-8
DOI 10.1007/978-1-4419-1099-8
Springer New York Dordrecht Heidelberg London

Library of Congress Control Number: 2009935053

Printed on acid-free paper

Springer is part of Springer Science+Business Media (www.springer.com)

In memory of Dr. Thomas R. Harwood, M.D.: A consummate physician, man of integrity, and wonderful father. I miss you everyday.

To the memory of Alma Zaccaro L'Abate and Giovanni L'Abate for providing me with whatever motivation I have received to "fare una bella figura," and to introduce me to the important values of my life, my music, and my Waldensian heritage "Lux lucet in tenebris."

Foreword

Self-help is big business, but alas not a scientific business. The estimated 10 billion—that's with a "b"—spent each year on self-help in the United States is rarely guided by research or monitored by mental health professionals. Instead, marketing and metaphysics triumph. The more outrageous the "miraculous cure" and the "revolutionary secret," the better the sales. Of the 3,000 plus self-help books published each year, only a dozen contain controlled research documenting their effectiveness as stand-alone self-help. Of the 20,000 plus psychological and relationship web sites available on the Internet, only a couple hundred meet professional standards for accuracy and balance. Most, in fact, sell a commercial product.

Pity the layperson, or for that matter, the practitioner, trying to navigate the self-help morass. We are bombarded with thousands of potential resources and contradictory advice. Should we seek wisdom in a self-help book, an online site, a 12-step group, an engaging autobiography, a treatment manual, an inspiring movie, or distance writing? Should we just do it, or just say no? Work toward change or accept what is? Love your inner child or grow out of your Peter Pan? I become confused and discouraged just contemplating the choices.

Make no mistake: Self-help can hurt as well as heal. Our research indicates that 10% of self-help resources are rated as harmful by clinical psychologists familiar with them. When scientifically dubious material is marketed to vulnerable people struggling with painful disorders, harm can and does occur. Such materials may waste their time and money. Such materials may dissuade them from seeking more effective and proven treatments. Such "guaranteed successes" may have people blaming themselves for their disorders and thwarting future efforts to recover. And, of course, harmful and even benign self-help materials tarnish the credibility of mental health professionals, as few laypersons can accurately differentiate between professional treatment and self-help nonsense.

How might the responsible practitioner reconcile the power and ubiquity of self-help, on the one hand, with its unregulated, Byzantine, and potentially harmful nature, on the other? By turning to Drs. Harwood and L'Abate's *The Self-help Movement in Mental Health: A Critical Evaluation.* These distinguished authors provide trenchant evaluations of the self-help literature, organize the morass into meaningful parts, and offer evidence-based self-support resources. The authors also tackle the thorny question of when self-help might prove unhelpful or contraindicated.

Mark Harwood and Luciano L'Abate tender a cornucopia of research-supported self-help initiated, guided, maintained, or monitored by professionals. They address bibliotherapy, distance writing online, support groups, health-related newsletters, and more for specific clinical disorders—anxiety, depression, addiction, eating disturbances, and personality disorders, among them. Something useful for every client or consumer to try; something practical for every practitioner to recommend.

The self-help revolution is here and it is growing. More people this year will read a self-help book, attend a 12-step group, or obtain psychological advice from the Internet than receive treatment from all specialized mental health professionals combined. Self-help is *the* major pathway to behavior change; self-help is *the* de facto treatment for most behavioral disorders. I implore you to use this book to select and harness self-help for the benefit of our patients and the populace. We professionals, by our behavior, can significantly enhance the effectiveness and safety of self-help.

John C. Norcross

Preface

This book aims to review the self-help (SH) movement in mental health (MH) through empirically based approaches in health promotion, prevention of illness, psychotherapy, and rehabilitation. Mental health is a vast field composed of multifarious aspects, including SH approaches that are self-administered or that can be administered by professionals, middle-level professionals, as well as volunteers. This review is conducted from an empirical standpoint, that is, how valid and reliable are claims made by advocates and supporters of this movement? What is the empirical evidence for SH? The basic question to answer in this review would be, How helpful is SH? Specifically: If it is helpful, under what conditions and with whom is it helpful? When might self-help not be helpful? When might self-help be contraindicated?

At this time, there are over 1400 entries in cross-indexing SH and MH in the PsycINFO search engine, enough information to review and to be condensed in the various chapters of this book. Even though there are many books published in this field, there is no comprehensive work that covers the field in the way (empirical evidence) this volume does, except for Norcross et al. (2000), where little attention was paid to empirical evidence. His paper (Norcross, 2006), however, brings up-to-date the literature on SH strictly in psychotherapy and not the entire MH field. Nonetheless, his suggestion to use films and self-help books as ancillary sources in psychotherapy did not provide any outcome evidence because these sources were not subjected to any empirical verification. Hence, his suggestion was impressionistic and in need of verification.

Among related secondary references available in the field SH in MH are (1) Clay, Schell, Corrigan, and Ralph (2005); (2) Kirk (2005); (3) Maheu et al. (2005); (4) Ritchie et al. (2006); and (5) Latner & Wilson (2007). Some sources are actually critically negative of the SH movement (Salerno, 2005).

Part I of this book contains three chapters. Chapter 1 defines various levels of SH and the two meanings of MH as a personal condition and as a discipline in its various applications. Chapter 2 includes the various levels of involvement in SH activities, from watching movies and reading to more active and even interactive activities, including advances that have taken place in the field of MH during the last generation, with the advent of the Internet, with its many implications for SH, the inclusion of low-cost approaches, and the increasing use of writing in homework assignments.

Part II contains all the Self-Support (SS) approaches that are initiated and maintained by participants themselves within a range of help from minimal or no help to regular interactions from external helpers. These approaches include distance writing in Chapter 3 that supports the position that distance writing will become the major medium of SH communication and healing in this coming century. The large field of bibliotherapy in Chapter 4 indicates how important this field is to the SH field. Chapter 5 covers the burgeoning field of online mutual groups and individual therapy. Chapter 6 covers the use of manuals for practitioners.

Part III includes approaches for Self-Change (SC), as distinguished from SH, that are initiated, administered, guided, maintained, and monitored by professionals, various levels of semi-professionals, and volunteers for particular conditions, including Anxieties (Chapter 7), Depressions (Chapter 8), Eating Disorders (Chapter 9), Addictions (Chapter 10), Personality Disorders (Chapter 11), Severe Psychopathology (Chapter 12), and miscellaneous medical conditions (Chapter 13).

In Part IV, on the basis of all the evidence reviewed in all the previous chapters, (Chapter 14), we outline relational competence theory that we think may answer some questions about who does and who does not benefit by SH and by SC. We close with a paradigm for SH in MH interventions based on a stepped approach, self-help first, talk second, medication, and hospitalization third, from the least to the most expensive approach.

The primary and direct audience for this work is mental health professionals, including policy makers at the federal and state levels, as well as graduate students in most mental health disciplines and graduate training programs in health education, prevention, psychotherapy, clinical psychology, couples and family therapy, psychiatric nursing, psychotherapists, religious and school counseling, social work, and psychiatry.

Wheaton, IL, USA   T. Mark Harwood
Atlanta, GA, USA   Luciano L'Abate

Acknowledgments

We are grateful to the substantial contribution made by doctoral student, Sarah Griffeth, M.A. Without Sarah's expert help with resources and organization, the quality of this work would have been compromised.

Contents

About the Authors

Dr. Mark Harwood began his training in psychology in September of 1987. In 1990, he received his Master's of Science degree in Counseling Psychology, with a specialization in Marriage and Family Therapy, from San Diego State University. His enthusiasm for this initial psychology training experience motivated him to enroll in a Doctoral Program in Clinical Psychology at UCSB where he studied under the direction of Dr. Larry E. Beutler, Ph.D. ABPP. Dr. Harwood quickly became involved in research on substance abuse and depression. He received extensive training in the areas of Schizophrenia, Dementia/neurological disorders, and aging. Mark's doctorate, with specialization in clinical psychology, was conferred in 1997. Dr. Harwood's specialization in neuropsychology and geropsychology continued with major rotations on the Brain Injury Rehabilitation Unit, Geriatric Outpatient Unit, and the Older Adult's Treatment Center at the Palo Alto and Menlo Park Veteran's Affairs Medical Center. His primary specialization in severe psychopathology and psychopharmacology included experience on the Stanford University Schizophrenia Research Unit and participation on the Stanford University's Multidisciplinary Medical Treatment Unit.

Following pre-doctoral internship, Dr. Harwood accepted a Post-Doctoral Research Fellowship with Dr. Beutler. Mark held both a Lecturer position and a full-time faculty research position at UCSB. He also held Adjunct Faculty positions at Santa Barbara City College and Antioch University, Santa Barbara. While at UCSB, Dr. Harwood lectured in the Combined Psychology Doctoral program and held the titles of Project Director, Associate Director of Psychotherapy Research, Clinical Supervisor, and Assistant Researcher. One of his programmatic training contributions involved developing and providing the instruction for two new doctoral level classes, psychopharmacology and neuropsychology, for the UCSB Combined Psychology program. Additionally, Mark taught doctoral level classes on psychopathology, human sexuality, psychiatric diagnosis, substance abuse, and geropsychology and provided all of the supervision for the neuropsychological assessments that came through the UCSB training clinic.

Dr. Harwood left the University of California-Santa Barbara to accept a faculty appointment with Humboldt State University in August of 2002—he received tenure in 2007. For a period of five years, between January 1st of 2000 and December 31st of 2004, Mark served as the Managing Associate Editor for the *Journal of Clinical*

Psychology, a top-ranked, peer-reviewed scientific journal. In 2007, Dr. Harwood moved to Wheaton College where he is presently the Director of Clinical Training and Associate Professor of Clinical Psychology.

Research Interests

Research interests include psychotherapy process research and the investigation of patient-treatment matching models (e.g., Prescriptive Psychotherapy) for individuals suffering from complex problems (e.g., co-morbidity of substance abuse and depression). More specifically, Dr. Harwood is interested in developing principles and strategies that help therapists match treatment elements/interventions to the predilections and predispositions of patients. For example, a growing body of research indicates that the dimensions of patient coping style (internalizing versus externalizing), reactance level (high versus low reactance), level of functional impairment, level of social support, problem complexity, and arousal level (high versus low distress) all provide useful information for guiding the selection of specific therapeutic interventions and ultimately improves the likelihood or magnitude of positive treatment outcome.

Additionally, Dr. Harwood is interested in research on geriatric depression and the problem of substance abuse among elders. Mark was the Principal Investigator for a recently completed research project funded by the California Endowment and partnered with the Area Agency on Aging. This project examined the prevalence of substance abuse (prescription medication and illicit drugs), depression, and anxiety among a culturally/ethnically diverse elderly population ($n = 967$) residing in Santa Barbara and San Luis Obispo counties.

Teaching Interests

Teaching interests include the following:

Psychopathology
Neuropsychology
Psychopharmacology
Substance Abuse
Geropsychology
Human Sexuality
Research Methods and Design
Forensic Psychology
Psychiatric Diagnosis
Psychological Assessment

Dr. Luciano L'Abate was born (9/19/28) in Brindisi, and educated in Florence, Italy. He came (1948) to the USA as an exchange student under the auspices of the Mennonite Central Committee to Tabor College in Hillsboro, Kansas from which he graduated with high honors in two years with majors in English and Psychology (1950). After receiving a UNESCO scholarship at Wichita (State) University where he received a M.A.(1953), he earned a Ph.D. from Duke University (1956). After working for two years as a clinical psychologist at the Pitt County Health Department (Greenville, NC) and teaching in the extension division of East

Carolina College (now University) (56–57), he received a USPHS postdoctoral fellowship in child psychotherapy at Michael Reese Hospital, Chicago, Illinois (1958–1959). After this training, he became Assistant Professor of Psychology in the Department of Psychiatry at Washington University School of Medicine, St. Louis, Missouri (1959–1964). Dr. L'Abate moved to Atlanta, Georgia, when he became Associate Professor and Chief Psychologist in the Child Psychiatry division of the Department of Psychiatry at Emory University School of Medicine (64–65). He later became a Professor of Psychology at Georgia State University since 1965, where he was Director of the Family Psychology Training Program and the Family Study Center. Retired from GSU as Professor Emeritus of Psychology on December 1990.

Diplomate and former Examiner of the American Board of Professional Psychology; Fellow and Approved Supervisor of the American Association for Marriage and Family Therapy; Fellow of Divisions 12 and 43 of the American Psychological Association. Life Member of American Orthopsychiatric Association. Charter Member of the American Family Therapy Academy. Past member of the National Council on Family Relations. Co-founder and past-president of the International Academy of Family Psychology. Charter Member of the American Association for the Advancement of Preventive Psychology. Worked for 25 years as Abstractor for *Psychological Abstracts*.

Formerly on Editorial Boards of national and foreign professional and scientific journals. In 2007 he was elected to the Editorial Board of *PsycCRITIQUES: An APA Journal of Book Reviews*. Consultant also to various publishing houses. Author and coauthor of over 300 papers, chapters, and book reviews in professional and scientific journals. Author, co-author, editor, and co-editor of 47 books, of which four books are in press. His work has been translated into Chinese, Danish, Finnish, French-Canada, German, Japanese, Korean, Polish, and Spanish languages. Four books have been published in his native Italy.

Awarded the 1983 GSU Alumni Distinguished Professorship in the School of Arts and Sciences. Named "Outstanding Citizen" by the House of Representatives in the State of Georgia in 1984. In 1986 received the "Outstanding Achievement and Service" award by the Tabor College Alumni Association. In 1987 received recognition by the Georgia Association for Marriage and Family Therapy for "Outstanding Contribution." Named "Family Psychologist of the Year for 1994" by Division 43 (Family Psychology) of the American Psychological Association. In 2003 received a medal from the President of the University of Bari (Italy) for "Outstanding Achievement." On October 28, 2006, he was awarded the Renoir Prize at the University of Lecce (Italy) for creative and outstanding contributions to psychological sciences. On August 16, 2007 he was awarded a Certificate of Appreciation from the Supreme Lodge of the Sons of Italy in USA. In 2009 he received the Award for Distinguished Professional Contribution to Applied Research by the American Psychological Association.

Lectured extensively in Australia, Canada, New Zealand, Japan, Germany, Spain, and Italy. Given workshops in many states of the Union, Australia, Canada, and New Zealand. Visiting professor to American and foreign institutions: in 1991 at the University of Santiago de Campostella (Spain) in May, in July 1991 at the University of British Columbia in Vancouver (Canada). In August 1991 he was the keynote speaker for the German National Conference in Developmental Psychology at the University of Cologne, and lectured at the University of Munich in Germany, University of Padova (Italy), and the Center for the Family in Treviso (Italy) in September of the same year.

In 1992 he was an invited Keynote Speaker for the 10th Anniversary Conference of the Japanese Association of Family Psychology at Showa Women's University (Tokyo), giving additional workshops on prevention for the Yasuda Life Welfare Foundation of Japan, and one workshop on "Love and Intimacy" for the Tokyo Family Therapy Institute. Invited to lecture at the Universities of Bari and Padova (Italy) in July 1994 and as keynote speaker for the Second International Congress of Family Psychology. In November 1994 keynote speaker for the annual conference of the Penn Council on Relationships, formerly the Philadelphia Marriage Council. In May 1996 lectured at the Universities of Urbino, Rome, Catholic University of Milan, Padova, and Bari. In October 1999, he lectured at the Catholic University of Milan, the Scientific Institute "La Nostra Famiglia" in Lecco, and the Universities of Bari and Padova. In October 2000, he lectured and gave workshops to mental health organizations and educational institutions in Warsaw, Krakow, Lublin, Poznan, and Rzeszow, Poland. In June 2002 and December 2003, he lectured in various clinical institutions in and around Milan (Italy), the Catholic University of Milan, and the Universities of Padua and Bari, as well as professional, post-graduate schools in Mestre (Venice) and Florence. In October 2006 he lectured at the University of Lecce, where he received the Renoir Prize for outstanding contribution to humanity. In October 2007 he lectured at the Catholic University of Milan, the University of Padua, and the University of Bari.

Full time clinical practice 1956-1964. Part-time clinical practice from 1965 to 1998. Consultant to Cross-Keys Counseling Center in Forest Park, GA from 1978 to 1998. From 1993 to 1998, Clinical Director for Multicultural Services in a mental health center for ethnic communities developed jointly by Cross Keys Counseling Center and a local Presbyterian Church (Doraville, GA).

In 1996 he founded "Workbooks for Better Living," to make available to qualified professionals low-cost, self-help mental health workbooks through the Internet <http://www.mentalhealthhelp.com> He has produced over 100 workbooks, 8 have been translated into Spanish and some in Italian. They will be published by Springer-Science in 2009 as a *Sourcebook of Interactive Exercises in Mental Health*.

After retirement from clinical practice (December 1998), he has taught one course on Personal Writing for senior citizens, and was a volunteer with the Diversification Program of De Kalb County Juvenile Court from 1999 to 2003. He is now involved in full-time writing and research.

Part I
Introduction to the Field of Self-help in Mental Health

Chapter 1
What Constitutes Self-Help in Mental Health and What Can Be Done to Improve It?

> *The challenge is to devise cost-effective, user-friendly interventions and to work with target populations involved to enhance their desire and ability to retain the program without, or with minimal, outside assistance. Such empowerment efforts increase stake-holders' sense of ownership of the program and the probability that the program will become incorporated into the setting's routine mode of functioning.*
>
> (Jason & Glenwick, 2002b).

The self-help (SH) movement in mental health (MH) is on the rise and its growth is necessary and inevitable. SH is an attempt by people with a mutual problem to take control over adverse circumstances in their lives. Formal SH efforts *in general* involve participation in organized groups for individuals with similar problems or in more differentiated and structured multi-service agencies. SH agencies include independent-living programs that help members to access material resources and gain practical skills, as well as drop-in community centers that provide a space for members to socialize, build a supportive community, and obtain advocacy and a gamut of independent-living services. SH agencies are distinguished from SH groups that work to help individuals gain control over or acceptance of their problems in that they are formal organizations providing services and often have a parallel focus on efforts directed toward changing social conditions. For example, some SH agencies are set up to assist poverty-stricken ex-patients and adopt the belief that members' problems result from social and economic inequities; however, these agencies also take the position that members must be responsible for making changes in their own lives and for reforming social structures. On the other hand, agencies may also reject the victimhood mentality and adopt the position that some poverty-stricken ex-patients (primarily addicts, criminals, and the attitudinally challenged/those with poor work ethics) are in their undesirable situation due to the sum total of the decisions they have made in their lives.

These agencies may offer mutual support groups as well as material resources to members that also promote the involvement of members in policy-making structures that affect their lives: board of directors of non-profit social service agencies, local MH advisory commissions, state MH planning services, and so forth. Indeed, this

T.M. Harwood, L. L'Abate, *Self-Help in Mental Health*,
DOI 10.1007/978-1-4419-1099-8_1, © Springer Science+Business Media, LLC 2010

movement might be one of the most significant MH developments in the last generation to the point that a Center for SH Research was created within the National Association of State Mental Health Program Directors. Forty-six states are funding 587 SH programs for persons with severe mental disabilities (Segal, 2005). Some 19 SH organizations in North America, Europe, and Asia offer a welcome check on the often culturally dependent conceptions about SH groups. The essential features of SH groups are (1) importance of member autonomy (ownership), (2) experiential knowledge, and (3) mutual interaction (Humphreys, 2004).

The foregoing overall definition of SH is directed toward dysfunctional populations. In that regard, Salerno (2005) argued that SH in that sense may seem like a godsend to some but like a joke to others. According to that author, SH is now a multi-billion dollar industry depending on "thinly credentialed experts" who dispense advice on everything from MH to relationships, to diets, to personal finances and business strategies. One potential downside of this movement is that instead of "empowering" individuals, they increase dependence on others. Fortunately, as we shall see, there is another *specific* definition of SH directed *particularly* toward functional populations that remain outside of Salerno's critique.

Traditional, individually delivered psychosocial practices are often cost prohibitive. Additionally, although psychotherapy is highly effective for depressive spectrum disorders and anxiety spectrum disorders, psychosocial treatment is not universally effective or it may produce only minimal improvement—in some cases patients are harmed (although this is typically due to unskilled and/or unethical practitioners). The foregoing illustrates the potential importance of self-help approaches as applied solo or in combination with existing, professional MH practices. For instance, there are many SH groups in North America, such as Alcoholics Anonymous (AA), Narcotics Anonymous (NA), Adult Children of Alcoholics (ACA), Overeaters Anonymous (OA) (Pearse, 2007), and Strategies for the Treatment of Early Psychosis (STEP). SH can also be applied for the improvement of physical and mental health, such as a group of young conservatives helping African villages cope with poverty and diseases (Bentley et al., 2007). In terms of treating psychiatric disorders, the self-help movement will proliferate and combine synergistically with traditional, individually delivered psychosocial treatments. It was inevitable that online SH would be used in the treatment of many psychological disorders, as discussed in Chapter 5 of this volume (L'Abate, 2008c).

Throughout this work it will be shown that there are many diverse uses for SH approaches (particularly online). But, what does the future hold for this promising approach? It has been projected that SH could be implemented in such fields as breast cancer (Klesges et al., 1987), dieting strategies (Segal et al., 1998), and mental health (Shaw et al., 2006). Though no one can project with absolute accuracy about this field's future, we can all be certain that it will, indeed, have a profound impact on our everyday lives. Even though self-help methods have been combined with therapies in its history (Watkins, 2008), it might be a contradiction in terms when combining SH with therapies, that is, how can one help oneself while depending on the help of someone else, which is what the term "therapy" implies? Therefore, some may wonder whether there is such a process of "pure" SH, since even a newspaper advertisement may begin the process of SH or a process of self-change (SC) (Klingemann & Klingemann, 2007; Sobell & Sobell, 2007). Self-help may be defined as a means of helping people to help themselves—this definition is consistent with self-help undertaken individually or with various levels of guidance from a therapist or para-professional. Homework, a common ingredient in CBT, may be considered a form of self-help; the patient must take initiative in the completion of the homework. Self-help is a method for not only providing individuals with the wherewithal to withstand the strains and stresses of everyday life in dysfunctional populations (e.g., patients) *in general* but also adding to already existing abilities and skills through enrichment and discovery for functional populations (non-patients) *in particular*. As Post (2007) amply demonstrated, volunteering and helping others in need can be extremely beneficial to those who help without expectations of any returns—the spirit of *agape*.

Nonetheless, SH in and of itself could include psychological benefits relevant to a sense of competence, self-acceptance, self-efficacy, and autonomy with a parallel decrease in anxiety and depression (Watkins, 2008, pp. 13–14, google.com). On the other side of the benefits coin, the wide range of possible and potential self-approaches makes it difficult if not impossible to evaluate their process and outcome in and of themselves (Watkins, 2008, pp. 15–16). SH implies self-care of self first and care of intimate others second, such as partners, children, family members, and close friends. By improving oneself it is inevitable that one's relationships with others, especially intimates, may also change for the better. Family and friends appear to be the most trusted and reliable in society's eyes regarding sources of help (Mond et al., 2007). Therefore, SH is attributed to already existing bonds between participants and those one cares for, along with the possible sense of satisfaction that can be experienced when helping loved ones, and not only family and friends (Meissen et al., 2002).

Morbidity among children, adult, and geriatric population seems on the rise along with psychiatric clinic referral rates (L'Abate, 2007c). What could be a viable solution to this problem? The delivery of self-help interventions over the Internet (Waller el al., 2005) may be a particularly effective method for reducing morbidity. Online SH groups could provide hope when participants realize they are not alone in their struggles. Additionally, online groups may prove to be rich sources of useful information for those suffering from a variety of problems (Glasser & Andria, 1999)—this topic will be discussed in greater length in Chapters 3 and 5 of this volume.

Another method that requires self-maintenance involves the use of popular books (i.e., bibliotherapy, see Chapter 4 this volume). This process requires participants to reflect on their own situation and use the book as a way to cope with their own troubles (Shechtman, 1999). A potential problem often identified with bibliotherapy is that the book, without corrective feedback, could increase the severity of the presenting problem; however, unless the individual is already struggling with a complex and chronic problem and social support is weak, this problem is relatively rare. Moreover, it is inappropriate to assign bibliotherapy without an appropriate level of therapist support for conditions or problems that are severe (chronic and complex)—likewise, a paucity of social support would indicate the need for therapist involvement. Continued exposure to problems through bibliotherapy could reveal new ways to think about problems; exposure may result in extinction or a diminution of symptoms (Morgan, 1976).

The foregoing introductory examples may illustrate many facets that enter into the meanings of SH and MH. The purpose of this chapter is to further define SH and MH and provide some clarification about how these two approaches operate separately and in unison. The two meanings for SH in general and in particular consequently lead to two definitions of MH, one as a condition of how we are (feel, think, and behave) and the second as a specialty discipline within psychiatry.

The Meaning of Self-Help

The primary aspect of MH treatment that will be considered in this volume is SH, defined as any approach or intervention focused on self-guidance and self-reliance along a continuum of approaches that rely to some extent on external professional and non-professional help. The historical roots of mental SH go back to Ash's (1920) original contribution. Rather than a dichotomy, SH and professional help constitute a continuum, ranging from absolute reliance on the self, completely outside of the direct or indirect presence of a professional, illustrated by self-change (SC) in addictions (Klingemann & Sobell, 2007), to a complete reliance on professionals for guidance, with a wide range of possibilities in between (McFadden et al., 1992).

Therefore, SH could be subdivided into (1) *self-care*, when the initiative is taken mainly by participants themselves, when participants help themselves on their own initiative to do or make something completely new that had not yet been attempted in the past, such as sleep hygiene, relaxation techniques, a vacation, new forms of social interaction, and spending time in natural settings that support restoration of optimal functioning (Smith & Baum, 2003), such as starting a new hobby or learning a new language or sport; (2) *self-support*, when various degrees of professionally initiated, monitored, guided, or interactive concerns are undertaken, when a new behavior or task is suggested or assigned by an external source, helping them through guidance and monitoring to make sure that the new behavior or task is maintained over time, as shown in Sections II of this volume; and (3) *self-change*, when individuals with deleterious conditions, such as addictions, decide to give up the addictions without any evident or visible professional or non-professional intervention (Klingemann & Sobell, 2007) or when a decision is made either by oneself or with help of an external source (often a spouse) to abstain from the destructive behavior and learn to adopt desirable behaviors, as shown in Section III of this volume (Hellerich, 2001). A continuum of SH is included in Table 1.1.

Table 1.1 A continuum of self-help and self-change approaches and levels of external support

Participants	External support
Complete self-care	No help necessary from anyone
Self-support	From various groups, AA, NA, DA, ACA, etc.
Self-help	With no or minimal volunteer help
" "	With semi-professional help part-time[a]
" "	With professional help part-time[a]
" "	With professional help full-time[b]
Self-change	No help necessary from anyone
" "	From groups with similar disorders
" "	With minimal volunteer help
" "	With semi-professional help part-time[a]
" "	With professional help part-time[a]
" "	With professional help full-time[b]

[a]Part-time may mean once-a-month visits, weekly phone calls, Internet interaction.
[b]Full-time may mean once-a-week individual psychosocial treatment.

To expand in Table 1.1, M.A. Sobell (2007, p. 154) proposed an important comprehensive model of the behavior change process that distinguishes among factors that favor or impede attempts to change or to stay the same. Attempting to change is determined by (1) *self-change*(SC) *without any help*, including "white-knuckles" resistance to temptation, engaging in alternative, positive activities, and even to the extent of relocating geographically; (2) *informal help*, including counsel from trusted friends, help from parents, help from a non-specific source, such as clergy, or reading about how others have changed; (3) *SH groups*, including AA, relational SMART recovery, mode-ration recovery, and other *self-support* groups mentioned above; and (4) *professional help*, which may include recommendations to engage in a 12-step program and other similar programs and public health or private professionals for a fee. As can be judged from this model, the costs of SH increase from almost no financial expenditure at the top to greater financial expenditure at the bottom.

This model illustrates also that not all helpers in the field of SH need to be doctoral-level professionals. In this field, middle-level professionals with a Master's degree or its equivalent may be effective—others may experience relief by clergy or para-professionals with a Bachelor's degree and by volunteers with minimal levels of education but with therapeutic personal characteristics such as maturity, responsiveness or empathy, personal knowledge, and enthusiasm that may substitute for educational training. This model, then, illustrates a progressive steps, hurdles, or sieves model proposed years ago (L'Abate, 1990) that could not be implemented then but that must be implemented now with so many more resources available, going gradually from the least expensive to the most expensive step. A caveat must be mentioned with respect to the foregoing. Specifically, chronic, complex problems, high degrees of functional impairment, co-morbidity, and paucity of social support all suggest the need for a doctoral-level clinician trained specifically in the treatment of difficult problems—for individuals suffering from more severe problems, it is simply not enough to be empathic, understanding, or mature; the therapist must be skilled in the selection of appropriate principles and strategies of change and the selection of effective interventions (Beutler & Harwood, 2000; Beutler, Clarkin, & Bongar, 2000; Harwood & Beutler, 2008).

SH, therefore, is a large part of the MH field that encompasses different populations of participants, different scientific and professional disciplines, and different degrees and levels of professional training and education, including a hierarchy of personnel, ranging from doctorate-level professionals to volunteers with a high-school education (L'Abate, 1990, p. 31, p. 102; 1992e, p. 44; 2002, p. 230; 2007c, p. 7). DeMaria (2003) and L'Abate (2007c) have argued that there is a divide between SH approaches and most private MH practitioners. The latter do not usually refer their consumers (clients, participants, patients, respondents) for follow-up or craft after-care plans for further psycho-education or enrichment, essentially for the purpose of learning additional skills, maintaining gains and solidifying already learned skills, and adopting less expensive coping strategies. Young et al. (2005) have argued that this divide is due to professionals who lack the competencies necessary for assigning effective after-care activities. If that is the case, then training program in psychology should include coursework on SH that involves the integration of clinical practices with SH components (Wollert et al., 1980). Presently, Italy is way ahead of the U.S. in combining practices that may reduce costs and hospital admissions (Burti et al., 2005). Although the research is mixed and dependent upon the diagnostic group, problem severity, and a host of other variables, a variety of investigations have shown that when self-administered treatments are compared with no-treatment or with therapist-administered treatments, the former and the latter were equally effective and significantly more effective than no-treatment (Scogin et al., 1990).

Mental Health as a Condition

Just as there are two different meanings for SH in general with dysfunctional populations and *particularly* with functional ones, there are two different meanings of "MH." One meaning relates to the level of health present in an individual, *MH as a condition*. The second meaning refers to the whole field of *MH as a discipline* dedicated to improving human functioning. The first definition of MH, according to the dictionary of psychology of the American Psychological Association (2007) is "a state of mind characterized by emotional well-being, good behavioral adjustment, relative freedom from anxiety and debilitating symptoms, and a capacity to establish constructive relationships and cope with the ordinary demands and stresses of life" (p. 568). At the end of this definition the reader is referred to two additional terms: "Flourishing" and "Normality." The first term is defined as "a condition denoting good mental and physical health, a state of being free from illness and distress, but more important, of being filled with vitality and functioning well in one's personal and social life" (p. 380). The opposite of flourishing is languishing, defined as "a condition of absence of MH, characterized by ennui, apathy, listlessness, and loss of interest in life" (p. 523).

The second term, normality, is defined as "a broad concept that is roughly the equivalent to MH. Although there are no absolutes and there is considerable cultural variation, some psychological and behavioral criteria can be suggested: (a) freedom from incapacitating internal conflicts, (b) the capacity to think and act in an organized and reasonably effective manner, (c) the ability to cope with the ordinary demands and problems of life, (d) freedom from extreme emotional distress, such as anxiety, despondency, and persistent upset, and (e) the absence of clear-cut symptoms of mental disorder, such as obsessions, phobias, confusion, and disorientation" (p. 631).

Sometimes MH is considered synonymous with well-being, a state of happiness, contentment, low levels of distress, overall good physical and MH, and a positive outlook on self and life, including also a good quality of life. But if MH is all of the above, then what is mental illness? Mental illness is defined as "a disorder characterized by psycho-logical symptoms, abnormal behaviors, impaired functioning, or any combination of these. Such disorders may cause clinically significant distress and impairment in a variety of domains of functioning and may be due to organic, social, genetic, chemical, or psychological factors. Specific classifications of mental disorders are elaborated in the American Psychiatric Association's *Diagnostic and Statistical Manual of Mental Disorders* (DSM-IV-TR, 2000) and the World Health Organization's International Classification of Diseases, also called psychiatric disorder or psychiatric illness" (p. 568).

The DSM-IV-TR, like its predecessors, includes a classification of "diagnostic categories without favoring any particular theory or etiology, with a great many details about any possible psychological and psychiatric symptom or syndrome imaginable and unimaginable, up to 300" (p. 303). The most important development of the latest revision lies in its acknowledgment about the relational nature of mental illness above and beyond its biological and evolutionary aspects (L'Abate, 2005).

Mental Health as a Discipline and How to Improve It

The field of MH as a discipline is composed of a variety of professions, including school counselors with master degrees, clinical psychologists with PhDs, physicians and psychiatrists with MDs, social workers with master level degrees, couple and family therapists possessing doctoral or Master's degrees, pastoral counselors with theology degrees and some with doctorates or MA level license, psychiatric nurses with nursing degrees and specialized training, and others. There are as many or even more schools of thought about what constitutes MH and how it should be improved; however, we shall restrict ourselves primarily to evidence and only secondarily to theories if and when necessary. No single profession owns the field of SH. Various professions are involved in mental health, each with its own contribution but all overlapping in their SH functions. When the use of SH services is coupled with traditional MH services, a synergistic effect rather than competition should ideally result (Hodges et al., 2003).

Based on substantial evidence selectively gathered in this volume and detailed also in a past, comprehensive publication (L'Abate, 2007c), SH approaches can substantially reduce the mortality and morbidity in the population—perhaps at a substantially lower cost than many current preventive, therapeutic, and rehabilitative practices. The net effect could be a boon to strained budgets in health, government, and social services. These approaches can inherently change practices in applied, clinical, preventive, educational, and rehabilitative settings. SH approaches have the capacity to dramatically alter human affairs by integrating public and private health ideologies and practices.

The delivery of MH services, particularly psychotherapy and other psychosocial care, is being increasingly limited by financial constraints. At least three trends will play an increasingly important role in the delivery of MH services in large agencies, such as health maintenance organizations. These constraints are (1) an increasing role for SH and bibliotherapy interventions (see Chapter 4 this volume), both in traditional and electronic formats; (2) MH services being offered in settings other than MH specialty clinics; and (3) an increasing emphasis on mechanisms for improving the quality and type of services offered, including quality improvement methods and pay-for-performance requirements (Clarke et al., 2006). A fourth avenue of service delivery in the not too distant future will be the advent of technology to deal with a host of neurological and psychological disorders that until now have been treated through medication and/or psychotherapy (L'Abate & Bliwise, 2009).

The field of MH consists of four different but essentially non-overlapping specialties relevant to SH that include most professions listed above: (1) health promotion, (2) prevention, (3) psychotherapy, and (4) rehabilitation.

Health Promotion

Promotion means any activity, operation, or procedure, including SH, that would improve physical and MH. Many SH activities may be self-initiated and may not need any help or prescription from a professional. A prescribed activity can be either self-administered or initiated and administered by someone else. When a prescribed activity is implemented by external sources it typically becomes a formal professionally delivered intervention. Hence, promotion means any approach, activity, or intervention designed to improve physical survival (morbidity and mortality) and enhance physical and mental enjoyment. Where is the line between SH and health promotion drawn? It will be difficult to draw this line, as the reader will discern in the course of reading this volume. Hence, SH overlaps with both physical and mental health promotion (L'Abate, 2007c); however, the contents of health promotion, as summarized here, differ from the contents of SH.

Health promotion was originally called primary prevention in the sense that it applies to mostly functional populations attempting to improve and push them to an even higher level of functioning. In this sense this specialty includes universal approaches that deal with normal rather than abnormal populations, i.e., "making even better what is already good." This specialty would include any educational enrichment that would provide an even wider range of experiences to already functioning populations. In so doing, it would attempt to lower the possibility of future breakdown, by increasing the level of an individual's already existing resiliency. Promotional approaches in this category include selected individuals, groups, or populations who seek to improve or promote healthier or more pleasurable lifestyles.

At this juncture there is no "universal" activity in health promotion. A universal approach can have two meanings: reaching the whole population or reaching those who might benefit from it. Each approach has—and should have—its limitations. For instance, the Good Behavior Game (GBG) for disruptive children (Embry, 2002), described below, could be applied only to schools and classes with some base-rates for disruptive behaviors to achieve preventive effects, not for schools or classes without disruptive behaviors. Writing, naturally, can be administered to literate participants. Kangaroo Care (described below), a form of close physical contact implemented specifically between caretakers with premature infants, shows potential as an intervention for many couples and families, as does Hug, Hold, Huddle, and Cuddle (3HC; L'Abate, 2001b). Omega-3 fatty acids obtained from eating fish or ingesting fish-oil supplements is beneficial to virtually all individuals (as long as mercury levels do not exceed safe levels). Omega-3 seems helpful to almost all persons, except those who might be on heavy doses of blood thinners, where Omega-3 has been shown to contain anticoagulant properties (Umhau & Dauphinais, 2007).

With most interventions, the basic issue lies in finding the limits of their applicability and potentials for negative side effects when larger scale studies are implemented. SH promotional approaches have a stronger chance of working at the community, state, or national levels without adverse effects (Klingemann & Klingemann, 2007). They are simple and concrete and do not require administration from personnel with advanced technical or professional training requirements to achieve optimal fidelity and dosage. Some evidence-based prevention or intervention strategies have such sharp boundaries of fidelity and other technical requirements for implementation that they lack practicality beyond research settings, where internal validity is far more important than external validity (Dane & Schneider, 1998).

Additionally, some promotional approaches might be used only when people have been exposed to a trauma or when they are likely to be exposed, meaning there could be risks associated with the approach itself. One could argue, for example, that expressive writing practice exercises (Chapter 3 this volume) might be a "required prophylactic activity" for people who have heart attacks or other acute medical events and where depression or negative rumination interact with health outcomes (Lepore & Smyth, 2002). However, one can no longer view this approach as a pell-mell for dealing with all ills of humankind (Solano et al., 2008).

The benefits of such prophylactic interventions could theoretically have a powerful impact on reducing secondary social problems, such as substance abuse or the illegal trade of prescription pharmaceuticals. Even with expressive writing there may be limits, as in the case of post-traumatic stress disorders, where increase in hurt feelings may be such that written disclosure without additional coping skills training may not be recommended (Gidron, Peri, Connolly, & Shaley, 1996; Smyth et al., 2008).

Defining the limits of any SH promotional approach, therefore, is necessary to locate and delimit conditions under which an approach could be considered effective or ineffective: Who will be helped? What approach will be more helpful than others? For instance, there are activities for children that would not be effective or may be irrelevant for adults, just as there are many interventions for adults that may be dangerous for children. Even negative findings do not necessarily mean that an approach should be ignored or eliminated; however, there may be certain conditions under which that approach is harmful or not effective. The emergence of new technologies will extend the application of promotional activities, as in the analogy of manual typewriters versus computers. The technology must be easy to replicate and as close as possible to what might be "anthropologically correct" in many different societies. There are foods and supplements easily available in the U.S. that would not be available in poor countries.

Promotional approaches suggest implications for a professional change from a financially costly, preventive, or therapeutic orientation to a promotional, public health ideology based on SH and SC (Hogan, 2007). Therefore, their existence raises many theoretical, social, practical, and economic questions. There are myriad SH approaches included in this volume that cost almost nothing, that are ubiquitous, that do not require professional time or presence, and that appear helpful. As assessed by beneficial consequences for their participants, these approaches might be more effective than individual psychosocial treatment even when this approach employs evidence-based practices (Gould & Clum, 1993).

When promotional approaches target specific, at-risk populations, they fall within the rubric of secondary prevention. Should they be excluded as promotional approaches? Of course, in dealing with human behavior, its deviations and deficiencies, we need as wide an armamentarium of verified approaches as we can find. What other criteria make for a promotional SH versus a preventive approach? Clearly, this is an important issue that needs to be debated with respect to its many ramifications.

A major issue with SH promotion approaches involves their definitions. For instance, exercise is a physical activity with well-known physiological and psychological advantages. However, is it a psychological or a physiological approach? The fact that many psychologists use it does not mean that exercise is an exclusive property of one profession over another. Most professionals are not required in the delivery of SH promotional approaches, making them available to more than one profession. Some approaches, by their definition, bypass professionals. But when there are no controls, neither institutional nor professional, what are the possibilities that an approach may be misused? Take, for instance, exercise addicts or "mindless" runners, who let these activities, negatively impact their lives (Calogero & Pedrotty, 2007). What are the responsibilities of a profession, professionals, or a scientific association? The field of SH, therefore, is vulnerable to misuse, and there is a need for quality and ethical control. Being easy to administer, inexpensive, and mass-oriented, who will control these interventions? Suggestions, some organizations, but no concrete answers exist at this time.

The decision about who will pay for promotional approaches is important but not critical for their implementation. Today, managed care is not likely to pay for SH promotional activities, let alone for preventive interventions, unless the payback in results are almost instantaneous. Managed care organizations (MCOs) have historically been concerned with the present year's bottom-line—prevention efforts will produce future returns. In other words, short-term profit outweighs an up-front cost expenditure that has been shown to increase longer term profits by a significant margin more than making up the costs of immediately financial outlay. Unfortunately, MCOs tend to be short-sighted and refuse to recognize the long-term benefits to patients and the MCO itself. Morbidity and mortality—crime, chronic illness, special education, etc.—are problems and programs borne by the public through taxes and fees (e.g., rising health care premiums driven by the demand for more psychotropic medications).

SH promotional approaches lend themselves to significant advertising and marketing participation by the private sector, because these approaches are universal and typically positive in focus rather than problem focused. To scientists and government policy-makers, the importance of these two new tiers, SH and promotion, may not be readily apparent (President's New Freedom Commission on Mental Health, 2003). If participation in an effective approach confers a marketing advantage to a sponsor, long-term maintenance and sustainability are greatly enhanced. One needs only to examine private sector involvement in breast cancer to see the impact of this conclusion.

SH and promotional approaches rely on various and different delivery systems also included in most MH approaches:

Novel Delivery Systems

Because of their inherent simplicity and product-like traits, SH approaches can be promoted via radio, TV, in-store promotions, and related marketing events. Effective prevention, intervention, and treatment need not be delivered by professionals or in person. Even the Surgeon General's report on MH (U.S. Department of Health and Human Services, 1999) or the President's New Freedom Foundation (2003) failed to include telephones, non-verbal communication, distance writing, computers, and the Internet as possible approaches in the delivery of services, such as prevention, therapeutic, rehabilitative programs, SH, and health promotion. These media are not yet part of traditional mainstream individual psychosocial treatment contact between patients and professionals. Traditional individual therapeutic approaches fall short in their access to potential patients and those who can benefit from self-help. Additionally, the traditionally underserved may experience obstacles in seeking treatment; however, most communities, even rural communities, have low-cost referral lists, and individual psychotherapy is often available for as low as $5 per session. Low-cost promotional approaches suggest that additional non-traditional avenues of interventions be introduced and systematically evaluated through psychotherapy process research, and, if found to be cost-effective, easy to distribute, and efficacious, they should be included in the professional training and practices of the future.

Working at a Distance from Participants

The notion that all patients do not require individual office-based treatment to help them is still relatively foreign if not repugnant to many MH professionals who prefer personal presence and talk to interactive distance approaches. By working at a distance from participants, we may increase objectivity and avoid personal whims and wills that may affect our judgment (L'Abate, 2008a, c). On the other hand, the therapeutic alliance may not be as robust, important nuances in communication may be lost, and the increased objectivity that distance may provide may come at the cost of decreased empathy, understanding, and the richness of human interaction that occurs in a mutually shared closed environment. Nevertheless, we believe that a variety of SH approaches may be effective from a distance. The amount of distance and personal contact with a professional is primarily dependent upon patient factors (e.g., the presenting problem, problem severity, social support). Feedback on homework assignments interspersed with scheduled in-person visits with a professional or otherwise may be necessary to check on progress and status. There is no substitute for in-person contact in determining whether or not a patient is deteriorating, improving, or simply not progressing (L'Abate, 1990, 2007c, 2008c, 2008d).

If one is interested in joining a SH public health model, MH professionals will need to learn to work with participants from a distance through intermediary means, such as computers, or new technologies (L'Abate & Bliwise, 2009), or intermediary personnel. This change may limit an effective but restricted model of individually delivered psychosocial treatment (L'Abate, 2001a, 2002) in favor of a model of interventions that relies on phones, distance writing, and the media in its different applications through computers (Chapter 3 this volume) and the Internet.

Homework Assignments

To better serve a large population of the underserved or unserved with effective physical and mental health interventions and approaches, MH professions will need to rely more on homework assignments (Kazantzis et al., 2005; Kazantzis &

L'Abate, 2007). This increased reliance on homework implies a transition from exclusive use of personal psychosocial contact as non-reproducible events to a reliance on replicable interventions as already found in empirically evaluated approaches (e.g., CBT-based programs) and most promotional approaches introduced here. This topic will be expanded in the next chapter of this volume.

Phones: Telephones are not novel means of communication. General marketers use telephone calls as their primary medium for immediate communication. For the layperson the phone could become another medium to disseminate many promotional approaches. Extensive research exists, for example, on using proactive rather than reactive phone calls to promote various preventive approaches. Mohr et al. (2008), for instance, found that telephone-administered psychotherapy significantly reduced the number of depressive symptoms and attrition rates.

Computers: There is no denying that computers are here to stay, they are part of our everyday communication throughout the world (Pulier et al., 2007; Seligman et al., 2005). Computers will very likely become the vehicles in healing. Some professionals argue that computers are not in the hands of the very people who most want and need help: children, handicapped and alienated adults, indigent couples and families, etc. On the other hand, one could argue that computers are increasingly available in clinics, hospitals, churches, and public libraries. Indeed, potential participants might be required to complete various questionnaires, tests, and written homework assignments administered via computers before they could see and talk with a professional (Gould, 2001). A cutting-edge program (Webpsych, 2009; www.innerlife.com) is currently being tested that includes patient-driven assessment and assigns empirically supported individualized treatments as necessary (ranging from no-treatment required to intensive, long-term, multi-person treatment). Empirically supported self-help approaches are immediately identified for both patient and clinician. Additionally, the clinician is provided with the empirically supported treatment manuals relevant to the patients presenting problem(s). Further, projected change trajectories are provided based on patients with similar characteristics, and actual change is plotted against average change—in this way, a clinician can track a patient's progress without ever seeing the patient in person. Additionally patients can track progress themselves to see if their self-help endeavors are producing returns.

As the foregoing suggests, computers allow for customized interventions—printing or displaying interventions or strategies personally tailored to the consumer. Substantial evidence shows that tailored interventions like these, as part of prescriptive promotional approaches, can improve therapeutic outcomes (Beutler & Harwood, 2000; Beutler et al., 2000; Harwood & Williams, 2003; Harwood & Beutler, 2008; Pulier et al., 2007).

Internet: This topic and its implications for SH promotions are too important to be considered briefly here. Its implications will be considered in detail in Chapter 5 this volume.

Technology: This growing field includes biofeedback, virtual reality, memory training, and transcranial magnetic stimulations, among others (L'Abate & Bliwise, 2009).

Vhat Constitutes Self-Help in Mental Health and What Can Be Done to Improve It?

15

n of Physical Health

ıal approaches deal directly with survival and physical health. The distinc-
ıen physical and mental health is inconsistent and weak, nonetheless, these
approaᴄ..es deal directly with longevity and mortality as dependent variables. There
are two types of prescriptive promotional approaches: (1) nutrition and (2) physical
and non-verbal activities.

Nutrition

Nutrition is necessary for survival. Today, a variety of nutritional practices exist
including traditional and non-traditional approaches.

Foods: Food is recognized as the first line of defense against sickness. Healthy
food intake is an area of controversy, and one must identify what constitutes myth
and what is a reflection of empirical findings (Fabricatore & Wadden, 2006; Finke &
Houston, 2007).

Diets: Americans are bombarded with information about a variety of diets, each
claiming significant weight loss and showing thin models or successful participants
on TV or in print media. Most claims made by marketers of diets are unsubstantiated
leaving it up to the consumer to discern which diet, if any, actually works (Katz, Yeh,
Kennedy, & O'Connell, 2007).

Omega-3 Fatty Acids: Epidemiological literature indicates that suicide, depression, post-natal depression, heart disease, inflammatory diseases, and possibly
human violence have a consistent inverse relationship to Omega-3 fatty acid (fish-
oil) consumption (Hibbeln, 2002). The evidence of beneficial effects from increased
fish or fish-oil consumption is well-documented (Umhau & Dauphinais, 2007).
Thus, psychological as well as other health conditions might be alleviated simply
by daily or weekly consumption of fish or fish oil.

Vitamins, Minerals, and Herbs: There is now sufficient evidence to recommend
supplementary vitamins and minerals (Giovannucci, 2007), but whether herbs can
be added to this recommendation is less clear. Akhondzadeh (2007) reviewed evidence from double-blind studies, which showed that the use of *Ginkgo biloba*, as
well as *Melissa* and *Salvia officinalis* either slow down symptoms or improve cognitive functioning in Alzheimer's disease participants. St. John's Wort (*Hypericum
perforatum*), lavender, and saffron may be helpful in lowering moderate levels of
depression. Valerian can still be used for mild sleep disorders, while feverfew and
butterbur can be used for migraine, with few, if any, side effects.

Primary Non-verbal Approaches

Many primary prescriptive approaches involve physical activities and movements,
such as exercise, yoga, expressive movements such as dance, and pleasant tasks such

as playing cards. Other non-verbal approaches, such as relaxation and meditation, of course, do not necessarily require movement.

Exercise: The value of physical exercise in promoting physical and mental health is so well recognized that it seems anticlimactic to include it in this classification (Minden & Jason, 2002; Stathopoulou et al., 2006). One wonders why, with its many physical and psychological benefits, this activity is not employed more often. Salmon (2001) addressed several limitations in the extant literature on the psychological effects of exercise. Nonetheless, he concluded that "...aerobic exercise training has antidepressant and anxiolytic effects and protects against the harmful consequences of stress...exercise training continues to offer clinical psychologists a vehicle for non-specific therapeutic social and psychological processes" (p. 33). The benefit of structured aerobic activity is not limited to adults; children experience improvements in behavior, attention, classroom focus, aggressive act, and other psychological and behavioral indices (Jarrett et al., 1998). Adolescents with mood and behavioral disturbance benefit from physical activity which in turn decreases obesity (Fabricatore & Wadden, 2006).

Calogero and Pedrotty (2007) made an important distinction between "mindful" and "mindless" physical activity, and listed various criteria for both. The former is a conscious process which varies in both pleasure and enjoyment, without compulsion or obsession. The latter is rigidly observed to the point of becoming painful and, in its extremes, destructive.

Relaxation Training (RT): A simple relaxation technique consists of five steps: (1) a mental device to prevent distracting thoughts, (2) a passive attitude, (3) decreased muscle tone, (4) a quiet environment free from distracting visual and auditory stimuli, and (5) concentration on internal or external stimuli. Relaxation includes a variety of methods and approaches, including progressive relaxation, meditation and mindfulness training, thematic imagery, and yoga-form stretching (Baer, 2003; McGrady, 2007). RT has been successfully applied to young children with developmental disabilities, adolescents, and, of course, adults. Due to page restrictions, we are unable to summarize the large body of positive literature about the effects of RT employed in a variety of clinical, medical, and non-clinical conditions and populations (Gatz et al., 2002).

The most effective relaxation technique may be relaxation response training (RRT). Since its inception (Benson, 1982), there is increasing evidence attesting to its effectiveness on a wide range of physiological and psychological antecedents. What is more relevant to the issue of universality in applications is the usefulness of RRT in high schools (Benson et al., 1994), middle-school curricula (Benson et al., 2000), in college students (Deckro et al., 2002), and in working populations (Carrington et al., 1980).

Meditation: In a recent review of research on the positive effects of meditation, Walsh and Shapiro (2006) surprisingly maintain that "Meditation is one of the most enduring, widespread, and researched of all psychotherapeutic methods"(p. 227). Again, space limitations do not allow for a more extensive and critical review of this approach or other approaches included in this classification. Detailed information can be found in McGrady (2007).

Expressive Movements: Dancing as another form of exercise is not only helpful to physical health but also pleasurable, involving auditory perception of music and integration of music with physical movements (Dulicai & Shelley-Hill, 2007).

Pleasant Activities: The list of potentially pleasant, pleasurable activities is practically endless. Pleasant activities may involve collecting subjectively or objectively valued items, reading, card- or game-playing, gardening, wood-working, bird-watching, watching movies, etc. The health benefits of these activities are incalculable (Anderson, 2007), and the Pleasant Events Schedule (PES) is a common treatment technique in CBT for depression.

Secondary Relational Approaches

This category includes the following approaches:

Close Physical Contact: Mother's Own Brazelton Neonatal Behavioral Assessment Scale (NBAS) and Kangaroo Care (KC) represent this area well. Human infants need considerable care and for an extended period of time in order to survive. Early engagement or bonding between the infant and mother improves developmental outcomes and enhances appropriate care-giving strategies. The NBAS was developed by Dr. T. Berry Brazelton in conjunction with a variety of child development specialists.

Originally designed for administration by nurses, physicians, or other clinicians, various investigators had mothers of newborns administer the Brazelton protocols (or very similar ones) themselves. With proper training the Scale teaches parents or caregivers how to better understand and engage the newborn. The effect sizes associated with the Brazelton or similar measures are modest (0.2–0.4); however, these effects are substantive considering that the intervention is only about 25 min in length and can be administered soon after child birth with reasonable results. The Scale is exciting and consistent with the Law of Parsimony in that it can be applied to a framework or theory which shows that various measures of the mother's biochemistry and an infant's biochemistry co-vary as described by the NBAS (Lundy et al., 1999).

Feldman, Weller, Sirota, and Eidelman (2003) illustrated another type of intervention for human neonates—though not with the wealth of longitudinal data of the NBAS. These researchers did employ the NBAS to assess developmental outcomes. They evaluated the outcome of Kangaroo Care (KC) which consists of a maternal–infant (skin-to-skin) body contact after a period of separation in premature infants. The results indicated that in comparison to a control group of parents who did not receive the intervention, couples in the experimental condition showed a significant increase in affectionate touching and proximity among all three family members (infant, mother, and father). In discussing the policy implications of this intervention, Feldman et al. suggested how this "low cost effective method" (p. 106), appeared to have no negative effects and should be subjected to a "large-scale longitudinal study" (p. 106).

Short-term random trials produce positive effects on pre-term infants (Chow et al., 2002). While approximately 200 reports exist on clinical outcomes of KC, only a small number of these reports are controlled. If it were to become standard practice, the implementation of the KC approach in neonate care would not only promote the child's well-being but also "sensitize the medical community to the social–emotional needs of high-risk premature infants and their parents" (Feldman et al., 2003, p. 106). Mothers using the NBAS or the KC intervention can be monitored through home visitation programs by nurses. These are brief procedures or routines conducted after birth that promise benefits for infant development (Feldman, 2007).

Extended Touch and Massage: Extended touch and massage is associated with improvements in physical health (Field, 1998; Jones and Mize, 2007). The major question with this approach is: Why it is not employed more extensively?

Affection: Children and adolescents placed in foster care or institutional care often receive very little tactile affection, in part because of concerns about perceived sexual behavior. Present data suggest a very tenable counter hypothesis: Deprivation of hugging, cuddling, and holding of children and teens by their adult caregivers might increase sexual behavior among these children. Ever since the trail-blazing work of Harry Harlow, research has consistently shown that touch is an important component of healthy development and early attachments (Gulledge et al., 2007).

Hugging, Holding, Huddling, and Cuddling (3HC): Basing this prescription on normative research cited above, this prescription was applied to therapy. One case study (L'Abate, 2001b) and three case studies (L'Abate & De Giacomo, 2003) indicate how this prescription consists of having participants hug, hold, huddle, and cuddle (3HC) each other in the dark without talking for 10–15 min every other day or on certain days of the week. The first case study included single mothers of the lowest socio-economic and educational background with three children from three different fathers. The second case study included another single mother from the same socio-economic and educational background with the father of her three children in the penitentiary for selling drugs. The third case was a family of upper-middle class with a higher educational and socio-economic status. The fourth was a couple of similar socio-economic background to the family. The intervention was anecdotally successful with all four case studies after a 1-year follow-up, except for the fourth couple that divorced but was reunited 3 years later.

However, this 3HC prescription should not be administered in certain conditions. For instance, it would be inappropriate to use it with incestuous or abusive families, even though it could be used cautiously at the end of treatment, as a method to evaluate whether such families are able to appropriately perform a task of this kind. Written instructions are easy to administer to couples and families once therapists have concluded that a family fits the criteria necessary for its administration.

Of course, in spite of the background research to support its administration, additional research is necessary to evaluate whether this simple 3HC prescription can be applied to a larger number of couples and families than could be managed by one researcher. Could especially well-functioning families profit from such an approach? How might this method of intervention be applied in a culture that is predominantly oriented toward performance with little time available for guidelines or directions for becoming more emotionally available to each other (L'Abate, 2005)?

3HC may not be limited to the home. At least one case report suggests positive effects in a school setting where a teacher and a counselor routinely hugged socially rejected or withdrawn children (Holly, Trower, & Chance, 1984). In addition to the benefits of touch and affection for physical health (Gulledge et al., 2007; Jones & Mize, 2007), this 3HC prescription found support in a survey (Gulledge, Gulledge, & Stahman, 2003), where participants rated hugging, as well as cuddling, among the top three of seven forms of physical affection. Of course, increased risks are involved when non-family members are involved in a program where physical contact is prescribed. Today, sexual abuse and molestation is rightfully taken seriously. On the other hand, many accused of sexual abuse or molestation have been found not guilty of these offenses; however, the negative fallout of the investigatory and legal process can be devastating to all involved. In other words, this is a sensitive area with a multitude of potential pitfalls—one must anticipate problematic issues and plan accordingly before considering implementation of the 3HC in a school environment involving teachers or counselors.

A prescription similar to 3HC, "Kiss, cuddle, squeeze," apparently has been used successfully with autistic children (Cullen & Barlow, 2002). What happens to children and teens who receive little if any physical affection? It is not ethical to conduct a random controlled group study to investigate this topic. Epidemiological research shows that children and teens who commit serious crimes tend to have a history of low physical contact and affection from their parents or other adults, and in controlled studies their violent behavior can be attenuated by massage (Field, 2002). Among children from difficult circumstances, excessive sexual behavior has been well-documented. One early report suggests a very interesting and parsimonious explanation: touch deprivation. Increased parental touch and affection may reduce excessive masturbation among children (McCray, 1978).

The research on 3HC and KC approaches underscores the importance of nonverbal communication (Burgoon & Bacue, 2003) and touch (Field, 1998), areas that have thus far been circumscribed to awareness-enhancing body-work exercises of an intra- rather than inter-individual nature. Touch may alter serotonergic functions—strongly connected to attention, aggression, and even addiction. The implications of this promotional prescription, supported by the research of Feldman (2007) and Field (1998), among many others, open new vistas about how clinical psychology, with its expertise in evaluation, could enlarge its clinical repertoires by including health promotion and public health. Clinical psychologists could assist larger numbers of people in need of help by evaluating the impact of these and many other interventions.

Intimacy and Fear of Intimacy: Intimacy is defined behaviorally, rather than through self-report, paper-and-pencil scales, as the sharing of joys, hurts, and fears of being hurt (L'Abate, Cusinato, Maino, Colesso, & Scilletta, 2010) which has opened a new field of research to find differences in how individuals want but are also simultaneously fearful of intimacy (Vangelisti & Beck, 2007). This topic is considered to be a model of relational competence theory reviewed in Chapter 14 of this volume together with forgiveness.

Forgiveness: Forgiveness is a derivation of sharing hurts and transgressions that need to be resolved in intimate relationships to produce definite, positive physiological outcomes (Root & McCullough, 2007). Fincham and Beach (2002) went as far as asking for a public health approach to spread the use of forgiveness using the Internet.

Spirituality: This approach can no longer be denied as being relevant to SH, because, as with prayer, it is a significant factor in health and illness (Potts, 1998; Sperry et al., 2007).

Tertiary Multi-relational Approaches

These approaches include more than one individual in dyads, groups, classes, and organizations.

Animal Companions: Perhaps half of U.S. households have a pet, typically a dog, a cat, or birds. Whether these companions promote physical and MH is still open to further research L'Abate (2007b). Undeniably, pets do have significant effects on the physiological functions of their owners (Wilson & Turner, 1998), to the point that they have become part of the field of animal therapy (Crawford & Pomerinke, 2003).

Friends and Social Support: With changes in the traditional family structure that have occurred in the last generation (Mitchell, 2006), friends and support groups are essential to prolonging and enjoying one's life (Rhodes, 1998; Sias & Bartoo, 2007).

Good Behavior Game (GBG): Disturbance, disruption, and disinhibition are the hallmarks of many childhood disorders that can have lifetime adverse effects. The GBG is an approach that can be easily implemented by teachers in elementary, middle, and high-school classrooms to deal with disruptive and impulsive behavior (Embry, 2002). The GBG is "fun" for students from kindergarten to high school, is inexpensive to implement, and has successfully produced definite decreases in disruptive behaviors, often with parallel improvements in academic achievement. In the review of some 20 studies, including 3 random long-term follow-up studies, the GBG had substantial effects on preventing the abuse of alcohol, tobacco, other drugs, and on preventing delinquency. GBG also reduces problematic symptoms of ADHD, oppositional defiance, and conduct disorders. Of course, results from the GBG have implications for placements in special education. Children who improve their behavior and achievement in special education classes may be mainstreamed back to regular classrooms. Considering its simplicity of administration by the teacher, the typical effect sizes associated with GBG (0.4–0.7) are substantial.

Class-Wide Peer Tutoring (CWPT): The recommended dose for CWPT is 3–4 times per week, about 20–30 min per session. This approach replaces passive seatwork where academic accountability is nearly a national obsession in education.

How did so many students matriculating from one-room schools do so well academically? That is something of a mystery, until one reads the scientific literature on CWPT. It works quite simply: Put two students in teams, set a timer. Have one of the children tutor another child quickly for about 10 min, then have them switch roles of tutee and tutor. Children give simple feedback and repeat questions for mastery. The team earns points with a pretest for completed work and post-test for work completed on the same day. Scores of studies have been performed on this procedure, with effect sizes ranging from 0.35 to 1.92 on diverse outcomes including academic engagement, achievements in reading, math, and science, and, perhaps, reducing the need for special education services (Greenwood, Horton, & Utley, 2002).

Self-Help Groups: SH groups can be viewed from three different perspectives from (1) an MH perspective, they are perceived in regard to their effectiveness as well as the processes and mechanisms responsible for the efficacy of clinical interventions, (2) an organizational perspective where their focus pertains to their growth and functioning as social systems, and (3) the perspective of social policy. Nonetheless, their important role as an integral component of an overall organized health-care system cannot be ignored much longer (Levy, 2000).

Usually self-help groups, such as AA, Weight-Watchers, or the like, are frequently ignored by mental health professionals who value their own interpersonal effects and verbal expertise over the expertise of "laypeople." Indeed, MH professionals should obtain additional information about the benefits of SH and the constructive role that SH groups can play in expanding the availability and continuum of beneficial MH services (Salzer et al., 2001). The increased frequency of war-related post-traumatic health disorders has promulgated the creation of specialized training programs for "disaster-related SH groups" (Young et al., 2006).

Mutual help groups for the mentally ill might be significantly different from psychotherapy groups on a variety of perceived social climate dimensions measured by the Group Environment Scale. Mutual help members may tend to perceive their groups as having more active members, greater group cohesion, more structure and task-orientation, ultimately fostering more independence. Members of psychotherapy groups may tend to perceive their groups as encouraging more expression of negative and other feelings and as showing more flexibility in changing the group's activities (Toro et al., 1987).

Positive Behavioral Interventions and Support: This kind of intervention offers a schoolwide approach to improving student behavior that may help reduce tensions schoolwide. Apparently more than 70,000 schools nationwide have adopted this approach (Cregor, 2008); however, no empirical evidence has been published to support claims by advocates of this approach.

From the above summary of research about promotion in self-help and mental health, it is clear that there are many available avenues with minimal costs and minimal external interventions to help functional as well as dysfunctional populations. The major issue here is one of motivation. How can we motivate people to help themselves, especially if they do not want to?

Prevention of Mental Illness

In the past, prevention has been divided into primary, secondary, and tertiary prevention; however, more recently (L'Abate, 2007c), what was called primary prevention is now considered health promotion, as just reviewed. Secondary prevention is conceptualized as simply prevention, while what was considered tertiary prevention is now labeled psychotherapy. Prevention includes any biological, nutritional, behavioral, and social intervention intended to lower the risk of future breakdown, disorders, diseases, or social problems. Prevention or what was called "secondary prevention" targets specific populations that are already at risk, such as adult children of drug addicts, alcoholics, adult children of criminals, physically, emotionally, and sexually abused children, recovered addicts or alcoholics, veterans of foreign wars, and many others (L'Abate, 1990, 2007c). Unfortunately, a great deal of prevention in the past century occurred on the basis of external research grants rather than from grass-roots, inexpensive initiatives that would provide evidence of effectiveness (L'Abate, 2007c). Furthermore, when prevention research was evaluated for "fidelity," that is, adherence to intervention protocol and how the intervention could be replicated easily, it was found that many prevention initiatives would need a great deal of external support (i.e., funding) to be replicated (Dane & Schneider, 1998). Another difficulty in prevention research involves evaluating long-term outcomes, a very difficult area to evaluate based on its complexity.

Psychotherapy

This term used to imply a somewhat prolonged professional relationship between a mental health professional and a client, patient, or participant. Winder (1957) defined psychotherapy more than 50 years ago and was given currency by being quoted in a recent work (Paul, 2007, p. 120):

1. There is an interpersonal relationship of some duration between two or more people.
2. One of the participants (the therapist) has had special experience and/or training in the handling of human problems and relationships.
3. One or more of the participants (clients) has entered the relationship because of their own or others' dissatisfaction with their emotional, behavioral, and/or interpersonal adjustment.
4. The methods used are psychological in nature.
5. The procedures of the therapist are based upon some formal theory regarding mental disorders, in general, and the specific problems of the client in particular.
6. The aim of the process is the amelioration of the difficulties that cause the client to seek the help of the therapist.

Please note at least three interesting aspects of this definition: (1) the intensity, or direction of the relationship is not specified; treatment could potentially occur over a period of a few minutes or it may occur at a frequency of 1 hr or more a week with a duration of months or even years; (2) the medium used in this approach, even though psychological in nature, is not specified; it could be verbal and face-to-face, non-verbal, or nowadays therapy could occur in writing through the mail, fax, or Internet; and (3) participation in therapy could involve an individual, individuals in a group, couples, groups of couples, families or groups of families. Therapy could include even classrooms, schools, and organizations. One positive aspect of this original definition is that it offers wide latitude in interpretations and applications as suggested by the foregoing.

Nonetheless, to make sure that the reader receives as much objective information as necessary, the APA dictionary (2007) defines psychotherapy as "any psychological service provided by a trained professional that primarily uses forms of communication and interaction to assess, diagnose, and treat dysfunctional emotional reactions, ways of thinking, and behavior patterns of an individual, family, or group" (p. 757). This definition includes various schools of psychotherapy, such as psychoanalytic, client-centered, cognitive-behavioral, humanistic, existential, or integrative, among many others. The second author (LL) has asserted that there are as many schools of psychotherapy as there are psychotherapists since the variability produced by individually administered treatment is so great that it is difficult if not impossible to repeat the same approach from one therapist to another or from one patient to another.

This variability has been addressed by trying to reduce it to greater uniformity of treatment according to empirically based principles. Note that all of the above refer to individually delivered psychotherapy between a professional and respondents. It does not include, but neither does it exclude, professional relationships based on the two non-verbal and written media, media that actually constitute the majority of SH approaches (L'Abate, 2008c).

An example of a treatment model based upon empirically based principles of change has been discussed elsewhere (e.g., Beutler & Harwood, 2000; Beutler et al., 2000; Harwood & Williams, 2003; Harwood & Beutler, 2008). Briefly, more than three decades of focused psychotherapy process research has contributed to the development of a model of patient–treatment matching. Several iterations of the model have been produced including Prescriptive Psychotherapy (PT; Beutler & Harwood, 2000), Systematic Treatment Selection (STS; Beutler & Clarkin, 1990; Beutler et al., 2000), and the most recent version (Webpsych, 2009 www.innerlife.com). Each of the foregoing iterations represents an improvement in the patient–treatment matching model as demonstrated empirically. More specifically, as the model has been refined and expanded, likelihood of change and magnitude of patient change has increased. At present, several patient dimensions associated with corresponding principles and strategies of change comprise the model employed by InnerLife. More specifically, six matching dimensions (i.e., patient predisposing dimensions), briefly described below, guide the selection of interventions based on empirically supported principles and strategies of change:

1. Patient coping style (represented by externalizing, impulsive, gregarious individuals versus internalizing, shy, self-blaming individuals—externalizers versus internalizers respectively, and an indicator of symptom-focused treatment versus insight-focused treatment, respectively).
2. Reactance level (the level of resistance to therapist direction based upon a patient's perceived threats to their independence and an indicator of the level of directiveness a therapist should adopt for each patient).
3. Subjective distress (operationalized as level of emotional arousal and an indicator of the need for clinicians to reduce or increase arousal, through the application of various interventions/techniques in an effort to maintain moderate levels of emotional arousal).
4. Functional impairment (an index of dysfunction in social and work environments and an indicator of treatment intensity).
5. Problem complexity and chronicity (related to functional impairment, a prognostic indicator, an indicator of treatment intensity, and an indicator of the need for multi-person treatment).
6. Social support (a prognostic indicator and an indicator of impairment and treatment intensity).

The interested reader is directed to www.innerlife.com, Harwood and Beutler (2008), or Harwood and Beutler (2009), for a more thorough discussion of empirically supported principles of change. We discuss, in the foregoing resources, the application of principles and strategies of change based on patient predisposing dimensions (indices of patient–treatment matching) to pre-treatment planning and the ongoing selection of interventions tailored to the unique needs of the patient and their presenting problem(s).

Rehabilitation

This term means restoring someone to a previous level of functioning, possibly helping participants achieve a higher level of emotional, cognitive, behavioral, and relational competence already present before an injury, breakdown, or trauma that has produced a lower level of functioning or impairment in any or most areas of functioning. It may consist of training or retraining skills or functions that were lost or impaired as a result of the injury or trauma (Corrigan et al., 2008). SH approaches would be included in this approach as well.

How Is SH Different from Promotion, Prevention, Psychotherapy, and Rehabilitation?

SH can be employed in all four mental health approaches. It can be differentiated from promotion, prevention, psychotherapy, and rehabilitation according to the following (L'Abate, 2007c, p. 6) criteria: (1) cost-effectiveness, (2) relative ease of administration, (3) mass-orientation or high accessibility, and (4) long-term outcome. Consequently, SH overlaps with health promotion and intertwines with and should be considered as a desirable component of prevention, psychotherapy, and rehabilitation. Furthermore, SH needs to be distinguished further according to additional criteria necessary for a specification of what SH means and implies according to the four criteria listed above.

Ease of Administration: Ease of administration means that the activity is either automatic, learned from societal norms, like nutrition, or self-identified pleasant activities. Some SH approaches may be initiated by others, but eventually external administration is dropped because the prescribed activity has been learned successfully. Clearly, the ease of administration shows that SH activities or interventions are easily replicable and concrete. Furthermore, no grant money or external funding is needed to implement them unless one wants to research their effects. Preventive activities or interventions, on the other hand, as already noted, are usually supported by research grants, and their complexity makes them difficult to replicate without external support (Dane & Schneider, 1998).

Cost-Effectiveness: Cost-effectiveness means that self-administrated interventions and limited influence by external administrators, laypersons, subprofessionals, or middle-level professionals, reduce considerably the costs of the approach. Even when an activity is administered by others, this intervention may still be less costly than preventive approaches, because it may be administered by lay-intermediaries or semi-professionals rather than by more expensive full-fledged professionals.

Mass-Orientation: Here is where the criterion of SH is fully acknowledged. SH approaches are truly universal, without limitations in ethnic groups, religions, or socio-economic backgrounds. SH activities are operative across the developmental lifespan and involve diverse strategies or approaches according to age and, perhaps, sex and gender. Though these approaches will not be organized in this volume according to developmental groupings (pre- and post-natal, school-age, adult, and multi-age), further refinements of this approach should include a developmental perspective together with community-wide approaches (Hogan, 2007).

Prolonged Results: If all three of the foregoing criteria are operational, then the outcome should produce prolonged results over time.

Low-cost SH approaches reviewed in this volume will include research supporting their use and prescription either self-initiated or administered by others, to promote physical and mental health (L'Abate, 2007c). Here is where SH overlaps a great deal with promotional approaches reviewed above. Policy and public health implications for self-help approaches are discussed elsewhere (L'Abate, 2007c).

This volume, therefore, includes inexpensive forms of self-help. Sometimes prescriptive approaches include activities and interventions proven to promote physical and mental health simultaneously. When we suggest that most self-help approaches are inexpensive, we mean that most SH promotional approaches reviewed here are financially within reach of most people. Prescriptive means that a recipe, as short as a sentence or as long as a paragraph, may be needed to explain the nature and extent of the approach, its dosage (i.e., frequency and duration), and limitations. In non-verbal approaches, such as dancing or sports, for instance, repeated modeling may suffice. In verbal approaches, such as SH support groups, the focus on talk is the only prerequisite.

Prescriptive SH promotional approaches might result in the greatest improvement for most people and at minimal cost. Promotional approaches can be used independently or in addition to traditional preventive, psychotherapeutic, and rehabilitative practices. Being easy and inexpensive, these approaches can be administered to well-functioning populations (i.e., primary prevention) to decrease the possibility of future breakdowns by strengthening levels of functionality and resiliency. With semi-functional populations at risk for a possible breakdown (secondary prevention), SH approaches can be added to traditional psycho-educational social skills training programs, and SH groups targeted with specifically selected interactive practice exercises, discussed in Chapter 3 of this volume (L'Abate, 2009b). With clinical and dysfunctional populations (tertiary prevention), these approaches can be prescribed and administered in addition to individual psychotherapy and pharmacotherapy if indicated (Baum & Singer, 2001; Sarafino, 1994).

SH promotional approaches have public health, preventive, and psychotherapeutic implications (Hogan, 2007). Prescriptive promotional approaches, because of their characteristics, make it possible to reach directly many populations with minimal cost, and often with little need for trained, technical, or professional personnel. Prescription and administration of these approaches are delivered regardless of age, sex, education or economic levels, social class, ethnicity, or religious background of participants.

Promotion of physical and mental health self-help has been cited by many authorities but has not been expanded upon as far as needed (Green & Kreuter, 1999). For instance, as Mrazek and Haggerty (1994) noted, "The current level of knowledge about mental health promotion activities that are occurring in this country is sparse" (p. 345). Their conclusion may be valid even today. For the foregoing reason, this volume represents and endeavors to update and summarize the research and practice of inexpensive self-help approaches for physical and mental health (L'Abate, 2007c).

Self-help approaches, as a whole, imply that some plan is followed according to specific, sequential steps that are not the same as conventional "universal," promotion, "targeted" prevention, "indicated" psychotherapy, or "selective" rehabilitation (Gullotta & Bloom, 2003; Mrazek & Haggerty, 1994). The difference in logic and theory, between promotion on one hand and prevention on the other hand, has important public health, safety, and economic consequences. Higgins (2001), for instance, argued that the distinction between promotion and prevention is crucial. Promotion means approaching health, as in self-help and health promotion, while prevention means avoiding pathology, as discussed above. However, self-help is intertwined in all four specialties of MH. All four disciplines need to impart and rely on SH as much as possible to avoid encouraging life-long dependence on others.

The MH continuum involves understanding SH from the viewpoint suggested by Higgins, starting from functional populations who want to *approach*, enrich, and add to their already existing functionality moving on to disordered populations that need

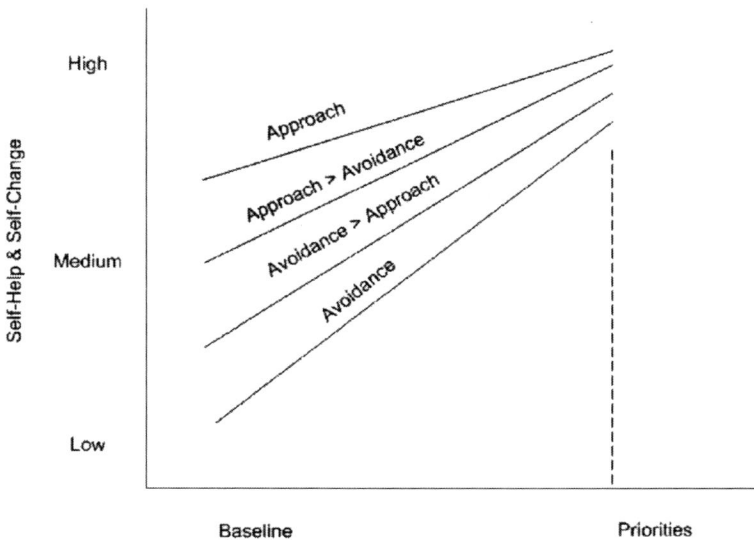

Fig. 1.1 A view of self-help and self-change

to *avoid* inadequate and dysfunctional behaviors by changing them and trying to include and approach more positive behaviors (Fig. 1.1). The baseline for functional populations is already high, while the baseline for dysfunctional populations is much lower, making it much more difficult to reach a priority of functionality. The slope of approach is less steep than the slope of avoidance because it is much more expensive and difficult to climb from an already low baseline to a priority of normalcy and functionality. Of course, SH may combine both approach and avoidance tendencies at the same time. One may approach exercise to avoid becoming obese. The ratio of approach to avoidance implies that a significant struggle is often present in the self-help movement in mental health. More of this is presented from a theoretical viewpoint in Chapter 14 of this volume.

Another relevant distinction contrasts survival with enhancement and enjoyment in life (Csikszentmihaly, 2004). Clearly, nutrition is necessary for survival, but what about enjoyment? Isn't enjoyment an important ingredient in life? Survival without enjoyment is similar to quantity of life without quality of life. Survival without any enjoyment makes for a very dreary life indeed! Consequently, most promotional and rehabilitation approaches are directly related to both survival and enjoyment, including the importance of play (L'Abate, 2009d). In their orientation toward sickness, prevention and psychotherapy do not even begin to direct their efforts toward enhancement and enjoyment because they do not include a playful component in their approaches. Perhaps prevention and even psychotherapy should add self-help approaches, including play, essentially incorporating enhancement and enjoyment in a more comprehensive model of change.

Self-help and promotional approaches aim for total population changes in morbidity and mortality. A typical prevention program, on the other hand, aims to increase protective factors or decrease risk factors for target groups exhibiting undesirable or destructive behaviors. Most prevention programs, even those well-grounded in exemplary research, usually do not meet the definition of inexpensive SH approaches. They are often costly, complex, and are not easily replicable or administered to mass populations (Dane & Schneider, 1998). Furthermore, participation in SH is usually voluntary and is eventually self-initiated, while prevention and psychotherapy, although voluntary, are often initiated and implemented by others, this is why they are not included here.

Relationships among self-help, promotion, prevention, psychotherapy, and rehabilitation are shown in Fig. 1.2 according to how many people can be included in each approach, starting with many people for SH and fewer people going as we move to the right of this figure, according to the four criteria mentioned above, cost-effectiveness, ease-of-administration, mass-orientation, and long-term results. The number of people involved in any approach diminishes as the level of dysfunctionality increases. Most people can use SH approaches. A smaller number of people do use promotional approaches. An even smaller number of people can and use prevention, while the smallest number of people avail themselves of face-to-face talk-based psychotherapy. However, the number of remissions from any of these approaches after termination suggests that many who failed in either of these approaches may need some form of rehabilitation, making this number greater than those who are undergoing psychotherapy (L'Abate et al., 2010).

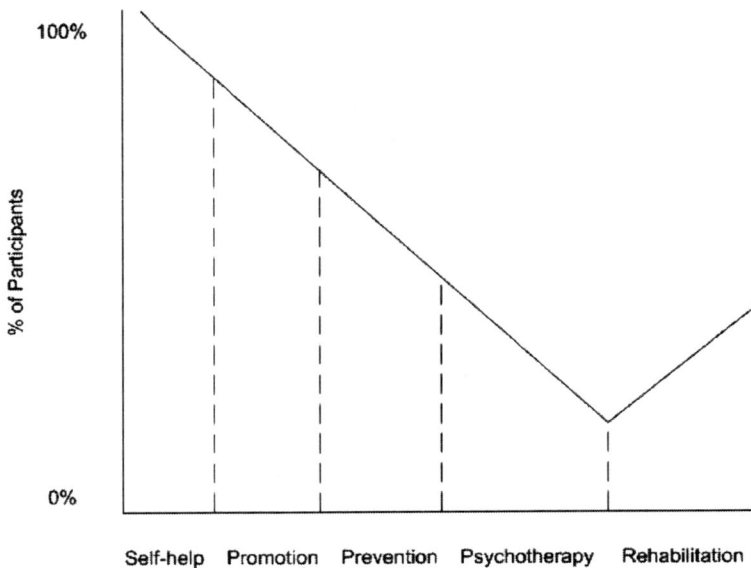

Fig. 1.2 An integrative model of self-help and various mental health approaches

Importance of Structure and Replicability in Self-Help

We are convinced about the need to verify our guesses, hunches, or hypotheses about how self-help approaches to mental health relies on how to improve them and also to see whether those guesses are correct (valid) or incorrect (invalid) (Scogin et al., 1996). The field of SH is so chockfull of half-baked ideas, interesting but unproven innovations, and downright charlatanry that it is crucial to safeguard the innocent but needy consumers to help professionals as well as consumers to distinguish between what is helpful from what is unhelpful or even dangerous. The mental health field is still plagued by fanciful fashions, grotesque fads, and bizarre ideas that have been promoted as gospel and applied to unsuspecting but needy and vulnerable participants. This is why it is important to evaluate the outcome of SH, where frequency of usage or attendance may still be the most reliable measure of outcome (Yeaton, 1994).

The foregoing requires that whatever is said and done about helping people needs to be verified by developers of programs, manuals, etc., and by the publishers of these programs and manuals. Additionally, independent investigations must be conducted to verify findings obtained by authors/publishers. Whatever needs to be verified must be set in a replicable structure, as done when creating enrichment programs for couples and families with *verbatim* instructions (L'Abate, 1977; L'Abate & Weinstein, 1987; L'Abate & Young, 1987) or when conducting psychotherapy outcome research involving manualized treatments and fidelity checks. Without replication there is no way to separate facts from false claims, reality from false impressions, anecdotal evidence from verifiable empirical evidence, and narcissistic self-interest from altruistic interest in the welfare of our clients, consumers, participants, or patients.

For instance, based on the second author's (LL) clinical impressions, he made an egregious error, based on his clinical experience, by claiming repeatedly that written homework practice exercises were cost-effective by reducing the number of therapy sessions (L'Abate, Ganhal, & Hansen, 1986); however, when he and his colleagues examined our 25 years of part-time private practice with individuals, couples, and families, we actually found the opposite. That is, practice exercise administration significantly increased the number of therapy sessions in participants who received written homework versus those who did not receive them (L'Abate, L'Abate, & Maino, 2005). These results were somewhat contradicted by Damian Goldstein in Buenos Aires using a problem-solving workbook with decompensating women with personality disorders in a charity hospital (L'Abate & Goldstein, 2007). Therefore, the jury is still out on cost-effectiveness of written practice exercises as homework. More discussion of this issue is presented in Chapter 3 of this volume.

An Experimental Checklist to Evaluate MH

Unfortunately, most psychological tests available in the market are oriented toward identification and specification of mental illness rather than of mental health; that is, dysfunctionality and psychopathology are the foci rather than functionality. A few notable exceptions exist including the California Psychological Inventory. Consequently, it is extremely difficult to accurately determine who should receive a promotional, preventive, psychotherapeutic, or rehabilitative intervention. In trying to achieve a modicum of identification, the second author has developed a structured interview designed to make this identification easier on the basis of one's history (L'Abate, 1992c), a theory-derived structured interview for intimate relationships (L'Abate et al., 2010), and the questionnaire in Table 1.2, instruments that are still at an experimental rather than validated stage. Therefore, this questionnaire should be used very tentatively before jumping at unwarranted conclusions.

Table 1.2 Constructive patterns: checklist of behaviors necessary to discriminate between levels of functioning in individuals, couples, and families*

Instructions:
Frequency means how often a behavior occurs from minimal (1) to maximal (5)
Duration means how long a behavior lasts from short (1) to long (5)
INTENSITY MEANS HOW STRONG A BEHAVIOR IS FROM WEAK (1) TO VERY
  STRONG (5)
SATISFACTION MEANS HOW MUCH PLEASURE A BEHAVIOR PRODUCES FROM
  LITTLE (1) TO GREAT (5).
CIRCLE THE NUMBER THAT BEST REPRESENTS HOW OFTEN, HOW LONG,
  HOW STRONG, AND HOW SATISFYING A BEHAVIOR LISTED BELOW IS FROM 1
  TO 5.
IF AN ACTIVITY IS NOT INCLUDED IN THIS LIST, THERE ARE TWO AVAILABLE
  SPACES WHERE SUCH AN ACTIVITY CAN BE ADDED. WRITE THE NAME OF
  THAT ADDED ACTIVITY.

Individuals:	Frequency	Duration	Intensity	Satisfaction
Nutrition:				
Weight, height, diet, vitamins and supplements, herbs	1 2 3 4 5	1 2 3 4 5	1 2 3 4 5	1 2 3 4 5
Physical activities:				
Exercise, sports, hunting, games	1 2 3 4 5	1 2 3 4 5	1 2 3 4 5	1 2 3 4 5
Pleasant and pleasurable activities:				
Hobbies, collecting, gardening and similar activities	1 2 3 4 5	1 2 3 4 5	1 2 3 4 5	1 2 3 4 5
Reading:				
Preferred books, magazines, newspapers	1 2 3 4 5	1 2 3 4 5	1 2 3 4 5	1 2 3 4 5
Television:				
How much time spent, programs watched, reliance on tapes, disks, etc.	1 2 3 4 5	1 2 3 4 5	1 2 3 4 5	1 2 3 4 5
Computer and Internet use:				
Enrichment: education extra-home, school/work interests	1 2 3 4 5	1 2 3 4 5	1 2 3 4 5	1 2 3 4 5
Friendships:				
Nature of friends and frequency of meetings	1 2 3 4 5	1 2 3 4 5	1 2 3 4 5	1 2 3 4 5
Correspondence:				
Writing versus computer-driven e-mails, etc.	1 2 3 4 5	1 2 3 4 5	1 2 3 4 5	1 2 3 4 5

Table 1.2 (continued)

Individuals:	Frequency	Duration	Intensity	Satisfaction
Use of car:				
Strictly for work and shopping purposes, joy riding/vacations	1 2 3 4 5	1 2 3 4 5	1 2 3 4 5	1 2 3 4 5
Abuse:				
Alcohol, smoking, drugs, Internet	1 2 3 4 5	1 2 3 4 5	1 2 3 4 5	1 2 3 4 5
Volunteering:				
Where, when, for how long?	1 2 3 4 5	1 2 3 4 5	1 2 3 4 5	1 2 3 4 5
Other _____	1 2 3 4 5	1 2 3 4 5	1 2 3 4 5	1 2 3 4 5
Other _____	1 2 3 4 5	1 2 3 4 5	1 2 3 4 5	1 2 3 4 5
COUPLES AND FAMILIES:				
Attending movies, plays, concerts, symphonies, or operas	1 2 3 4 5	1 2 3 4 5	1 2 3 4 5	1 2 3 4 5
Camping and hiking	1 2 3 4 5	1 2 3 4 5	1 2 3 4 5	1 2 3 4 5
Cooking together	1 2 3 4 5	1 2 3 4 5	1 2 3 4 5	1 2 3 4 5
Eating together	1 2 3 4 5	1 2 3 4 5	1 2 3 4 5	1 2 3 4 5
Eating out	1 2 3 4 5	1 2 3 4 5	1 2 3 4 5	1 2 3 4 5
Playing cards or board games	1 2 3 4 5	1 2 3 4 5	1 2 3 4 5	1 2 3 4 5
Shopping together	1 2 3 4 5	1 2 3 4 5	1 2 3 4 5	1 2 3 4 5
Vacations	1 2 3 4 5	1 2 3 4 5	1 2 3 4 5	1 2 3 4 5
Watching at home together vs. apart:				
movies, CD-ROM, TV	1 2 3 4 5	1 2 3 4 5	1 2 3 4 5	1 2 3 4 5
Other _____	1 2 3 4 5	1 2 3 4 5	1 2 3 4 5	1 2 3 4 5
Other _____	1 2 3 4 5	1 2 3 4 5	1 2 3 4 5	1 2 3 4 5

Feel free to add any comments that may relate to the activities listed in this form by adding more information about these activities.

*Please note that this questionnaire is still experimental and it has not been validated.

Concluding Remarks

The SH field, as shown in this chapter and in chapters to follow, intersects all four mental health approaches listed above because it can be applied by oneself, or in conjunction with all the approaches listed briefly above as an adjunct, additional, integrative, or even alternative source to widen available avenues of change for participants, professionals, and various levels of helpers. The two basic questions that remain unanswered are (1) "Why do some people, regardless of level of functioning or dysfunction, choose to take advantage of SH resources, and (2) Why do some people fail to recognize the importance of self-help and instead reject its use?" (Klingemann & Sobell, 2007; L'Abate, 1990, 2007c; Robins, 1993).

The primary motivation to seek SH might be understanding of need, but need interacts with so many other internal and external factors that it becomes almost impossible to arrive at helpful SH decisions without engaging in a trial-and-error process (Goering et al., 2006; Segal et al., 2002). One useful approach to the identification of the form of self-help that is the patient's or participant's best fit is to begin with the least expensive form of self-help and gradually work up to more expensive approaches. The following suggestion is proposed to indicate the utility of a stepped care model that involves a progression through increasing successive hurdles or sieves in an effort to identify the most appropriate form of self-help/level of intervention. Of course, problem complexity and chronicity, functional impairment, financial considerations, level of social support, and subjective distress are all important considerations in the selection of the appropriate level of entry in a stepped care model. In general, one should not rely solely on self-help unless they are experiencing sub-clinical levels of psychiatric disorders, are able to function well and in a planful manner, and are not dangerous to self or others. Additionally, a psychologist is typically needed to reliably determine if the individual is at sub-threshold levels and is functional and not dangerous. Some Internet programs are in development to provide a patient-driven method of obtaining this information (e.g., WebPsych, 2009; www.innerlife.com). With that said, a stepped care model specific to self-help might look like the following:

1. Employ self-help before promotion
2. Promotion before prevention
3. Prevention before individual psychosocial treatment
4. Rehabilitation after either Steps 1, 2, or 3 are completed or failed

Self-help is no doubt a useful resource in many instances. Future research efforts will help us identify better forms of self-help and provide important information with respect to how self-help is best utilized for each individual or patient. Whether or not self-help approaches are considered preventive (both in the prevention of progression from sub-threshold to clinical problems or the prevention of relapse), or palliative (as in an adjunct to treatment, and integral part of treatment, or the primary method of treatment with minimal therapist contact), they should always be considered as a component in the treatment process.

Chapter 2
The Self-Help Movement in Mental Health: From Passivity to Interactivity

Introduction

This chapter expands and updates on Norcross' (2006) original proposal to integrate self-help with psychotherapy through the reading of self-help books, autobiographies, and viewing of relevant self-help films. This relatively passive approach can be expanded with active and interactive SH interventions in promotion, prevention, psychotherapy, and rehabilitation through: (1) distance writing (DW) in its various approaches, which will be considered in greater detail in Chapter 3 of this volume, (2) homework assignments, and (3) low-cost approaches to promote physical and mental health. These new approaches suggest a paradigm shift in mental health from traditional individually delivered psychosocial treatment to distance writing (DW) approaches that may mean interacting with participants online without ever seeing them directly (L'Abate, 2008a; 2008b,c).

Since publication of Norcross's proposal a great many evolutionary advances have occurred in the field of MH. Except for community interventions, health promotion, prevention, psychotherapy, and even rehabilitation have been traditionally based on the individually delivered psychosocial treatment paradigm of the last century. In this century, these MH interventions will slowly but inevitably and inexorably change into a DW paradigm in its many interactive forms (L'Abate, 2001a; 2002). This relatively new DW paradigm is based on the increasing use of the Internet, as Norcross notes in his proposal, and in recent advances in the use of homework assignments in prevention, psychotherapy, and rehabilitation, and especially the growth of low-cost approaches to promote physical and MH as discussed in the previous chapter (L'Abate, 2007b).

The utility of the foregoing Internet, distance writing approaches to those suffering from complex and chronic problems is unknown. In many cases where problems are complex and chronic, a structured in-patient environment is often required initially and the need for medication management is likely as well. Additionally, for those who suffer from complex chronic problems (i.e., long-standing/recurring, highly distressing, often accompanied by widespread functional impairment and a lack of social support), a multi-pronged/multi-person treatment is typically recommended. Further, research evidence supports the notion that clinical skill is most

T.M. Harwood, L. L'Abate, *Self-Help in Mental Health*,
DOI 10.1007/978-1-4419-1099-8_2, © Springer Science+Business Media, LLC 2010

important when treating individuals suffering from serious complex, chronic problems (e.g., Beutler & Clarkin, 1990; Beutler et al., 2003; Beutler & Harwood, 2000; Beutler, Clarkin, & Bongar, 2000; Harwood & Beutler, 2008; Harwood & Beutler 2009).

Whether or not the Internet can provide the conduit necessary for the effective application of clinical skills (including the accurate identification of empirically based principles and strategies of change) and the seamless application of interventions based on these principles and strategies and relevant patient in-session cues is an empirical question; however, it seems that many elements necessary to the successful therapeutic process (close human in-person interaction, accuracy of clinical judgment) based on patient cues are lacking in Internet or distance writing methods. Relatedly, the likelihood that the written word will be less efficient than the spoken word in communication does not augur well for this treatment format among patients with complex and chronic problems. Another concern centers on the formation of a robust therapeutic alliance. More specifically, how strong will the alliance be among patients treated from a distance, and how will ruptures in the alliance be repaired through the Internet and distance writing?

It is unclear if the Internet will improve treatment efficiency or effectiveness (i.e., reduce time in treatment, produce an increase in the likelihood of change and magnitude of change, improve satisfaction with treatment, or if we can identify which patient types/psychiatric disorders respond best, etc.). Likewise, we do not know if these distance treatment methods will prolong the change process in general or among those with more serious psychiatric conditions. Undoubtedly, the Internet and distance writing has application to rural populations and others who are typically underserved (e.g., prison populations, the homebound)—for these reasons, the Internet and distance writing, as well as other forms of self-help treatment require quality investigation into their efficacy, effectiveness, the patient characteristics that suggest these methods are a good match, and the refinement of treatment formats and methods.

The Passive–Active–Interactive Dimension in Self-Help

These terms do not apply solely to participants, they apply more directly to professional helpers, ranging from the reflective "hum, hum" of client-oriented non-directive counseling to the directive stance of behavioral therapists (Kazantzis & L'Abate, 2007). For instance, in defining SH, Norcross (2006) includes reading self-help books and autobiographies and viewing films related to a variety of clinical and non-clinical conditions. Lists about these three approaches include rankings by a large number of psychologists who use them in their professional practices. Additionally, Norcross et al. (2000) compiled a veritable encyclopedia of SH resources available in MH, and there is no reason to replicate them here. Self-help resources identified by Norcross (2006) include books/novels and autobiographies,

Internet resources, and national support groups. The interested reader should consult Norcross (2006) to discover and possibly use that helpful information.

Norcross (2006), even though reporting some of the resources available in the earlier publication (Norcross et al., 2000), did not report on the evidence in support of the ancillary use of these approaches in psychotherapy. The absence of evidence for his proposal seems strangely contrary to the need to support professional practices with evidence rather than with just personal consensus, opinion, or talk. Nonetheless, his 16 practical suggestions to integrate self-help into psychotherapy are right on target and should be heeded by MH professionals who use or plan to use SH information and materials in their clinical, community, and preventive practices. Consequently, we are in Norcross' debt for furnishing an ample and distinct background for his introduction and later expansion and updating in this area. He provided such a completely thorough review of the literature with a full-scale rationale for the introduction of self-help approaches in MH interventions that it is included here in Table 2.1.

Table 2.1 Norcross' (2006) practical suggestions to enhance the effectiveness of self-help approaches

1.	Enlarge our conceptualization of change mechanisms
2.	Cease devaluating self-help
3.	Broaden the definition of self-help
4.	Capitalize on the multiplicity of self-help benefits
5.	Familiarize yourself wih self-help
6.	Assess clients' self-help experiences
7.	Help administer difficult self-help programs
8.	Offer tangible support when linking clients with self-help resources
9.	Recommend research-supported self-help
10.	Rely on professional consensus in the absence of research evidence
11.	Tailor recommendations to the person, not only to the disorder
12.	Recommend self-help for life transitions (as well as disorders)
13.	Employ self-help during waiting periods and maintenance
14.	Address common concerns
15.	Collaborate with self-help organizations
16.	Incorporate self-help methods and referrals into training

Shaked (2005), on the other hand, performed an analysis of 10 contemporary best-selling personal SH books published between 1997 and 2002 to assess the degree to which they met both scientific and ethical standards. She used, however, a new and untested instrument to examine its utility in evaluating SH books by both MH professionals and lay readers. A qualitative method, informed by grounded theory, was used to explore and to assess the books. Open coding yielded 33 concepts and 3 categories, namely: scientific rigor, ethical adherences, and book contents. The books were then rated on a 5-point Likert scale, using a new model for content evaluation. Results suggested that most SH books lack empirical support and integrated ethics to a moderate extent. Contents of these books indicated that most were written by authors with doctorates in psychology, who are likely to produce another best seller and did not delineate their theoretical orientation. Religion/spirituality was salient along with some mention of psychological theories and emphasis on advice-giving. Anecdotes and case studies were not used consistently, nor were questionnaires, other self-assessment exercises, proverbial sayings, or highlighted text. These books were well-organized, although bibliographies and appendices varied in quality. These results indicate the importance of RCT investigations of SH books and other self-help materials or resources.

Note that in this volume we are trying to fulfill Norcross' recommendations as much as possible. Instead of conceiving of SH as connected solely to psychotherapy, as he did, SH is conceived as forming a tier of interventions with characteristics of its own, independent from but intertwined with traditional MH interventions. These characteristics may run hand in hand along a continuum of community and prevention approaches consisting of universal promotions, targeted preventions, necessary psychotherapies, and obligatory rehabilitations, as discussed in the previous chapter; (L'Abate, 1990; 2007b; Mrazek & Haggerty, 1994).

From Passivity to Activity

Self-help interventions may be able to stand alone, depending, for instance, on whether they are directed toward functional populations in mental health promotion, or toward at risk or sub-clinical targeted populations, such as adult children of alcoholics in prevention, or toward clinical or chronic populations in crisis, as in psychotherapy, or injured populations, as in rehabilitation. The introduction of SH approaches in these four categories would produce and obtain a synergistic outcome. SH may, and often should be paired with traditional individually delivered psychosocial interventions; however, SH should demonstrate empirically positive outcome properties of its own before coupling it with any kind of professionally delivered intervention or treatment plan.

No matter how interesting and even absorbing the reading of self-help books, or autobiographies, or viewing films may be, they are *passive* activities. They are based on receptively experienced input and internal processing rather than on the expressive output side of information processing. They do not demand an active involvement and investment on the part of participants; however, therapists may assign interactive, homework assignments, or these self-help approaches can be integrated into the therapeutic process where they demand active participation by the patient. In some cases, these activities may be quite valuable in the pre-contemplative and contemplative phases of any intervention, perhaps encouraging potential participants to seek professional help. During treatment these formerly predominantly passive activities may become a focus of primary involvement in the therapeutic process.

The passive-receptive nature of reading self-help books, autobiographies, and viewing films, for instance, stands in stark contrast to the many studies about the level of active involvement required by therapists as well as by participants for change to occur. The level of activity on the part of therapists and of participants, for instance, predicts a more positive outcome. More specifically, there is a correspondent relationship between level of activity from both therapist and patient and degree of positive outcome (Bergin & Garfield, 1994; Hubble, Duncan, & Miller, 1999; Snyder & Ingram, 2000). It is logical to extrapolate from the foregoing that the same outcome would be present among self-help mental health interventions. Of course, it all depends on the type of activity we are talking about. Activity per se does not make for a positive outcome (one should never mistake activity for accomplishment). It is important to specify the nature of the activity (positive–negative, frequency, duration, intensity, and satisfaction), how it is prescribed (individually delivered, online, mail, fax, etc.), how it is received by participants, and how it is implemented by both helpers and participants, as defined in the Questionnaire presented in Chapter 1 of this volume.

From Activity to Interactivity

In addition to the three approaches advocated by Norcross that could be considered relatively passive and self-absorbing, there are relatively new advances in the field of SH that require an active and even interactive involvement by both helpers and participants. These advances were not considered in Norcross's otherwise interesting and important proposal. These advances require an "interactive" involvement by participants to become part and parcel of the process of change since they involve participation with actions rather than solely with words (Bohart & Tallman, 1999).

In addition to the ever increasing role of the Internet in providing information to help people in need of greater knowledge about their perceived troublesome conditions, a topic considered briefly by Norcross, there are at least four interactive SH advances that were not covered by Norcross. These advances possess significant implications for the evolutionary progress of MH interventions because they are evidence-based rather than based on the subjective impressions or personal opinions of therapists, let alone participants: (1) the advent of DW as an additional or alternative approach to traditional individually delivered psychosocial interventions, (2) an increase in the use of targeted homework assignments to increase and widen the scope and effect of individual psychosocial treatment interventions, (3) the rise of low-cost approaches to promote physical and MH, and (4) the growth of technology in psychology, psychiatry, and MH (L'Abate & Bliwise, 2009).

Growth in the Use of the Homework Assignments in MH

A taxonomy of counseling goals and methods (Frey & Raming, 1979), based on content analyses and multi-variate taxonomic procedures, produced seven goal clusters. The cluster most relevant to the advances in self-help psychological interventions considered here was "Transfer of Therapy Learning to Outside Situations." The other six clusters are still relevant to MH interventions in general but not to this particular chapter. The primary goal of any MH intervention, whether self-initiated or prescribed, be it in the home, community, school, clinic, or hospital, is to ensure that whatever positive behaviors or relationships are confronted, considered, and discussed in those settings will generalizes to the patient's environment. These are the specific settings that serve to help demonstrate whether any self-help or professional help has been beneficial in a general sense.

In line with this goal, in the last few years the evidence in support of homework assignments to increase transfer of change from the office to the home has grown exponentially (Kazantzis et al., 2005). Administration of homework, for instance, may be minimal in non-directive and psychoanalytical psychotherapies, but achieves much wider applications in most other psychotherapeutic schools, involving a wide range of clinical conditions. The most relevant conclusion that can be made about homework assignments is that they have not received the widespread, systematic applications they deserve as part of mainstream MH practices. Unfortunately, many homework assignments are administered in a helter-skelter fashion without clear goals or prescriptive purposes—the work of Beutler and Harwood (2008), Lambert and Whipple (2008) are notable exceptions to this professionally irresponsible practice.

The last few years have experienced resurgence in the literature about homework assignments involving a variety of populations with both clinical and non-clinical conditions (Kazantzis et al., 2005; Kazantzis & L'Abate, 2007; L'Abate, 1977, 1986; L'Abate & De Giacomo, 2003; L'Abate & McHenry, 1983). Better treatment outcome is associated with specific therapist behaviors (i.e., setting concrete goals, checking to see if the patient understands the assignment, and discussing barriers to completing homework), characteristics of the homework task (i.e., using written reminders of the homework, providing a workbook that contains assignments, due dates, and the materials needed to complete the homework), and client involvement in the discussion and determination of the homework to be completed (Detweiler-Bedell & Whisman, 2005).

Most homework assignments (Kazantzis & L'Abate, 20007) rely in large part on written instructions and, in some cases, writing assignments. Thus far, homework assignments, in spite of their being used by many psychotherapeutic schools, have not produced a model for their systematic administration, perhaps with the exception of Brown-Stanbridge's model (1989) that relies solely on verbal instructions rather than on writing. Nonetheless, the therapeutic potential for homework assignments in MH treatment is immense and in need of full exploitation—after all, homework extends treatment beyond the clinician's office and into the real world. Additionally, therapy time is increased when a patient becomes involved in homework; however, this increase in therapy time does not result in a correspondent increase in treatment costs.

Low-Cost Approaches to Promote Physical and MH

Another advance relevant to the evolution of self-help in MH interventions lies in low-cost approaches to promote physical and mental health (L'Abate, 2007a). These approaches are based on substantial evidence of positive outcomes in survival and mortality reviewed already in Chapter 1 of this volume.

The major implication of this advance lies in its helping to identify levels and types of functionality for the appropriate administration of homework to strengthen average or even superior functioning in mental health interventions. The large numbers of individuals who can benefit from both promotion and prevention make individually delivered psychosocial interventions unrealistic for a large portion of those in need. Identification of functional and semi-functional populations may prove difficult on the basis of most self-report paper-and-pencil tests available on the market. As already noted in Chapter 1, most psychological tests are designed toward identifying and measuring the type and extent of psychopathology and dysfunctionality with little attention to the measurement of average or superior functioning.

It is important to differentiate between the assessment of functionality based on actual behaviors across contexts (using scales or measures such as the GAF, DSM-IV-TR, 2000; STS-CRF, Fisher, Beutler & Williams 1999; www.innerlife.com, Webpsych, 2009) and the indirect assessment of functionality based on most personality or symptom inventories that tend to focus on pathology. In line with this type of reasoning, an assessment of the activities listed in Table 1.1 was developed to assess behaviors among individuals, couples, and families. The contents of that questionnaire are consistent with the positive psychology movement that emphasizes strengths and sources of resilience rather than the dysfunctional aspects of our lives. This list has not yet been validated, but it is presented as a replicable form that should allow one to determine levels of functioning. Responses to this list would allow the development of a plan to help participants (individuals, couples, families, and groups) with cost-effective and therapeutically effective forms of intervention. Additionally, the foregoing positive-based assessment must be supplemented with measures of pathology/impairment to determine problem severity, complexity, and chronicity.

For instance, participants scoring within the most functional range of scores and without a presenting problem or chief complaint, could be administered any of the self-help activities presented in this volume or any of the non-clinical practice exercises introduced in Chapter 3 of this volume. Participants scoring somewhere in the middle range of scores and presenting with a presenting problem, similar to what might be seen in adult children of alcoholics, could be administered targeted practice exercises directed toward a specific conflict area. Participants scoring at the lowest range of scores with a clinically relevant presenting problem or chief complaint in clear distress could be assigned to individually administered crisis-intervention psychotherapy, with the eventual assignment of self-help approaches relevant to their condition.

Of course, the most professionally responsible method to determine where a patient should enter a stepped-care model of treatment is through clinical interview, reliable and valid measures of diagnosis, distress, and impairment, coupled with measures of resiliency and areas of functionality. For example, patients found to be sub-clinical, with adequate resources and good functioning, are candidates for prevention-based interventions. Patients with moderate levels of functioning, mild to moderate clinical diagnoses, and some sources of social support may be considered good candidates for self-help interventions that are adjunctive or integral to psychotherapy with various levels of therapist involvement. Finally, patients exhibiting complex, chronic, and severe problems along with high levels of functional impairment and low levels of social support would generally be better served through intensive, longer-term, multi-person, and multi-format psychosocial treatment that may involve pharmacotherapy and various sources of self-help (e.g., AA).

Toward a Technology for MH Interventions

Technology has been a major influence in American society and has become important in most aspects of our lives (Klein, 2007; Marx & Mazlich, 2007). This technology, regardless of whether or not some psychotherapists like it, will continue to exert substantial influence in the directions that clinical psychology, psychiatry, and MH take in general (e.g., www.innerlife.com). The implications of this technology as a revolutionary force in MH will most likely be immense. Biofeedback, virtual reality therapy, working memory training, and transcranial magnetic stimulation, among other interventions, seem destined to supplement or supplant semi-professionals and professionals in administering treatments in ways that were inconceivable heretofore (L'Abate & Bliwise, 2009). The potential ramifications for service delivery provided by technology include enhanced cost-effectiveness, increased access to care, and step-by-step progression from least to most expensive approaches. Possible challenges in the areas of insurance coverage and professional training loom but are not without solution (L'Abate & Bliwise, 2008). These devices will be coupled, on a large scale, with validated SH approaches at some point in the future.

Implications of Recent Advances for MH Interventions

On the basis of the advances summarized above, one admittedly extreme implication relevant to the conduct of MH interventions would consist mainly of administration of written or non-written homework assignments interspersed with rare, infrequent psychosocial treatment sessions. The purpose of these sessions would be four-fold: (1) to check on homework outcomes after completing each assignment or practice exercise; (2) to assign new, relevant homework; (3) to gauge if progress is being made in treatment and determine if adjustments to the treatment plan are indicated; and (4) to make sure that the patient is improving instead of deteriorating. In some cases, these checks could be performed online once the correct identity of participants is assured; however, we suggest that patients periodically visit their treating clinician so a thorough, reliable and valid assessment of progress and patient status can be performed. In other cases, individual treatment sessions interspersed with homework assignments may be significantly reduced. In the foregoing instance, the valued and expensive presence and talk of a therapist could become contingent on participants completing homework assignments, and therapists can become more available to individually treat severely impaired patients (L'Abate, 2008a,c).

The foregoing might seem preposterous to many MH professionals who value their personal presence and their words. However, it could be argued that because the presence and expertise of the professional is so important, these qualities could be used sparingly and selectively, not just on the basis of words but on the basis of deeds: how well do participants complete prescribed SH homework assignments and how can the therapist's time be better utilized?

A less extreme result of the technological advances relevant to self-help psychotherapeutic interventions involves the already mentioned stepped care approach consisting of successive sieves or stages or steps moving from the least to the most expensive interventions (L'Abate, 1990; 2007c). For instance, after an informed consent form about homework and distance writing is signed by participants, homework could consist first of the most concrete, easy-to-complete behaviors/tasks, including those already existing and listed in Table 1.1. Second, assignments of activities that are the most frequently performed and enjoyed by participants could progress to more difficult and complex homework with workbooks specific to the individual functioning of partners and family members. Individual psychotherapy, for instance, could occur while participants complete practice exercises specific to either individual or relational conflicts or disorders.

Conclusion

The overriding goal of self-help psychotherapeutic interventions is to help assure and increase the generalization of positive behaviors from professional offices or venues to the patient's many environments and contexts. Secondary goals include the following:

1. Improve the effectiveness of treatment(s) by augmentation as an adjunctive form of therapy or to act as an integral component of treatment.
2. Provide for mental and physical health promotion.
3. Reduce the likelihood of relapse.
4. Free up valuable therapist time for those suffering from severe problems.
5. Instill a sense of self-efficacy.
6. Provide for prevention (reduce the likelihood that sub-clinical problems will reach the clinical threshold).
7. Increase the likelihood and magnitude of positive change.
8. Reduce time in therapy and the corresponding cost of treatment.

The likelihood that the foregoing will occur is increased by the administration of homework assignments and a range of relatively low-cost self-help programs or materials. If self-help materials are to be employed and recommended by a therapist, that clinician should make sure the materials are safe, empirically supported, and relevant to the problem(s) at hand. If there are no available empirically supported self-help materials available for a particular problem and/or patient, then the clinician should make a judgment about assigning what is available. If the decision is to assign, the patient should be fully informed of the lack of empirical support for the self-help procedure being prescribed or suggested. In such cases, if the patient accepts the self-help material, it is important for the therapist to monitor the patient on a regular basis to determine status on functioning, mood, and other indices of mental health.

Generally speaking, if an individual is contemplating self-help psychotherapeutic treatment, they should undergo a clinical intake/diagnostic interview. The reasoning behind this is that most individuals who are considering purchasing a self-help resource are experiencing some sort of distress or impairment—a clinician is able to determine the extent of a problem and assign the appropriate level of care indicated for the individual. That is, a clinician may determine that self-help alone is appropriate; however, this should be accompanied with instructions to contact the therapist if symptoms, functioning, or mood worsen (a referral list should also be provided).

Although not all patients may be able to engage in therapy delivered individually (e.g., cost or time considerations may be prohibitive), low-cost referral, phone check-ins, support groups, and a range of resources are available and with a little creativity and motivation, an acceptable and appropriate treatment plan should be available to virtually all individuals. In the vast majority of cases, we suggest at least minimal therapist involvement, perhaps no less than on a monthly basis, to help ensure that the patient is not experiencing deterioration, to monitor homework or discuss self-help readings, and to make adjustments in treatment if necessary. This should continue until the patient is asymptomatic. Booster sessions may be considered for a period of time following termination, and the therapist should let the patient know that they may return for treatment if the need arises.

Part II
Self-Support Approaches: Initiated, Guided, Maintained, and Monitored by Professionals (for Participants)

As already indicated in Chapter 1, we need to differentiate among the many, perhaps overlapping, meanings of *Self-Support* (SS) included in this and in the next section III of this volume: (1) *initiated* means that the helper, professional or otherwise, is the one who suggested and started the intervention, hoping and making sure that participants understood fully what was being suggested and started with their own approval, formal agreement, and full participation to follow through if there was something that was going to be assigned or administered, including a formal evaluation and an Informed Consent Form; (2) *guided*, means the helper is responsible for being available to participants on a regular basis, once a new SS activity is initiated by participants with reminders as simple as a weekly phone-call or an e-mail note indicating interest, continuous availability, and reliability on the part of the helper; (3) *maintenance*, means that the availability is present over time, that could range from a few weeks, few months, and, if there is a follow-up, even years; and\break (4) *monitoring*, means that the helper needs to be informed about the progress that is occurring in participants, including checking on completed homework assignments and interactively *correcting* or improving on whatever homework has been assigned, completed, and return to the helper for evaluation and corrective feedback. These different meanings, therefore, cover a continuum of possible behaviors on the part of helpers, at whatever levels of professional, semi-quasi-professional competence, or even lay-person volunteers, as discussed in Chapter 1 of this volume.

Chapter 3
Distance Writing: Helping without Seeing Participants

An interactive SH approach that is becoming more and more frequent and that has been always important is distance writing (DW). Online therapy has already emerged in the area of SH therapy as the fastest growing method, as discussed in Chapter 5 of this volume (L'Abate, 1986, 1990, 1992e, 2001a, 2002). Participants can receive therapy sessions with e-text and/or voice with video and can also complete online questionnaires, handouts, workout sheets, or practice exercises at their own pace (Greg, 2007). DW, as a progressive step in the evolution of SH, owes its phenomenal growth to the Internet and is now an everyday occurrence (Lange et al., 1993; Ritterband et al., 2003a; Ritterband et al., 2003b; Watkins & Clum, 2008).

Information about help of any kind, and how to get it, is now at the fingertips of almost anyone who can write using a computer. Now even the phone can take over many functions of the computer. Information and help is continuously exchanged through SH groups, chat-rooms, formal and informal, structured and unstructured treatments in health promotion, prevention of illness, psychotherapy, and rehabilitation. The use of the Internet implies an interactive involvement in the process of acquiring and exchanging information. To retain such information and incorporate it in one's daily living that information needs to be *in writing*, either in printed form for reception or in one's handwriting or typing for recording reactions and responses. If the Internet is indeed the most revolutionary development in the last generation, it will require reception and printing of written information to remember and express that information to keep records and documentation.

With the Internet, DW is progressively entering the SH/MH field as the major medium of intervention and service delivery in this century, especially with the use of online communications (Lepore & Smyth, 2002; Pulier et al., 2007; Seligman, Steen, Park, & Peterson, 2005) and the increased use of homework assignments in promotion, prevention, psychotherapy, and rehabilitation (Kazantzis & L'Abate, 2007), as discussed in Chapter 2 of this volume. Instructions for most homework assignments must be administered through writing to qualify as easily replicable procedures without the expensive presence of a professional and F2F talk. The Internet has produced the creation of "Electronic Tribes" of single-minded individuals connected online around a mutual interest or topic, making virtual reality a second reality of its own with its own dangers, including white-collar crime,

T.M. Harwood, L. L'Abate, *Self-Help in Mental Health*,
DOI 10.1007/978-1-4419-1099-8_3, © Springer Science+Business Media, LLC 2010

fraudulent identity theft, pornography, terrorism, and extreme racist groups, among others (Adams & Smith, 2008). On the other hand, the Internet represent an uncharted territory open to unending possibilities to help people in ways that were unforeseen a generation ago (L'Abate, 1992a, 2001a, 2002, 2003; 2004a, 2004b, 2008b; L'Abate & De Giacomo, 2003).

Reliance on DW occurring outside the presence of a professional, therefore, may represent the next evolutionary step for change in the delivery of SH/MH services: from an individually administered psychosocial treatment paradigm between participants and professionals remnant from the past century to written, more impersonal but interactive contacts exchanged at a distance online. Consequently, reliance on DW, as the next step in the evolution of MH interventions from traditional individual one-on-one treatment to the Internet, suggests a completely different paradigm. Ultimately, in its extreme, this DW-based paradigm implies not ever seeing participants F2F or talking with them, as it happens every day online.

DW includes a variety of approaches, depending on their level of structure (Table 3.1).

Table 3.1 Classification of distance writing

A. *Focused*, as in autobiographies to be mailed or sent online (Demetrio & Borgonovi, 2007)

B. *Open-ended*, as in personal information gathered through diaries or journals (Levine & Calvanio, 2007).

C. *Expressive*, as in "Pennebaker's Paradigm" writing about hurts and traumas heretofore not shared with others for 15–20 min a day for four consecutive days (Esterling et al., 1999; Kacewicz, Slatcher, & Pennebaker, 2007; Lepore & Smyth, 2002).

D. *Guided*, as in answering written questions in writing to either A, B, C, or D.

E. *Programmed* as in interactive practice exercises or interactive practice exercises for targeted clinical participants (children and youth, single individuals, couples, and families) and non-targeted conditions for life-long learning for non-clinical participants.

F. *Dictionary*, as an offshoot of programmed writing.

A Classification of Distance Writing

This classification about various types of DW is presented in Table 3.1.

From the classification presented in Table 3.1, in addition to expanding on those types included in that Table 3.1, two approaches will be highlighted: (1) a classification of SH interactive practice exercises and (2) dictionary-based writing.

Open-Ended Diaries, Journals, and Personal Information

Diaries have become a veritable source of personal information that have promoted a great deal of research during the last decade (Bolger, Davis, & Rafaeli, 2003) as well as interventions (Levine & Calvanio, 2007). The diary method, especially, has achieved a great deal of attention in the last decade as a credible method of research and as an adjunct to prevention and psychotherapy (Alaszewski, 2006; Mackrill, 2008; Thiele, Laireiter & Baumann, 2002)

Historically, Allport (1942) promoted the use of personal documents as a legitimate source of information and study. Rogers (1951) published extracts from a client's diary about her experiences in psychotherapy. As Mackrill (2008) concluded his review of the literature:

> . . .the diary is not merely a method that records data about the clients' ongoing therapy. The diary is a secondary form of intervention that affects and some would argue contaminates the data concerning the psychotherapy. Research has suggested that writing about emotional experiences and thereby confronting emotionally upsetting events may be associated with improved mental health (p. 15).

Focused Autobiographies

Results from the "nun study" (Snowdon, 2001) indicate the importance of writing down chronologically important events in one's life. A review of research supporting the positive effects of writing an autobiography is found in Demetrio and Borgonovi (2007).

Expressive Writing

Expressive writing (The Pennebaker Paradigm) is a more focused, time-limited activity about undisclosed traumas (15 min a day for four consecutive days). More than 50 well-constructed studies suggest that widespread use of this approach might dramatically reduce the social and personal costs of depression, anxiety, separation, loss, and addictions (Esterling et al., 1999; Kacewicz, Slatcher, & Pennebaker, 2007; Pennebaker, 2001; Williams & Chung, 2001). Its initially individualistic approach has been extended to relational breakups (Lepore & Greenberg, 2002), job loss and re-employment (Soper & Von Bergen, 2001), and to academic performance (Lumley & Provenzano, 2003). Honos-Webb et al., (2002) supporting this paradigm, did also raise some questions about the universality of this and other writing paradigms. Expressive writing may reduce health care utilization in healthy participants, such as college students, but not in populations defined by medical diagnoses or those exposed to stress (Harris, 2006). Furthermore, one would question its use with severely dysfunctional populations, for example schizophrenics, where expressive writing may be counter-productive (Smyth et al., 2008; Solano et al., 2008) unless perhaps, introduced through the use of computers (Bloom, 1992).

An interesting recent study (Romero, 2008) involves helping participants to forgoing of destructive thoughts, feelings, and behaviors by engaging instead in constructive responses following an interpersonal offense or transgression, that is: forgiving. Romero (2008), in addition to an up-to-date review of the relevant literature, compared two different types of expressive writing tasks with a control writing task to determine whether writing about an interpersonal offense promotes forgiveness of the offender. Participants who empathized with the offender and identified benefits of forgiveness experienced decreases in avoidance and increases in prospective taking. Participants who wrote about their thoughts and feelings or about daily events did not experience such forgiveness outcomes. This study represents an important link between expressive writing and the field of forgiveness as an important if not crucial aspect of SH/MH, as discussed in Chapter 14 of this volume.

Programmed Writing

A parallel advance in the field of MH, in line with the use of DW and homework assignments, has been the growth of SH, MH interactive practice exercises. Programmed writing (PW) means systematically written homework assignments on a specific topic contained in SH, MH interactive practice exercises (L'Abate, 1986, 1990, 1992e, 2001a, 2002, 2004a, 2004b; L'Abate & De Giacomo, 2003; L'Abate & McHenry, 1983). These practice exercises involve participants by asking them to answer in writing a systematically programmed series of questions, tasks, and prescriptions in order for them to receive the next practice exercise. With the plethora of such interactive practice exercises available commercially in the USA (L'Abate, 2004a, 2007c), practically any clinical, semi-clinical, and non-clinical condition can be matched with a SH series of practice exercises linking evaluation with treatment in a way that cannot be accomplished verbally. As such, PW can be directed toward specific problem areas, such as externalization and internalization personality disorders in children and adults, or conflicting couples or families.

Interactive practice exercises because of their low cost, mass administration, and versatility in prevention, psychotherapy, and rehabilitation could be administered for either functional or dysfunctional conditions. They can be administered online as computer-assisted interventions, qualifying as secondary prevention where the contents are targeted at problematic topics, concerns, or at-risk populations (Table 3.2). They can serve as auxiliary adjuncts to the process of psychotherapy and rehabilitation.

SH/MH interactive practice exercises are to psychological interventions what medications are to medicine and psychiatry, matching a specific condition with a specific protocol, although the same workbook, unlike medication, cannot be repeated as often. The availability of different interactive practice exercises for the same condition, however, makes it possible to address the same condition repeatedly from different viewpoints. For instance, there are at least six interactive practice exercises to deal with depression in its different manifestations (L'Abate, 2004a, 2008c). In addition to practice exercises for traumatic stress (Vermilyea, 2000), there are at least two other practice exercises about post-traumatic stress disorder for children and adults (L'Abate, 2008c).

Through the use of interactive practice exercises, it is now possible to reach typically underserved populations, such as incarcerated felons (L'Abate, 2008c;

Table 3.2 A classification of interactive practice exercises in distance writing

---

1. *Composition of Participants*: singles (adults, children, youth), couples, families, groups.
2. *Reason for Referral*: concern(s), diagnosis(es), single versus dual or multiple, problem(s), symptom(s).
3. *Level and Type of Functionality*: DSM-IV or Reason for Referral
   (a) Functional; No diagnosis
   (b) externalizations: Axis II. Cluster B
   (c) internalization: Axis II. Cluster C
   (d) borderline: Axis II. Cluster A
   (e) severe: Axis I.
4. *Specific* practice exercises for particular symptoms or syndromes versus general conditions as in life-long learning.
5. *Symptom*-free versus symptom-related & diagnosis-linked.
6. *Theory*-derived, theory-related, theory-independent.
7. *Format*: (1) fixed (nomothetic); (2) flexible (idiographic); and (3) mixed (nomothetic and idiographic).
8. *Style*: Linear versus circular (paradoxical).
9. *Derivation*: Single versus multiple score tests, i.e. BDI versus MMPI-2.
10. *Content*: clinical addictions, affective disorders, Axis I and Axis II: Clusters A, B, C, etc. and non-clinical for life-long learning in individuals, couples, and families.

McMahan & Arias, 2004; Reed, McMahan, & L'Abate, 2001), shut-ins, and handicapped people in their homes as well as military personnel, missionary families, and Peace Corps volunteers overseas. Practice exercises generated by this interactive approach involve participants with verbal or written feedback from professionals (L'Abate, 2007c; L'Abate & Goldstein, 2007). Many practice exercises include most clinical conditions derived directly from many psychological tests and lists of symptoms from the Diagnostic and Statistical Manual of Mental Disorders published by the American Psychiatric Association for individuals, and from relational tests for conflicting couples and families. There are also practice exercises for non-clinical conditions and life-long learning for individuals, couples, and families without a diagnosable psychiatric condition (L'Abate, 2008c).

A meta-analysis of 6 interactive practice exercises for physical health and 12 for MH yielded effect sizes of 0.25 and 0.44 respectively (Smyth & L'Abate, 2001). These low and medium effect sizes, although not very high, must be considered within the context of their administration. These interactive practice exercises were administered to individuals or couples at a distance with little if any contact with professionals, thus reducing costs of professional time to a minimum. The results from these administrations (L' Abate, 2004b, 2008b) demonstrated that we can indeed change behavior and relationships at a distance without ever seeing or talking with participants F2F.

Additional research relevant to the evidence necessary to support the use of interactive practice exercises as SH in community interventions, prevention approaches, and the psychotherapies was performed by L'Abate, L'Abate, and Maino (2005). In going over 25 years of part-time private practice, this research divided individuals, couples, and families into two groups: one group received F2F TB therapy without interactive practice exercises, a second group received self-help practice exercises involving DW as homework assignments in addition to F2F TB psychotherapy. On the basis of the frequent claims of cost-effectiveness made for self-help interactive practice exercises, it was expected that the second group of participants would show a lower number of psychotherapy sessions. Results demonstrated this expectation to be completely incorrect. The second group showed a significantly greater number of therapy sessions than the first group. On the other hand, problem-solving series of practice exercises administered to women hospitalized with personality disorders in Buenos Aires showed a significantly shorter length of hospitalizations and lower remission rates for participants who completed that workbook (L'Abate & Goldstein, 2007).

These contradictory results indicate how it will be important to evaluate the outcome of any intervention with and without interactive practice exercises, or evaluating the sole effect of just homework administration without any other interventions, as already performed (L'Abate, 2004b) but in dire need of replication. Future evaluations need to include the nature (structure, contents, topic, etc.) of interactive practice exercises themselves, the setting where this administration is occurring (school, community center, clinic, outpatient, hospital, etc.) and, of course, the type of concern addressed by a particular series of practice exercises.

In addition to this evidence, ten research studies completed in L'Abate's laboratory more than 25 years ago, found varying positive and negative effect size estimates, averaging a medium effect size. These estimates demonstrated that it is possible to improve behavior from a distance, using interactive practice exercises without ever seeing participants F2F or talk (L'Abate, 2004b). These results have been supported by the research by Cusinato (2004), Maino (2004), and Maino et al., (2004). Consequently, is it possible to change one's behavior from a distance through writing? The answer certainly is positive with respect to PW with adults as well as with teens and children, though interactive practice exercises to change child or teen behavior differ in structural characteristics from interactive practice exercises for adults, couples, and families (L'Abate, 2008c).

SH interactive practice exercises, however, must not be confused with SH books, as discussed in Chapter 4, or manuals as discussed in Chapter 6 of this volume. SH interactive practice exercises require interactive involvement with written systematic homework assignments. SH books, on the other hand, require only that participants passively read. Unlike self-help interactive practice exercises, there is no way to know what effect passive reading may have on participants, either as a process, even though there is extensive literature to support their use (Norcross et al., 2000). As Lewis, Amini, and Lannon (2000) commented: "Self-help books are like car repair manuals: you can read them all day long, but doing so doesn't fix a thing" (p. 177).

These contradictory results raise a question about the outcome of written practice exercises as a function of interacting with different personality disorders and different clinical settings, let alone with severe psychopathology. Nonetheless, if promotional approaches are to be effective at all levels of socio-economic status in SH, they will need to rely on two, still professionally underused, media: the non-verbal and the written. An even more egregious error may lie in claiming the usefulness of the dictionary in helping participants "think" through a variety of definitions for many practice exercises created over the last two decades, as described above (L'Abate, 2007a, 2008b, 2010).

According to Clum and Watkins (2008) in regard to devising effective SH programs, these authors concluded:

> In one real sense we have no better idea today (about) how to write a self-help book than we did 30 years ago...As empiricists, therefore, we must conclude that we simply do not know how to present therapeutic content in ways to maximize behavior change: (p. 421) ... Additionally, no information is provided on the venue of the treatment approach – e.g., book, tape, or Internet – likely to prove more effective. We do not know what steps are important and in what order they should be presented. This deficiency is largely related to the lack of formal assessment of the many self-help offerings that exist in a given domain, a deficiency that is at least particaly remediable (p. 422) ... Assessment is an effective change agent for several reasons. Assessment informs whether the individual seeking change is using the recommended strategies to produce that change (p. 424).

These authors went on to expand on the importance of assessment as a way to produce change. However, they did not consider two important issues in trying to produce change for the better through DW in SH:

(1) DW as the most important medium of communication and healing, and in some cases more cost-effective than talk. For instance, the major approach reviewed thoroughly is bibliotherapy, as reviewed in Chapter 4 of this volume (Watkins and Clum, 2008). However, from the best that can be surmised, this approach is based strictly on passive reading and little if any interaction with a professional helper. For instance, there is only one passing reference to written self-help materials for smoking cessation (pp. 273–278) but not to DW as a medium of communication and healing.

(2) A continuous interaction at a distance from a professional, who responds routinely and interactively to the completion of practice exercises on a weekly or biweekly basis. This process involves feedback loops which are considered in Watkins and Clum's work for self-administered treatments (pp. 52–54), goal attainment (pp. 60–61), its function (p. 63), and personalized use (pp. 260–261). Furthermore, this feedback is apparently administered verbally rather than in writing, making it difficult to keep a record of what is happening during this process.

L'Abate has argued (2004b, pp. 3–64) that when a practice exercise is administered to individuals as homework, there are at least two new feedback loops that are missing in most talk-based treatments: (a) having to respond in writing to items and questions contained in a written practice exercise, a requirement to think about relevant to one's life and not just emote, (b) receiving feedback about one's answers from a professional helper, either verbally or in writing. In couples, there are at least two additional loops: (a) comparing one's answers with those of a partner by oneself, and (b) comparing, contrasting, and discussing those answers face-to-face with a partner even before receiving feedback from a professional helper (L'Abate, 2010).

What is important in Clum and Watkins' foregoing statement is the function of the initial assessment/evaluation and linking specific evaluation with specific treatment, something advocated from day one (L'Abate, 1986, 1990, 1992e) but which has still a long way to go. Instead of passively inert qualities, most psychological and psychiatric tests can be linked dynamically to treatment through dictionary-based writing as well as through psychiatric diagnosis and reasons for referral.

Dictionary-Assisted Writing

According to this DW approach, participants are asked to define with the help of a dictionary, give two examples, specify, and rank-order which behaviors, signs, or symptoms apply directly to them and are more applicable to themselves than other behaviors, signs, or symptoms. Standard practice exercises consequently are assigned according to the rank-order of behaviors, signs, or symptoms endorsed initially by participants. In this fashion, through programmed DW, it is possible to link evaluation or diagnosis with SH/MH interventions in ways that are difficult to replicate by talk alone (L'Abate, 2007a). Quite a few practice exercises produced over the years of clinical practice (L'Abate, 2010), require the use of the dictionary because this process might be necessary and helpful to think more clearly especially in dealing with people whose impulsivity lands them in jail or worst, or whose emotional upsets land them in a hospital or worst (L'Abate. 2007a). Whether this belief is supported by evidence remains to be seen, as discussed further below.

A recent study with undergraduates at the University of Padua failed to show main effects or interactions of dictionary administration versus no dictionary (Eleonora Maino, personal communication, June 10, 2008). Of course, one single study is not sufficient to validate or invalidate an original claim. More evidence will be necessary to support or impugn the possibly erroneous nature of that claim; that is, to help participants to think in better ways than it would be possible without a dictionary. Without a dictionary many participants would flounder and eventually give up. The dictionary, therefore, would serve as a prosthetic tool to help participants think more clearly and more directly. Whether this hunch is valid or not needs to be verified by some one rather than its author.

Whether the dictionary or no dictionary is necessary, however, the process that follows Clum and Watkins's foregoing recommendations, also remains to be seen because of its recency and inherent novelty. For example, in addition to the approaches listed in Table 3.1, one DW step in the process of acquiring and expressing information interactively lies in the use of the dictionary, which is available in most homes, college, and public libraries. Instead of receiving and answering to a test instrument, say for instance, the Beck Depression Inventory (BDI), which implies a pell-mell diagnosis of depression attributed to participants, why not ask participants as homework to follow progressively these three steps?

First, define in writing items in the BDI (or items in any other single item test that for this matter) using a dictionary. Second, give two examples of how each item applies to each participant's personal experience. Third, rank-order items according to how they apply to each participant's experience with depression, going from extremely applicable to not applicable. Instead of a totally undifferentiated global diagnosis, now the term "depression" becomes more specific and unique to each participant's personal and individual experience. *The first two steps are nomothetic, they apply to all participants. The third step is idiographic*, it applies to a specific participant and to no one else. Now depression becomes a more specific condition that is experienced uniquely by individual participants and not shared with anyone else. The same approach can be used with non-clinical instruments for individuals, couples, and families (L'Abate, 2008).

This rank-order becomes a treatment plan because participants can now complete a standard practice exercise that requires them to answer in writing, of course, questions related to history, origin, frequency, duration, intensity, personal and relational functionality of a particular symptom rated as most important by participants. After completion of this first practice exercise, further homework follows the same sequence derived from the rank-order. Here, then is how evaluation is linked directly to treatment in ways that would be impossible to implement through talk, what has been called *prescriptive evaluation* (L'Abate, 1990), linking evaluations with interventions in ways that are practically impossible to achieve through talk.

A recent application of the dictionary dealt with definitions of hurt feelings that anecdotally produced significant emotional reactions in Italian undergraduates, requiring the signing of an Informed Consent Form. The first series of practice exercises dealt with the nature of hurt feelings. A second series of practice exercises deals with the causes of hurt feelings (L'Abate, 2008b). We will have to see what results will come out from administering the same homework to addicts and inmates (Eleonora Maino, personal communication, June 10, 2008). We expect explosions and anger in this kind of population, if the hypothesis is correct that these as well as troubled individuals in general avoid and have avoided hurt feelings most of their lives through denial, repression, and suppression (Bonanno et al., 2005; L'Abate, 2008b, in press; Roemer et al., 2005). Consequently, the jury about the use of the dictionary in writing is still out (L'Abate, in press, a).

Very likely, the use of the dictionary might work with some participants better than others, with certain practice exercises better than others, and with certain populations better than others. We cannot claim that any method of intervention will produce pell-mell effects on everybody. We need to specify how a particular approach will work with specific individuals, under what relational conditions, and at what cost. For instance, low literacy is a recognized barrier to efficient and effective health care. In MH, low literacy may have additional detrimental effects. Chronic mental illness may lead to deterioration in literacy by limiting opportunities for reading and writing, as well as for formal education and vocational training (Sentell & Skumway, 2003). Therefore, the dictionary may be a possible avenue of entrance and possible enhancement of people who have difficulty with words and with writing, and especially with emotionally leaded terms like hurt feelings.

The Importance and Dangers of Addressing
Hurt Feelings in Writing

We are all subject to being hurt by and to hurt those we love and who love us. We may be hurt physically by strangers, of course, either accidentally or by design. However, those hurts do not count as much as those produced to and by those we love (L'Abate, 2010; Vangelisti, 2009). We need to be aware and discriminate between memories implanted by others, such as psychotherapists or psychiatrists (Travis & Aronson, 2007), and memories of painful events that have been forgotten or suppressed. Here is where the line between fantasy and reality needs to be double-checked, because, as Travis and Aronson amply demonstrated, at the slightest hint, we tend to make up easily quite a few stories that bear no resemblance to reality. Hurt feelings would be the kind of topic wide-open for supposedly buried events that never happened. It is crucial that professional helpers be familiar with this literature, reviewed critically by Travis and Aronson (2007).

In functional individuals and relationships, hurt feelings are admitted, approached, disclosed, expressed, and shared with loved ones (family and friends), verbally, non-verbally, as in crying together, or in writing, allowing these feelings to dissipate and disappear over time through a process of intimacy, the sharing of joys and hurt feelings as well as fears of being hurt. In dysfunctional individuals and relationships, hurt feelings are avoided through more ridicule, put downs, and abuse (Bonanno et al., 2005; L'Abate, 1997; Roemer et al., 2005). Consequently, in these individuals and their immediate, proximal relationships hurt feelings are kept inside to fester and damage individuals and their intimate relationships. There is little if any intimacy in these dysfunctional relationships, except at funerals or weddings (L'Abate, 2005). These feelings are at the bottom of the psychotherapeutic experience and become manifest through all three media: verbal, non-verbal, and in writing. Once these are expressed with a sympathetic listener, professional or otherwise, these feelings no longer need to be denied, repressed, or suppressed, freeing the individual from a taxing and debilitating condition. These feelings are components of two models that are part of a theory of relational competence.

Why are these feelings included here and what do they have to do with SH and SC? Because most individuals who are able to benefit from SH and SC are very likely emotionally wounded individuals, as helpers, we need to recognize this characteristic if we want to help them properly and appropriately.

Rationale for the Usefulness of DW

For some years, De Giacomo, his collaborators, and I have been involved in studying the effects of selected phrases that seem relevant to participants (De Giacomo et al., 2007, 2008, submitted for publication, a and b; L'Abate & De Giacomo, 2003). At the same time, Duane M. Rumbaugh, my former boss at GSU, a noted primatologist, was proposing a salience theory of learning that essentially debunks Skinner's mechanistic and simplistic response–reinforcement model. Rumbaugh posited an Amalgam of underlying internal sensations that become salient when matched with related and relevant environmental stimulations. Additionally, philosophers like Fredrick Schick wrote about the Ambiguity of language while Ludwig Wittchenstein wrote about the Arbitrariness of language. Consequently, we expanded Pennebaker's notion (Pennebaker & Chung, 2007) about going from an analogic to digital process when we talk or write. This model is derived from Pennebaker's expressive writing paradigm and from his even more exciting research on word usage. The progression from analogic to digital is a model strongly supported by Pinker's work (2007). This progression indicates that language and, of course, writing involves a digital process, putting into words unspoken experiences that are essentially analogic at the internal experiential level (De Giacomo, L'Abate, Pennebaker, & Rumbaugh, 2008).

What does this mysterious unconscious consists of? This *ambiguous, undefined, amorphous amalgam* is the depository of our salient, pent-up, avoided, denied, repressed, and suppressed hurt feelings inevitably accumulated during the course of our lifetime, as argued by De Giacomo et al. (2008).

Consequently, when we ask people to write or talk about a topic such or traumas in Pennebaker's paradigm or hurt feelings, as done by Eleonora Maino, what are we doing? We are tapping and giving digital words to a heretofore ambiguous, ill-defined, unclear mass of salient memories and feelings that have not yet have had the chance to be expressed and shared with loved ones. This unconscious, semi-conscious, pre-conscious, and at times conscious mass consists of hurt feelings, a topic that has been consistently avoided by scientific researchers and MH professionals. We may want to approach pleasure and we may try to avoid pain but we may not succeed in the pursuit of either goal (L'Abate, 2010).

Putting 2 and 2 together from various sources, such as Ambiguous, Analogic Amalgam, or Amorphous, an ill-defined or undefined amorphous mass constitutes what Freud called our unconscious along a dimension of awareness, ranging from extreme unconscious, to semi-conscious, to pre-conscious, and to conscious (Bargh & Williams, 2007; Fitzsimons & Bargh, 2004; Kinsbourne, 2005; L'Abate, 2010; Laird & Strout, 2007; Ohman, 1993, 2000; Stegge & Terwogt, 2007; Wiens & Ohman, 2007).

Discussion

The bottom line about DW is whether it produces positive or negative changes in participants who use it. In addition to a meta-analysis of self-help, MH practice exercises that produced significant effect sizes (Smyth & L'Abate, 2001), professional experience with programmed writing has been usually focused on decreasing the impulsivity of acting out youth and incarcerated inmates (L'Abate, 1992e, 2010). Some participants had been seen F2F also professionally, therefore it would be difficult to evaluate whether any changes that might have occurred for the better were due to the relationship or to written practice exercises. However, the second author worked with two inmates never seen F2F. Both were evaluated before and after termination of written homework practice exercises. Both showed positive changes, at least psychometrically and by self-report, one in lowering impulsivity and the other decreasing the initial level of depression that was the reason for referral. In other words, behavior, functional and dysfunctional, can be improved through DW without ever seeing participants F2F, as it is already occurring every day on the Internet (L'Abate, 2010).

If DW can be demonstrated to be cost-effective over talk, then we can expect and predict that given two different methods to help troubled people positively, we should choose the least expensive first, such as distance writing, before initiating, instituting or switching to the more expensive method such as talk (L'Abate, 2007a, 2008b, in press).

Conclusion

There is no doubt in our minds, therefore, that DW will become the predominant medium of intervention in SH/MH promotion, prevention, psychotherapy, and rehabilitation in this century because talk is too expensive and too difficult to record, replicate, analyze, and codify. This conclusion and prediction does not mean that talk is not important. On the contrary, it means that to help people in need or in trouble we need to rely on as many media and approaches as are available to us and to them. All three media, verbal, written, and non-verbal are equally important, and we should use all three as much as necessary, sensitively, and responsibly (L'Abate, 2002, 2008d). The two decades from the 1960s to the 1970s in the last century were devoted to talk. The next two decades from the 1980s to the 2000 were devoted to writing. The fifth decade, from the 2000 on to an end, is devoted to the heretofore missing, third non-verbal medium of communication and play across the life cycle.

Chapter 4
Bibliotherapy

Introduction

> ... our task as psychologists is to help people learn to help themselves (Watkins & Clum, 2008, p. x).

> Bibliotherapy is the primary means of media-based self-help, although computer-based approaches are on the rise. Many forms of bibliotherapy exist, but problem-focused approaches that prescribe cognitive-behavioral techniques have received the most empirical attention... Self-help materials may be less efficacious when consumed in isolation from others (e.g., therapists, family members, etc.). (Watkins, 2008, p. 20).

Self-help books have the potential to reduce the burden placed on mental health practitioners by providing easily obtained, potentially effective, self-administered forms of treatment. Of course, bibliotherapy is not appropriate for all patients or presenting problems—more about this later; however, among mild to moderate forms of disorders such as anxiety and depression, bibliotherapy may be especially useful in the early stages of treatment. In general, bibliotherapy is more effective when it is accompanied by some level of therapist contact. Therapist involvement may include a review of self-help materials, an exploration of how bibliotherapy applies to the patient and their presenting problem, periodic monitoring of patient status/progress, determining if a higher step in a stepped-care approach needs to be implemented, and recommending evidence-based materials.

Bibliotherapy is typically initiated, administered, guided, maintained, and monitored by professionals for their patients. In general, bibliotherapy is a helpful intervention; however, as Scogin (2003) points out, many extant self-help books (and other self-help materials or programs) cannot be considered evidence-based treatments. Additionally, publishers and authors of self-help materials should bear some of the burden involved in establishing empirical support for the materials they develop and market to therapists and the general public (McKendree-Smith, Floyd, & Scogin, 2003; Scogin, 2003). In the same vein, therapists should be familiar with the research support associated with various self-help materials—if bibliotherapy or other form of self-help is indicated, evidence-based materials or programs should always be employed first.

According to extant research, it appears that the results of bibliotherapy vary based on the patient's behavioral type. For instance, some research suggests that

T.M. Harwood, L. L'Abate, *Self-Help in Mental Health,*
DOI 10.1007/978-1-4419-1099-8_4, © Springer Science+Business Media, LLC 2010

realistic types may benefit the most from this method, while enterprising types might not be as successful (Mahalik & Kivlighan, 1988). Bibliotherapy may be especially useful among patients who are high in resistance levels. For example, a therapist may circumvent patient resistance by offering a choice of useful, empirically supported books or by *suggesting* specific books and other forms of written materials, such as manuals that target the particular problem for which help is sought (Beutler & Harwood, 2000; Beutler, Clarkin, & Bongar, 2000). The use of audio cassettes has also been integrated with the treatment of depression and has been shown to have a considerable effect on the level of depression exhibited by patients (Neumann, 1981). With the amalgamation of audio and visual cues, it is expected that the use of self-help methods online would prove to be an exceptional tool in relieving levels of depression, not only in patients but in the population at large, as discussed in Chapter 3 of this volume.

Watkins (2008, p. 2) defines the term "bibliotherapy for interventions that are actually delivered in written form." In essence, bibliotherapy is a subset of a broader term known as "media-based self-help," which refers to interventions delivered across the aforementioned modalities. According to Watkins, bibliotherapy "...remains the largest category of media-based self-help," acknowledging that "...some level of practitioner contact inevitably takes place" (p. 5). She goes on to consider the advantages of self-help, such as financial and psychotherapeutic benefits. Limitations of some forms of self-help include the absence of specific therapeutic motives and treatment delivered by qualified professionals in favor of questionable approaches, such as books written by celebrities, motivated by commercial and financial reward. Women appear to be the most frequent consumers of bibliotherapy-based SH. There is danger of trivializing professional help in favor of supposedly miraculous "cures," even though many SH books written by professionals, let alone celebrities, have been dismal failures (Rosen et al., 2008). Nonetheless, self-administered treatments for specific problems have steadily increased over the last 30 years (Clum, 2008, p. 46), with their success depending a great deal on the target populations and target syndromes (Clum, 2008, p. 49).

An area that is relevant to all types of self-help interventions relates to the nature of the feedback process participants receive from facilitators to chart, monitor, guide, and support their progress. Clum (2008, p. 53) acknowledges, "Feedback systems such as described in ...psychotherapy processes have not been systematically incorporated into therapist-assisted treatments or self-administered treatments." This is why self-help written practice exercises reviewed in Chapter 3 of this volume were called "interactive" because without feedback interaction with a concerned helper, participants may lose interest, flounder, and eventually drop out (L'Abate, 2004b, 2008b).

There are various theories about self-regulation that are relevant to self-help and self-change, including self-control, self-efficacy, and personal commitment; however, as Febbraro and Clum (2008) concluded (p. 72), "There are several limitations to self-regulation theories." One problem may lie in the fact that many of these so-called theories are actually simplistic models that do not rise to the level of an elaborated theory (L'Abate, 2007c). This is why we will be presenting a more comprehensive theory to account for self-help and self-change in Chapter 14 of this volume.

Regardless of theory, most researchers emphasize the importance of repeated measures that involve pre-treatment assessment to assist in the selection of appropriate principles and strategies of change, reliable and valid assessment of symptoms throughout treatment, an end-of-treatment assessment, and follow-up assessments. There are two basic therapist-initiated practices that effectively enhance motivation for change and patient self-efficacy (Febbraro & Clum, 2008, p. 68). More specifically, patient change is enhanced if a concise and collaboratively developed written treatment contract is signed by the therapist and patient(s) and homework compliance and success is carefully monitored and documented (Kazantzis & L'Abate, 2007).

Because we are limited to one chapter devoted to bibliotherapy, we are going to rely rather heavily on the various excellent contributions contained in Watkins and Clum (2008) that reviewed in detail the extant literature on bibliotherapy. The interested reader is directed to Watkins and Clum (2008) for a more nuanced treatment of bibliotherapy than can be supplied here.

Integrating Bibliotherapy with Treatment

Self-help materials are recommended frequently by mental-health practitioners. For example, surveys by Norcross (2000; Norcross et al., 2003) indicate that 85% of clinicians recommend bibliotherapy. Additionally, self-help groups are recommended by 82% of clinicians. Finally, films, web sites, and autobiographies are recommended by clinicians 46%, 34%, and 24% of the time, respectively. Unfortunately, few guidelines for the recommendation of self-help books and methods for their utilization in therapy exist; however, Campbell and Smith (2003) help fill the void and discuss effective methods that therapists can use to integrate self-help books into psychotherapy. These authors suggest a collaborative, systematic, integral method for incorporating bibliotherapy in treatment. More specifically, Campbell and Smith discuss three of the most realistic uses for bibliotherapy: (1) adjunctive versus integrative, (2) nonfiction versus fiction, and (3) clinical use versus support/informational use.

Bibliotherapy employed as an adjunct to psychotherapy includes homework-reading assignments for clarification, provision of information, direction, or practice activities. Bibliotherapy is adjunctive to treatment for patients who cannot attend sessions on a regular basis—these patients may be frail elderly, distal to the therapist's location, or physically challenged. When employed as an integrative element in psychotherapy, bibliotherapy is actively related to the patient's presenting problems. For example, the evocative material contained in the book can be used in treatment to manage time more efficiently (i.e., target critical areas highlighted by the reading). Additionally, visual (reading) and auditory (discussion) learning modalities are employed. Finally, therapist-assigned readings can help in the transfer of treatment gains to everyday life and bring therapy outside the clinician's office (Campbell & Smith, 2003).

When bibliotherapy involves nonfiction, the primary category of self-help books, content focuses on the provision of information, decision making, and problem solving. This nonfiction information lends itself to edification aimed at changing behavior, thinking, and producing insight. On the other hand, fictional bibliotherapy is effective at bringing about change through identification with a specific character in the book—in this way, patients have the opportunity to vicariously experience the life of another and relate these experiences to their own life (Campbell & Smith, 2003). Fictional bibliotherapy does not have the same amount of empirical support as non-fictional; however, it appears to be effective in reducing stress levels (Cohen, 1993; as cited in Campbell & Smith, 2003).

Bibliotherapy for clinical use involves the treatment of specific disorders or problems that are the foci of treatment (e.g., depression, anxiety, eating disorders, substance abuse, and sexual dysfunction). Additionally, anger management, relationship problems, or defiance in childhood or adolescence may be the focus of bibliotherapy (Campbell & Smith, 2003). These authors recommend that bibliotherapy used for clinical purposes should be monitored closely and brought up in session on a frequent basis—bibliotherapy should be part of the formal treatment plan.

Fit between patient and self-help book is an important consideration. Additionally, treatment compatibility is an important issue with bibliotherapy lending itself very well to cognitive-behavioral treatment approaches. Campbell and Smith (2003) recommend asking if the recommendations and solutions are (1) within the patient's capability, (2) evidence-based, (3) consistent with the goals and procedures of treatment, and (4) appropriate and applicable for the patient's presenting problem(s). An additional question involves whether the self-help book is at a reading level that is consistent with the patient's reading ability (Martinez, Whitfield, Dafters, & Williams, 2008).

Campbell and Smith (2003) recommend specific books based on the Norcross et al. (2003) study. More specifically, the ten top-rated books recommended by Campbell and Smith cover the following treatment categories: (1) abuse, (2) ADHD, (3) addictive disorders, (4) anxiety disorders, (5) communication and people skills, (6) death and grieving, (7) eating disorders, (8) love and intimacy, (9) depressive disorders, and (10) trauma/PTSD. The interested reader is directed to Campbell and Smith (2003) for titles and author information for the foregoing categories. According to Mains and Scogin (2003), self-help books that have received high levels of empirical support include (1) *Feeling Good* (Burns, 1980), (2) *Control your Depression* (Lewinsohn, Munoz, Youngren, & Zeiss, 1986), (3) *Parent Effectiveness Training: The Tested Way to Raise Children* (Gordon, 1975), and (4) *1-2-3 Magic: Effective Discipline for Children 2-12* (Phelan, 1996). It is important to note that many of these specific book editions are out of print; however, recently updated versions of each one are easily obtained through outlets such as Amazon.com.

Bibliotherapy for Anxiety Disorders

In general, the anxiety disorders occur most often among females. The female to male ratio for panic disorder without agoraphobia and for specific phobia is two to one—for panic disorder with agoraphobia, the female to male ratio is three to one. On the other hand, adult males and adult females are diagnosed equally with obsessive-compulsive disorder. The anxiety disorders are potentially debilitating and they are often the source of a great deal of distress. Fortunately, there is a great deal of published self-help material about panic attacks, fears, and phobias, including over a dozen books that overall follow a cognitive-behavioral approach (Hirai & Clum, 2008). The advantage of published self-help materials lies in their availability and relatively inexpensive cost. Additionally, these materials can be accessed anytime and anywhere furnishing consumers with motivational information that includes case studies, self-help handouts for homework assignments, and in some cases audiotapes. Further, there are more than 20 studies on the treatment of anxiety disorders that support the use of computerized programs administered through the Internet. As Hirai and Clum (2008, p. 78) concluded, "Given that approximately 54% of the population in the United States (is) using the Internet, with an increase of 26 million in a period of 13 months (US Department of Commerce, 2002), computers and the Internet have considerable potential to become major self-help treatment modalities in the near future." In their review of self-help therapies based on findings from more than 60 studies, Hirai and Clum (2008) concluded that

> The future of self-administered programs in the treatment of anxiety problems lies in the use of advanced communication technology. Such programs offer the types of advantages available for users of videos or books that come only when an effort is made to conduct a study of their effectiveness. Computerized SH programs on the internet, on the other hand, can provide the formal treatment material, pre-, during-, and post-programs assessment, as well as regular contact via e-mail. Such programs can also provide interactive and programmable functions, including tailoring the programs to specific needs of the clients, providing immediate assessment feedback, and augmenting the treatment experience using audio and visual displays. Future consumers of SH interventions await the development and evaluation of such approaches (p. 100).

A problem with commercially available self-help materials is that systematic evaluation of their effectiveness is not easy to obtain. Thus, the results obtained from controlled studies tell us little about a meta-analysis of SH treatments for anxiety disorders. For example, Mains and Scogin (2003) concluded that effect sizes for self-help treatments ranged from medium to large.

Rapee, Abbott, Baillie, & Gaston (2007) conducted randomized clinical trial comparing the efficacy of pure self-help materials for social phobia. The pure self-help condition utilized the book *Overcoming Shyness and Social Phobia: A Step-by-Step Guide* (Rapee, 1998). Specifically, these investigators compared the effects of a pure self-help written materials condition to a group therapy condition, a self-help combined with group therapy condition, and a wait list control condition. Group treatment was led by a mental health professional. The findings supported the use of pure self-help written materials in the treatment of social phobia. For example, a higher percentage of those in the pure self-help condition no longer met diagnostic criteria for social phobia when compared to the wait-list controls (20% versus 6% respectively). When the self-help materials were augmented, percentage of those no longer meeting criteria for social phobia post-treatment was 19%. Among those in group treatment, 22% no longer met criteria for social phobia at post-treatment. Overall, there was no difference at post-treatment between those who received pure self-help alone when compared to those who received self-help that was augmented and those who received group therapy. Rapee et al. conclude that pure self-help for social phobia is not as efficacious as it is for other anxiety disorders; however, the finding that some benefit from this approach supports a consideration of this approach when planning treatment for social phobia.

For panic disorders, Mains and Scogin (2003) indicate that therapist contact is preferable to solo self-administered treatment. In the SH treatment of panic disorders, even minimal therapist contact seemed to produce significantly superior outcomes compared to therapist-directed interventions and even group therapy (Hirai & Clum, 2008), more specifically, "...bibliotherapy plus minimal therapist contact produced improvements significantly superior to therapist-directed interventions... The fact that only five studies compared therapist directed interventions to self-help programs limits the confidence one can have in concluding that self-administered interventions are comparable to therapist directed interventions... Whether therapist contact is necessary to enhance the effectiveness of SH treatments remains unanswered given the limited number of studies directly examining this variable" (p. 82). According to Hirai and Clum (2008), "Little evidence exists indicating that one type of SH venue is superior to another in treating panic... [Additionally,] duration of self-help treatment does not appear to effect strength of treatment effects" (p. 83). Self-help interventions based on therapist-administered treatment programs of proven effectiveness for panic disorder have been shown to be effective when compared to wait-list or self-monitoring conditions (p. 84). Overall, therapist-directed exposure treatment offers a distinct advantage in treating individuals diagnosed with social phobia when compared to self-administered treatments, which in turn are more effective than no treatment (p. 88).

For individuals suffering from agoraphobia, self-administered materials may be exceptionally important. More specifically, self-administered treatments for agoraphobia may reduce the likelihood that patients will become dependent on their therapist (Chambless, Foa, Groves, & Goldstein, 1982; as cited in Mains and Scogin, 2003). Additionally, self-administered treatments may increase the patient's sense of self-efficacy and help the patient generalize treatment gains. Multicomponent cognitive-behavioral bibliotherapy (Gould, Clum, & Shapiro, 1993; Hecker, Losee, Fritzler, & Fink, 1996; Lindren et al., 1994; as cited in Mains & Scogin, 2003), exposure-based bibliotherapy (Ghosh & Marks, 1987; McNamee, O'Sullivan, Lelliott, & Marks, 1989), and computer-administered vicarious exposure (Kirkby, Daniels, Harcourt, & Romano, 1999) all produced reductions in agoraphobic symptoms—gains were maintained at follow up. Finally, bibliotherapy appears to be more effective than audio-therapy (McNamee et al., 1989), and home-administered bibliotherapy or lab-assisted cognitive bibliotherapy is as effective as therapist-delivered bibliotherapy (Ghosh & Mark, 1987; Gould et al., 1993; Hecker et al., 1996; Lidren et al., 1994).

In sub-clinical populations with specific phobias (e.g., snakes or spiders), "Overall, SH approaches appear more effective than no treatment when used to treat sub-clinical phobic reactions". On the other hand, among patients who earned a formal diagnosis of phobia, therapist-directed exposure therapies seem more helpful than self-help approaches (p. 88). Additionally, SH approaches for sub-clinical presentations of social phobia and anxieties in general seem as effective as therapist-directed ones; however, those who earn formal clinical diagnoses appear to profit more by therapist-directed treatment (pp. 91–92). The efficacy of self-help for post-traumatic stress disorder is unknown at this time due to the limited number of empirically rigorous studies; however, writing exposure shows some promise as an inexpensive adjunctive or integral self-help approach, as discussed in Chapter 3 of this volume.

The efficacy of self-help treatments for obsessive-compulsive disorder, generalized anxiety disorder, and test anxiety is questionable at present—the body of research literature supporting self-help for these problems has not yet reached a critical mass (pp. 94–98). In general, across a variety of self-help approaches for the treatment of OCD, good outcomes appear to occur in less than 50% of patients (Mains & Scogin, 2003). Higher levels of OCD severity, poor levels of motivation, and higher disability levels impacted outcome negatively. One possible explanation for the paucity of supportive research for these conditions may stem from a failure to develop effective self-help approaches for these problems (L'Abate, 2008b), a conclusion supported by Hirari and Clum (2008, p. 100).

Bibliotherapy for Depression

Self-help books have the potential to reduce the burdens associated with depressive spectrum disorders. For example, bibliotherapy may allow therapists to concentrate on patients suffering from more severe forms of depression and other disorders. If a patient is suffering from mild to moderate depression, bibliotherapy may be enough to resolve the depression. On the other hand, bibliotherapy may augment individual therapy and increase the effectiveness of treatment—change may occur earlier and the magnitude of change may be greater when bibliotherapy is integrated with treatment. The foregoing applies to any psychiatric disorder that has associated bibliotherapy products.

When treating depression, a common method of intervention is bibliotherapy (Karpe & Scogin, 2008). According to one survey, between 60 and 97% of practicing psychologists prescribe bibliotherapy as part of their treatment for depression

(Mains & Scogin, 2003). The efficiency of bibliotherapy for depression or other
mood disorders has been well-documented (e.g., Cuijpers, 1997; Hrabosky & Cash,
2007). In a meta-analysis involving bibliotherapy for depression (Cuijpers, 1997),
an overall effect size of 0.83 was obtained—this compares favorably to the overall
effect size (0.73) obtained by Robinson et al. (1990) in their review of psychosocial
treatments for depression. On the other hand, bibliotherapy may not be appropriate
for all forms of depression or all patients—at least one study demonstrated greater
improvement at post-treatment for patients who received individual psychotherapy
compared to those receiving bibliotherapy alone (Floyd, Scogin, McKendree-Smith,
Floyd, & Rokke, 2001). Obviously, patient characteristics, how bibliotherapy is
incorporated in treatment, severity of depression, co-morbidity, and social support
are elements that must be considered with making treatment recommendations,
including recommendations for bibliotherapy. Martinez et al. (2008) recommend
the use of self-help materials in the early stages of intervention for mild to moderate
depression and within a stepped-care model.

With depression, in its various degrees of severity effecting more than 25% of the
American population, and the sometimes prohibitive costs of professional help, it is
imperative to find inexpensive but effective ways to provide treatment to as many
individuals as possible. In addition to self-help books, there are myriad computer
programs, automated telephone systems, audiotapes, and videotapes dedicated to
this disorder. Unfortunately, the majority of these approaches may be most effective with Caucasian females rather than women or men belonging to other racial
or ethnic groups (Karpe & Scogin, 2008, p. 110). Combining modes or formats of
therapy with bibliotherapy may increase the likelihood and magnitude of change
in depressive spectrum symptoms; however, when bibliotherapy is combined with
appropriate medication, synergistic results are not always forthcoming. More specifically, the combination of bibliotherapy with pharmacotherapy offered no significant
incremental benefit over medication alone (Holdsworth, Paxton, Seidel, Thomson,
& Shrubb, 1996). Ultimately, the combination of bibliotherapy and antidepressant
medication may be most effective for patients who are struggling with major depression (Mains & Scogin, 2003). Fortunately, the large effect size of 0.83 associated
with bibliotherapy for depression indicates that in a large number of cases (particularly mild to moderate depression), self-help approaches are typically as successful
as individual psychotherapy (Karpe & Scogin, 2008, p. 116).

Results from computer-administered treatments indicate that they can serve independently or as an adjunct to individual therapy. When computer-administered
treatments for depression are employed in an adjunctive role, they are likely to
decrease costs by reducing the number of treatment sessions with professionals
(Karpe & Scogin, 2008, p. 119). On the other hand, as discussed in Chapter 3 of
this volume, L'Abate et al. (2005) found that written homework practice exercises
significantly increased the number of visits with individual, couple, or family therapists. No matter whether treatment is administered individually and in-person, or
conducted at the distance from a professional through the Internet, effective evaluation is essential, beginning at pre-treatment and ongoing thereafter to track change
and maintenance of gains.

Bibliotherapy for Childhood Disorders

Elgar and McGrath (2003, p. 129) start their chapter with an enthusiastic endorsement of self-help approaches for childhood disorders because these approaches "circumvent barriers to traditional delivery models of health care." These authors follow up their almost unqualified endorsement by listing all the research on bibliotherapy and instructional materials for childhood disorders (pp. 134–143). These studies cover almost as many issues as one can conceive, from depression, bedtime resistance and night waking, parenting skills, post-operative pain, self-harming behavior, fear of the dark, chronic headache, disruptive behavior, inattention and hyperactivity, aggression, adoption, abuse, nocturnal enuresis, cystic fibrosis, asthma, encopresis, conduct disorder, cancer, and other psychiatric conditions. Although self-help treatments cannot replace more aggressive forms of treatment, self-administered treatments offer an alternative for less severe cases (Mains & Scogin, 2003).

Ackerson, Scogin, McKendree-Smith, & Lyman (1998) developed a bibliotherapeutic approach for adolescent depression. The major goals of the Ackerson et al. approach are (1) to provide the child and family with self-management skills, (2) to disseminate information about the problem or condition, and (3) to create and maintain a healthy social support network (Mains & Scogin, 2003). As the foregoing suggests, some self-administered treatments are developed for the parents—the parent learns and applies the treatment to the child. For behavioral disorders such as hyperactivity, ADHD, and conduct disorder, manuals may be especially helpful—benefit may accrue when medication for childhood ADHD is combined with parent manuals (Mains & Scogin, 2003).

The childhood disorders area is replete with instructional manuals for children and their parents. Additionally, electronic self-help devices for children and their parents are available and a variety of support groups exist to provide help for parents and their children struggling with childhood disorders. Nonetheless, despite this enthusiasm and the rich variety of available materials, the short-term and long-term benefits of all these approaches remain in need of systematic evaluation (Elgar & McGrath, 2008, p. 154). Nevertheless, there is a stronger evidence-base for manual-based and multimedia-based treatments than for inspirational literature and support groups (Elgar & McGrath, 2003).

Bibliotherapy for Eating Disorders

Eating disorders are relatively common among college-age women; however, the lifetime prevalence rate for anorexia nervosa is only 0.5% and the lifetime prevalence rate for bulimia nervosa ranges from 1 to 3% (DSM-IV-TR, 2000). Despite their relatively low base-rate, especially among individuals suffering from anorexia nervosa, these disorders need to be taken seriously due to their lethal nature and concomitant medical complications. One of the problems associated with the treatment of eating disorders involves their durability and a general requirement of longer-term treatment. Unfortunately, for many individuals suffering from an eating disorder, the expense and time commitment renders individual treatment impractical. Fortunately, numerous commercially produced books are available that cover the entire gamut of eating disorders (see Chapter 9 this volume) (Winzelberg et al., 2008).

These self-help materials are most appropriate for less severe forms of bulimia nervosa and binge eating disorder; however, they are not recommended for the treatment of anorexia nervosa unless the self-help treatment is integral to therapy or employed as an adjunct to intensive individual and group therapy. Additionally, because of the potentially lethal nature of anorexia nervosa, medical monitoring is a requirement for any individual struggling with this severe form of eating disorder. In addition to bibliotherapy, self-help groups for eating disorders are quite common for women across the country. In some cases, limited professional guidance may be combined with both bibliotherapy and group support.

Winzelberg et al. (2008) include a summary of structured, controlled, and uncontrolled self-help interventions for bulimia nervosa (BN) and binge eating disorder (BED; pp. 167–171). These authors conclude their review of the literature by suggesting that, "...self-help approaches for women with eating disorders and those at risk for developing an eating disorder are widely used, feasible to deliver and effective" (p. 179). An Internet-based CBT approach for the treatment of bulimia nervosa was recently examined (Fernández-Aranda et al., 2009). A variety of interventions were part of this Internet-delivered treatment with bibliotherapy as one component. Following an initial evaluation, patients worked independently for 4 months; periodic (once-a-week) Internet-based interactions with their "coach" and two face-to-face evaluations during the course of therapy were required. The investigation did not examine components of treatment but examined the programs efficacy overall. Findings suggested that an online self-help approach could be a useful treatment option, especially for patients who present with a less severe form of eating disorder. Finally, some prognostic indicators of successful outcome included higher scores on the Eating Attitudes Test and the Eating Disorder Inventory perfectionism scale and a higher minimum body mass index. This topic is covered in more detail in Chapter 8 of this volume.

Bibliotherapy for Sexual Dysfunctions

There are definite advantages and disadvantages to self-help approaches with sexual dysfunctions (van Lankveld, 2008, pp. 188–190). For instance, self-administered treatments may be preferred by individuals who are apprehensive about self-disclosure of their sexual problems or habits—privacy is more easily secured with self-help via bibliotherapy. Economic and societal advantages are obvious and patients may experience a reduction in shame and embarrassment by the avoidance of self-disclosure. Furthermore, many sexual problems can be resolved with minimum intervention. On the other hand, serious, intrapsychic or interpersonal complicated sexual dysfunctions are likely to be refractory to self-help approaches.

Serious, deep-seated, emotionally based sexual dysfunctions will need specialized therapist-administered attention. Additionally, some sexual dysfunctions are physiological in nature and require medical attention by appropriate specialists. Males experience physiologically based sexual dysfunctions at a higher rate than females. If physiologically based, no amount of psychosocial intervention is likely to be helpful. Older adults experiencing sexual dysfunction should be referred for physical evaluation including a pelvic exam. Among younger adults (under the age of 50), it is usually safe to initially assume a psychiatric etiology for the sexual dysfunction—psychosocial treatment can be delivered and assessment of change should be periodic. If change is not forthcoming following a sufficient trial of psychosocial treatment, medical referral is recommended.

Additionally, van Lankveld includes an overview of outcome studies of bibliotherapy for sexual dysfunctions ranging from premature ejaculation, preorgasmia, organic, and primary and secondary dysfunctions (pp. 194–197). Most studies on bibliotherapy for sexual dysfunctions have produced some of the largest effect sizes found for self-help interventions (p. 198). The most frequently used self-help methods for sexual dysfunction consist of systematic desensitization, self-administered sex-exam, sensate focus, mutual masturbation, stop–start technique, vibrator, and video-therapy. Computer-assisted sex therapy via the Internet is still in its early stages of development and in need of controlled studies to evaluate its effectiveness (van Lankveld, 2008, pp. 235–236). Some forms of bibliotherapy on sex and sexual dysfunctions are very user-friendly—one example, *The Guide to Getting it On* (Joannides & Gross, 2009), is an excellent educational resource and is now in its sixth edition and available for less than $15. It consists of 928 illustrated pages of information on everything from treatments available for sexual dysfunction to behaviors that promote healthy sexual functioning.

Bibliotherapy for Insomnia

Sleep disorders are common but many go untreated by a professional (Currie, 2008). Currie (2008, p. 219) provides a simple self-scoring, self-diagnostic test for insomnia. Other objective criteria symptomatic of insomnia include, sleep onset latency, waking shortly after sleep onset, the number of awakenings, total sleep time, and satisfaction with sleep quality (p. 224). The Internet provides access to numerous top-selling self-help books that could be used with minimal or maximal therapist support depending on the seriousness of the problem.

Nine studies on the bibliotherapeutic treatment of insomnia are included in Currie's (2008, pp. 226–228)—review of the literature covers commercially available sleep-related books and manuals, relaxation tapes, written instructions, brochures, specific instruction on sleep hygiene, and the thought-stopping technique. Currie also includes a detailed table of changes in sleep following SH bibliotherapy (p. 230). Some investigations comparing individually delivered psychotherapy (Currie, 2008, p. 233) with self-help groups indicate that similar outcomes are achieved from both treatment formats. Core issues impacting on the effectiveness of self-help approaches include participant compliance and consistent adherence to a specific plan and program (p. 233). Currie concluded that

> ...self-help materials for insomnia ere efficacious in helping individuals to reduce time to fall asleep, decrease the duration and frequency of awakenings, and increase sleep quality. The magnitude of change is not as large as in person treatment for insomnia but post-treatment improvement are sustained at follow-up assessments. Furthermore, most sleep parameters show additional improvement over time (p. 235).... Although self-help approaches for insomnia show promise, there are still important gaps in our knowledge base (p. 236).

Bibliotherapy for Problem Drinking

There are at least four levels of drinking: (1) complete abstinence, (2) low risk, (3) hazardous/harmful, and (4) dependence on drinking to the point that one cannot live one day without it (Kypri & Cunningham, 2008). As will be discussed in Chapter 10 of this volume, alcohol dependence is the result of an addictive behavior that supercedes other activities, responsibilities, and obligations through denial of its existence (Serritella, 1992a). The widespread individual and societal consequences of alcoholism and the high prevalence rate are indications that no existing mental health service can effectively accommodate the treatment of this disorder alone. Alcoholics Anonymous and other self-help organizations are necessary adjunctive or alternative forms of treatment. Self-help approaches for problem drinking vary from cognitive-behavioral therapy to motivational interviewing and include treatment through correspondence (Kypri & Cunningham, 2008, pp. 247–249).

The literature on self-help is not lacking in controlled studies on self-administered interventions for problem drinking (Kypri & Cunningham, 2008, pp. 253–256); however, attrition continues to be a problem in virtually all studies on substance abuse. Drop out rates for alcoholics may exceed the average due to denial and impulsivity, especially when problem drinking occurs within the context of Axis II, Cluster B personality disorders. Self-help approaches are based on the FRAMES system, relying on assessment-based feedback, emphasizing individual responsibility for change, providing direct advice to reduce drinking, offering a menu of strategies to achieve goals, adopting an empathic style, and promoting self-efficacy (Kypri & Cunningham, 2008, p. 262). These authors concluded their review thusly: "From an evidence-based prospective, self-help interventions for problem drinking can best be described as promising...more research is needed... to develop and evaluate effective self-help interventions for the many problem drinkers who will never seek intervention" (p. 261).

As will be seen in the section on smoking cessation below, self-administered treatments for problem drinking are promising because they have great potential to reach a large number of individuals. Additionally, a sense of enhanced self-control may be obtained through the utilization of self-administered treatments. Moreover, not all individuals are comfortable talking about their alcohol abuse—self-administered treatment may be more appealing for these individuals.

A meta-analysis on bibliotherapy for alcohol problems involving 22 studies and spanning three decades rendered moderate support for bibliotherapy (Apodaca & Miller, 2003). More specifically, the investigators found modest support for the efficacy of bibliotherapy; episodes of at-risk and harmful drinking decreased and a small to medium effect size (0.31) was obtained for the bibliotherapy condition compared to a no treatment condition. A weighted pre/post effect size of 0.80 was obtained for bibliotherapy among those who self-referred to treatment for problem drinking. Among those who were identified as problem drinkers through health-screening, a weighted pre/post effect size of 0.65 was obtained. When examining the signal elements in bibliotherapy's efficacy, direction on the use of free-time activities appeared to contribute to successful outcome 3 months into treatment. Pace drinking, goal setting, and coping without alcohol were associated with treatment gains at 1-year follow-up. Finally, based on the findings from Apodaca and Miller, bibliotherapy appears to be a cost-effective and clinically useful method for the reduction of problem drinking, especially among those who self-refer but also for those identified through screening.

Self-administered treatments for problem drinking alone may not be effective in treating alcohol abuse (Mains & Scogin, 2003). The research literature in this area is mixed and not all research supports self-administered interventions as a stand-alone treatment for problem drinking. A study that compared bibliotherapy alone to assessment only and physician advice only found no differences in alcohol use between conditions. Further, advice and counseling both improved the efficacy of a manual on alcohol abuse (Mains & Scogin, 2003).

Bibliotherapy for Smoking Cessation

Cigarette smoking is the single most preventable cause of premature morbidity and mortality in the United States (Doweiko, 2009). Approximately half a million individuals die prematurely as a result of smoking each year. Self-help approaches to smoking cessation have the potential to reach a large population of individuals addicted to smoking. Public health interventions may reach a larger population of smokers; however, their effectiveness is negligible. On the other hand, clinical interventions have higher success rates but access is limited to a relatively small population of smokers. Self-help approaches offer a good compromise between public health and clinical interventions (Curry, Ludman, & McClure, 2003; Mains & Scogin, 2003). When individual self-help approaches are compared to group treatments, immediate abstinence rates favor group programs; however, with time recidivism rates for group treatments rise steadily to as high as 80% while the abstinence rates for individuals who utilized self-help increase over time.

There is no question that smoking is one of the primary risk factors leading to heart disease, cancer, and stroke. Fortunately, there are a variety of commercially available self-help pharmacological approaches to help stop smoking, such as nicotine gum, transdermal patch, nicotine inhaler, and nicotine nasal spray. Some of these nicotine-replacement therapies and bupropion have demonstrated success in smoking cessation—when compared to placebo, these pharmacological interventions double cessation rates (Curry et al., 2003). These approaches have apparently helped produce abstinence rates ranging from 20 to 24% (Schare & Konstas, 2008, p. 184). One problem with pharmacological interventions is that it is difficult to assess their effectiveness under real-world conditions—poor compliance and discontinuation are issues that compromise, to some degree, the utility of these approaches.

Self-help behavioral therapies to quit or reduce smoking include written leaflets, brochures and books, audio- and videotapes, telephone counseling, and Internet (Schare & Konstas, 2008). Most of these self-help materials employ cognitive-behavioral interventions. For example, typical CBT interventions would involve the self-monitoring of smoking activity and specific emotional, cognitive, or behavioral "triggers" that induce craving. Most of the self-help literature provides information on how to improve social support, develop healthy ways to relax, and methods for stress management (Curry et al., 2003). There are more than 300 extant smoking cessation manuals, including *Kicking Butts* and *7 Steps to a Smoke Free Life*.

Unfortunately, as discussed further in Chapter 6 of this volume, it is difficult to quantify the difference between manuals requiring passive reading, manuals requiring definite and specific action, and manuals bordering on workbooks with handouts, worksheets, or practice exercises under the supervision, guide, monitoring, and interactive feedback of a facilitator, para-professional, or professional. Furthermore, it is difficult to evaluate efficacy when drop-out rates are very high. Consequently, Schare & Konstas (2008, p. 283) indicated that "The efficacy of popular smoking cessation programs as they appear in current published book form is simply questionable." When bibliotherapy for smoking cessation is combined with personalized adjuncts such as tailored materials, written feedback, and outreach telephone counseling, quit rates improve (Curry et al., 2003). Additionally, prognostic indicators for successful outcome in smoking cessation treatment include high motivation levels, less severe forms of addiction, higher self-efficacy, and better social support (Curry et al., 2003).

Bibliotherapy for Weight Loss

Obesity is considered by many to be an epidemic in the United States. In spite of self-made changes in weight loss and other approaches considered in Chapter 9 of this volume, dieting has become a popular pastime in American culture. A passing acquaintance of the second author had amassed a library of 46 diet books, which represents only a small percentage of the diet books available today in the English language. Apparently, none of the books had produced any changes in the diet and weight control of this person. When a suggestion to track food intake was made, a violent reaction followed. This anecdote is presented to illustrate that a great deal of weight control or weight loss may be due to underlying emotional, character, and personality factors that need to be taken into consideration when dealing with self-help and especially self-change for weight loss. We discuss these factors throughout this volume and specifically in Chapter 14.

The problem of obesity has reached such epidemic proportions that even federal agencies, such as the Center for Disease Control, or private agencies, such as the American Obesity Association have expressed their concerns for the serious health consequences of being overweight. Watkins (2008) summarized prevalence rates and demographic information for obesity. Additionally, Watkins touched on the controversial definition of what constitutes obesity (body mass, weight alone, or both), the fine line between obesity and being overweight, and the health implications involved. Morbidity and mortality rates for obese individuals who fail to exercise surpass those of smoking (Watkins, 2008, pp. 290–295).

The major signal variable that has emerged from an excellent literature review by Watkins (2008) is adherence to any given diet; that is, the longer one maintains any specific diet, the better the outcome (p. 314). There are pros and cons about each of the major commercial diet programs, to be reviewed below; however, weight-loss program consistency is paramount in successful weight loss. A number of important resources about diet and weight control are presented by Watkins (2008, pp. 322–323).

Given the serious nature of obesity, prevention through cost-effective Internet programs has become a high priority item in this field. The effectiveness of these programs relies on the nature and frequency of feedback given to participants. It is important that feedback be provided individually, even on the Internet. Additionally, success appears to be dependent upon frequent reminders, consistent e-mail messages, and scheduled phone calls from live helpers who might have experienced the same condition (Winett et al., 2008).

Bibliotherapy for Diabetes

Rates of diabetes are correspondent with weight; however, it is important to keep in mind that diabetes can occur for a variety of reasons—being overweight is simply a primary risk factor. Although diabetes is a physical disease, psychological, social, and societal consequences are enormous. As a result of the foregoing, a multi-layered ecological perspective on self-help has been applied to diabetes by Fisher et al. (2008). The Fisher model considers individual biological and psychological factors, family, friends, small groups, culture, community, and policy. This perspective is relevant and complementary to a hierarchical theory of relational competence for self-help and self-change that is summarized in Chapter 14 of this volume.

Fisher et al. (2008, pp. 362–367) also included a thorough summary of recent research on minimal contact interventions providing resources and supports for the self-management of diabetes. These interventions include computer-based individual dietary assessment, realistic goal setting, ongoing follow-up and support for engagement in self-management, continuity of care, with inclusion of primary physician care, individual delivery of psychosocial interventions based on cognitive-behavioral therapy, including cognitive reframing and support for the initiation of exercise, telephone counseling, Take Charge of Diabetes, a multimedia CD-ROM program consisting of five modules, computer kiosks in waiting rooms, Internet education, and many other community-oriented interventions.

In addition to the above, this ecological perspective also includes community resources. Unfortunately, the enormity of the problem and complexity of the Fisher program makes it difficult to draw definite conclusions about the outcome of this very interesting ecological perspective.

Bibliotherapy in Primary Care

Vincent et al. (2008, p. 392) identified five barriers for the use of self-help resources by primary care physicians: (1) lack of knowledge, (2) limited availability, (3) few guidelines for the use of SH materials, (4) cost, and (5) lack of culturally sensitive self-help materials. One additional barrier not mentioned by Vincent et al. might be fear of liability for recommending a questionable self-help treatment to a patient. Unfortunately, many primary care physicians are usually too busy to sufficiently concern themselves with SH or self-care. In general, primary care physicians view the direct responsibility for SH and self-care as residing outside their training and their specialties (Vincent et al., 2008). On the other hand, primary care physicians do possess sufficient authority, clout, and care to recommend and prescribe SH and self-care if they are sufficiently knowledgeable about what is available for their patients. Consequently, it would be important to know what their opinions are concerning self-administered treatments (Vincent et al., 2008, p. 392). Physicians are generally satisfied by referring or even prescribing SH or SC interventions, especially if another medical specialty is involved, such as psychiatry. They may have some general knowledge about SH but usually no more than informed laypersons. As a group, physicians are interested in knowing more about self-help, especially if this information and its dissemination do not take too much time or energy. Internet-delivered self-help is one example of a SH approach that is attractive to physicians (Vincent et al., 2008).

Vincent et al. (2008, pp. 394–397) listed effect sizes for self-administered treatments in primary care that included leaflets, self-help manuals, booklets and audiotapes, computer programs, and Internet-based tailored self-management versus peer support. Examples of self-management programs appropriate to primary care settings include (1) *Beating the Blues* for depression, (2) the *PACE* program for exercise and diet, (3) Interactive Voice-Response Systems, (4) Web-based systems,

(5) *FearFighter.com* for anxiety, (6) *MoodGYM* for depression, and (7) the Diabetes Network Project.

As is customary in medicine and as recommended by various sources cited in this volume, a stepped-care approach fits into the medical model. Such an approach may begin with a minimal form of intervention/treatment—if this proves insufficient, the next step represents a more aggressive treatment. Of course, the severity of the disorder guides the professional's selection of the appropriate step to initiate treatment. A stepped care model is recommended throughout this text and covered in Chapter 14 of this volume.

Vincent et al. (2008, pp. 408–409) also consider in detail the various advantages and disadvantages of different approaches to disseminate self-administered interventions in primary care, providing a valuable resource for health professionals who are involved or who want to become involved in this field. Consequently, the future of self-help and self-change in primary care is bright when they are coupled with the authority and respect usually present in that field.

Discussion

In retrospect Clum and Watkins (2008, pp. 419–436) indicate how their contribution is limited to bibliography while being aware of the substantial contribution that computer/Internet-based treatment programs can make. Outcome data vary from one condition to another while drop-out rates and relapses are still significant and cannot be ignored. Motivation for self-help and self-care is still a major issue that has not found a consistent and reliable solution; however, practice exercises for individuals resistant to treatment are found in L'Abate (2010). Clum and Watkins (2008) suggest devising more effective self-help programs in a way that has been covered in Chapter 3 of this volume. One area that is of concern to all professionals involved in self-help and self-care is "targeting interpersonal behavior" (p. 427), including expressed emotion. Clum and Watkins might be happy to know that in addition to practice exercises matching *DSM-IV-TR* categories (see Chapter 3 of this volume), a sourcebook (L'Abate, 2010) includes at least three series of practice exercises not only about emotional competence and development in general but also about hurt feelings in particular, which are assumed to be involved in the development and maintenance of a great many conditions reviewed in most chapters of this volume (L'Abate, 2009b).

Concluding Remarks

Bibliotherapy is a potentially useful, efficient, cost-effective method of treatment. When bibliotherapy is used most effectively, some degree of therapist involvement is required. Bibliotherapy may function as an adjunct to treatment or as an integral component of treatment. As adjunctive to treatment, bibliotherapy primarily extends therapy to the environment that exists outside the therapist's office. For example, bibliotherapy can be used in myriad ways as homework, it can function as a substitute for the therapist for those who cannot attend sessions on a regular basis, and it can serve as an ongoing resource providing "booster-sessions" beyond those scheduled by a clinician. As an integral component of treatment, bibliotherapy may function as a focal point in the process of change within formal treatment. For example, written material may evoke powerful emotions and hot-cognitions that might have taken a significant amount of time to identify in therapy alone. Patients may identify with the protagonist or a variety of characters in a written work—this identification may elicit rich material for therapeutic work. Thus, the skillful use of written material in the therapy session can help a patient make greater progress in treatment by helping to introduce important topics in the therapy session. This effect may be especially true of resistant patients who tend to perceive therapist-directed change efforts as attempts to control patient behavior. Bibliotherapy may effectively provide patients with personally meaningful material that they can work through in sessions and between sessions.

The only population of individuals that does not appear to consistently require therapist involvement with bibliotherapy is those who present with mild to moderate, uncomplicated, transient conditions—typically sub-clinical problems. In this scenario, bibliotherapy may constitute a pure form of self-help; however, the determination of sub-clinical presentation is best achieved through professionally administered psychological and diagnostic assessment. The foregoing would constitute the first activity in a stepped-care model, that is, one must determine if a specific level of formal treatment is indicated or if bibliotherapy appears to be a sufficient method of treatment. Further, any individual who is prescribed bibliotherapy alone should be reassessed at some point to determine if there has been sufficient improvement or to make an appropriate treatment recommendation if deterioration is evident. The reassessment point is a clinical decision and should be guided by information based on formal assessment data, contextual factors (e.g., social support), and clinical interview.

Presently, the empirical support for bibliotherapy is insufficient except for a few well-established volumes. We agree with McKendree-Smith et al. (2003) and Scogin (2003)—that is, publishers and authors of self-help materials should bear some responsibility for establishing empirical support for the products they market and develop. Essentially, it is unethical and professionally irresponsible to make claims about published self-help materials in the absence of a sufficient body of research to back up these claims. Even if specific claims are not made by the authors or publishers are not explicitly stated, they are implied in titles, marketing and advertising efforts, and touting of the author's expertise.

We recommend some form of quality/claims control, much like what is required for nutritional supplements, for any published and publicly available self-help material. For example, a statement indicating the presence of empirical support along with a brief summary would help consumers make appropriate choices in the products they purchase. If no empirical support exists or if the support is mixed or otherwise insufficient, a disclaimer should be clearly stated on the cover or advertising materials for any written self-help product. Truth and accuracy in advertising is an important safeguard in the burgeoning self-help industry. Just as patients may be harmed by sham treatments and therapies that have not received sufficient evaluation, false claims about specific bibliotherapies may result in serious consequences for patients and others. Among bibliotherapies that have received evidence-based support and are employed in a manner appropriate to the patient's presenting problem, their clinical utility has generally been well-established.

We thank Watkins and Clum for furnishing much of the information about bibliotherapy contained in this chapter. Their excellent and detailed volume is an important contribution to the field of SH and SC.

Chapter 5
Online Support Groups and Therapy

Introduction

A large segment of the population does not receive needed psychiatric services. The reasons for this unfortunate situation are manifold and include (1) restricted access to psychiatric services for rural communities or prison populations, (2) an over-burdened mental health care system, (3) social stigma, (4) financial constraints, (5) time constraints, (6) educational deficits with respect to treatment options and pathological symptoms, and (7) a general tendency to resist entering therapy inherent in some diagnostic categories (e.g., social phobia).

Printed self-help manuals have been available for decades; however, for many their efficacy is still in question (Rosen, Glasgow, & Moore, 2003, as cited in Andersson et al., 2006). In recent years, Internet-based self-help interventions coupled with minimal text-based (Ritterband et al., 2003), telephone or face-to-face therapist contact, or provision of information (Nicholas, Oliver, Lee, & O'Brien, 2004; Gray, Klein, Noyce, Sesselberg, & Cantrill, 2005) has become increasingly popular. Internet-based therapy and support groups have the potential to address each of the barriers to mental health treatment and, as the following information will illustrate, it can do so in a cost-effective, timely, and therapeutic manner. The variety of Internet-based psychiatric services range from information/psychoeducation to empirically supported treatment delivery. In some cases, therapists guide treatment via the Internet through email or chat rooms. In other instances, therapist guidance is delivered over the telephone. Finally, minimal face-to-face therapist contact, either in group or individual formats, may be part of the primarily Internet-based treatment protocol. The Internet increases the possibilities for dissemination of information that may help prevent sub-clinical conditions from developing into clinical conditions. Additionally, Internet-based systems of treatment may help guide patients to the best treatment(s) freeing up valuable time for clinicians to engage in more face-to-face psychotherapy.

For individuals suffering from severe forms of depression, anxiety, or other functionally impairing psychiatric diagnoses, the lion's share of the Internet-based interventions discussed in this chapter may be best viewed as an adjunct to therapy.

T.M. Harwood, L. L'Abate, *Self-Help in Mental Health*,
DOI 10.1007/978-1-4419-1099-8_5, © Springer Science+Business Media, LLC 2010

As the need for mental health treatment grows and cost constraints continue to limit what clinicians are able to offer, the Internet can fill a needed niche for a large segment of the population. Additionally, aftercare or prevention of relapse may be enhanced through Internet-based support groups or the delivery of psychotherapeutic advice and interventions. Although the Internet may not be the preferred method of treatment for many (Proudfoot, 2004), there is enough evidence to suggest that the Internet can be a useful tool for cost reduction, resource reallocation, prevention, treatment, outreach, and relapse reduction. Indeed, numerous investigations have supported the efficacy of Internet-based treatments along with minimal therapist contact for various conditions (Carlbring & Andersson, 2006). In fact, most computer-assisted psychotherapeutic treatment programs are intended for use with some degree of human contact and professional guidance (Marks, Cavanagh, & Gega, 2007).

In this chapter, we have covered selected online and technology-based treatments, support groups, and information resources—a wide range of additional online resources exist; however, we are unable to provide a comprehensive coverage here. Instead, we provide a listing of a variety of websites that the clinician and patient may find useful in locating diagnosis-relevant information, treatments, and support. Consumers are encouraged to access only quality sites—to this end, we have provided a brief section on quality assurance. Additionally, in the interest of patient safety and best practices, some level of clinician involvement is encouraged for the lion's share of mental health issues. This may simply involve a consultation or clinical interview by a qualified professional to ensure that the individual receives appropriate treatment if treatment is warranted. Relatedly, some Internet resources help to determine if treatment is necessary or if self-help resources are appropriate for sub-clinical versions of disorders; however, the quality and empirical support for these Internet sites and some of the recommended resources are still in the evaluation process. Further, except for a handful of Internet-based self-help sites, most investigations into the efficacy or effectiveness of these sites have used samples comprised of individuals suffering from disorders of mild or mild-to-moderate severity and almost all sites employ minimal to moderate therapist contact in the treatment protocol.

Telemedicine

In general, telemedicine involves the delivery of healthcare services via telephone or video conferencing; however, online computer-assisted services may also be offered. It has been used successfully in the treatment of a number of psychiatric disorders and medical conditions. For example, Schoenberg et al. (2008) conducted an investigation of a computer-based cognitive rehabilitation teletherapy program for individuals who suffered moderate to severe closed head traumatic brain injuries. Schoenberg et al. concluded that their computer-based teletherapy cognitive rehab program was similar to face-to-face speech–language therapy with respect to functional outcomes and total cost of administration. Telemedicine is most effective when delivered along with advice from a trained professional—this is the usual method employed in the delivery of telemedicine.

Telemedicine may be delivered within a clinic setting, via home-based computer, or anywhere that computer technology and telephone access is available. This technology, like other technologies discussed in this volume, can assist in the provision of 24/7 guidance, reach patients who are housebound, rural, or resistant to seeking traditional mental health services (Marks et al., 2007). As cited in Schoenberg et al. (2008), telemedicine has been successfully employed in stroke rehabilitation (Clark et al., 2002), neuropsychological screening (Schopp, Johnstone, & Merrell, 2000), and the delivery of cognitive therapy (Day & Schneider, 2002). In any event, telemedicine has the potential to speed access to effective treatments, improve treatment outcome, reduce treatment costs and relapse rates, and make teaching more effective.

Child and Adolescent Telepsychiatry Service (CATS)

Child psychiatrists are in demand—the medical specialty with the greatest shortage is child and adolescent psychiatry. The shortage is most severe in rural and low-income communities (Savin, Garry, Zuccaro, & Novins, 2006). According to Pesamaa et al. (2004), telepsychiatry has garnered a strong body of literature with at least two randomized clinical trials demonstrating the efficacy of this treatment format. For example, an investigation by Elford et al. (2000) indicated that diagnoses and treatment plans rendered by psychiatrists were similar 98% of the time when the results of in-person interviews and telemedicine were compared. Further, Nelson et al. (2000) found that telemedicine was efficacious in the treatment of child depression.

Telemedicine has had its critics; however, patient reports indicate that, for some, telemedicine provides the distance needed for disclosure of sensitive and treatment relevant information (Savin et al., 2006). In a similar vein, telemedicine allows access to care that would otherwise be costly, time-consuming, and disruptive for patients residing in rural and underserved areas. That is, providers and patients are both spared the disrupting effect of trips and the expense in cost and time necessary for treatment (Savin et al., 2006).

The CATS model involves minimal contact with mental health professionals. As employed in Rapid City, South Dakota, a community with more than 60,000 individuals and only one part-time psychiatrist (Savin et al., 2006), a clinic is available twice monthly with appointments lasting approximately 2 hrs. Eighty minutes are typically spent on initial evaluation and forty minutes are spent on treatment planning, follow-up/after-care, and general administrative matters.

Despite the negative reactions of critics and fears of those developing and implementing CATS, it was found that patients were generally receptive to the services provided by CATS. Further, clinicians in Rapid City provided favorable reports indicating that CATS helped them manage case loads and reduced their sense of professional isolation. Savin et al. (2006) indicate that the high patient and provider satisfaction coupled with the convenience of CATS supports the use of telemedicine. Telepsychiatry is a modality that assists in the treatment of underserved populations and enhances teaching and collaboration with other mental health professionals. Telephone-based guided self-help has received support from other investigators as well (e.g., Palmer, Birchall, McGrain, & Sullivan, 2002; Wells, Garvin, Dohm, & Striegel-Moore, 1996).

Telemental Healthcare for Military Populations

Military personnel are often deployed to remote locations where access to mental health care is generally difficult. Additionally, the stressors involved in remote and often long-term deployment may increase the need for mental health services. For these populations, video conferencing (telemental health care, TMHC) is an option when professional, in-person mental health services are unavailable. In the Grady and Melcer (2005) investigation, the effectiveness of TMHC was compared to face-to-face care (FTFC). It was reported that those receiving TMHC had higher Global Assessment of Functioning (GAF, DSM-IV-TR) scores compared to those in the FTFC condition. Moreover, the mean change in GAF scores was significantly greater in the TMHC condition than in the FTFC condition. Finally, compliance rates with medication plans and follow-up appointments were significantly better for TMHC (Grady & Melcer, 2005). In an earlier study on TMHC, Grady (2002) found that telemental health care services could be provided at a cost that was comparable or reduced compared to TAU.

Telemedicine for Depression and OCD

Two telemedicine programs have been successfully employed in the treatment of depression and obsessive-compulsive disorder. *Cope* for depression (Osgood-Hynes et al., 1998) may be accessed via telephone from the patient's home. *BTSteps*, a telephone-delivered treatment for OCD (Greist et al., 2002), is also appropriate for in-home access. Both of the foregoing telemedicine programs use interactive voice response and a manual to assist calls (Marks, 2004). In a recent meta-analysis, Mohr, Vella, Hart, Heckman, and Simon (2008) found that telephone-administered psychotherapy produced clinically significant reductions in depressive spectrum symptomology (pre/post effect size $d = 0.82$) and compared favorably with the findings from other meta-analyses involving face-to-face therapy (pre/post effect sizes ranged from $d = 0.71$ to 0.73). Moreover, attrition rates were lower than those reported in traditional face-to-face psychotherapy.

Online Support Groups

Computer-assisted cognitive-behavioral therapy has empirical support (based on open studies and randomized clinical trials, RCTs) in the treatment of panic disorder and phobias, generalized anxiety, obsessive-compulsive disorder, and non-suicidal depression (Marks, 2004). Computerized treatments may be accessed through the Internet or by telephone.

Some recent research on psychotherapeutic Internet chat groups has provided some interesting findings with respect to Internet group members' linguistic behaviors (Haug, Strauss, Gallas, & Kordy, 2008). For example, Haug et al. found that interaction or activity between chat group members, other than the therapist, exerted the most important effect on group member satisfaction. When these results are viewed in light of research findings on face-to-face group therapy, a patient activity level that may be characterized as outgoing is important for a successful group experience for members of both face-to-face and online groups.

Haug et al. (2008) developed an activity index from the Linguistic Inquiry and Word Count (LIWC, Pennebaker & Francis, 1996), which can be utilized as an indicator of patient satisfaction or dissatisfaction with an Internet group session. This index may help therapists to craft individualized treatment plans to maximize outcome. These investigators point out that algorithms may be programmed into the system to quantify specific words or phrases allowing therapists to receive automatic feedback on activity levels for each patient. Such feedback may be used to identify patients at risk for drop-out or to modify treatment plans.

Internet Support for Eating Disorders

Some investigations support the notion that guided self-help results in a larger magnitude in treatment effects when compared to self-help alone (Carter & Fairburn, 1998; Loeb, Wilson, Gilbert, & Labouvie, 2000). Further, guided self-help appears to produce treatment effects similar to those obtained from the therapist-delivered standard treatment (Bailer et al., 2004; Carter & Fairburn, 1998; Peterson et al., 2001; Thiels et al., 1998). With respect to eating disorders, Ljotsson et al. (2007) conducted a randomized clinical trial of Internet-assisted cognitive behavioral therapy. More specifically, these investigators employed a self-help version of CBT coupled with Internet support in the treatment of *bulimia nervosa* and binge eating disorder. Ljottson et al. employed the self-help book *Overcoming Binge Eating* (Fairburn, 1995) with a standard CBT developed for eating disorder treatment. The CBT portion of the treatment protocol involved homework relevant to each chapter in Fairburn's book and email contact with graduate students designed to monitor homework and assist if needed. Graduate students followed the manual developed by Fairburn (1999) for the self-help program. Participants were provided with online chat-room access where they could discuss treatment and support each other. Ljotsson et al. (2007) found that their version of Internet-assisted self-help coupled with CBT-based self-help books (Fairburn, 1995, 1999) was both feasible and efficacious.

Internet Support for Anxiety Disorders

One research group conducted a series of investigations on a 9-week Internet-delivered cognitive-behavioral treatment for social phobia (Andersson et al., 2005, 2006; Carlbring et al., 2007). The first study employed two group in-vivo exposure sessions coupled with minimal therapist email contact. The Andersson investigation found the Internet-based self-help program to be effective in the treatment of social phobia and reported mean Cohen's d effect sizes of 0.87 and 0.70 for between groups and within groups respectively. In the Carlbring et al. study, the treatment program was similar; however, group in-vivo exposure was not employed and therapist email contact was supplemented with therapist telephone contact. Again, findings supported the use of Internet-based treatment, this time with only supplemental weekly telephone contact (Carlbring et al., 2007). In both of the foregoing investigations, treatment gains were maintained at 1-year follow-up.

A randomized clinical trial investigation of Internet-delivered self-help versus face-to-face therapy in the treatment of panic disorder, with or without agoraphobia, was conducted by Carlbring et al. (2005). The Internet-based intervention consisted of a ten-module self-help program for panic disorder with an intended treatment duration of 10 weeks. The self-help intervention included minimal therapist contact via email (the mean total time spent on each participant was 150 min). The face-to-face intervention consisted of ten CBT sessions designed for panic disorder delivered in an individual format at a frequency of one session per week. Based on the method of evaluating clinical significance suggested by Jacobson and Truax (1991), results suggested that both treatments were equally effective with both conditions receiving within group effect sizes in the high range (Cohen's $d = 0.78$ and $d = 0.99$ for Internet and live treatment conditions, respectively). The between group effect size was small (Cohen's $d = 0.16$) and favored the live treatment condition. Treatment gains were maintained in both conditions at 1-year follow-up (Cohen's $d = 0.80$ and 0.93 for Internet and live treatment conditions respectively). In a later randomized study on the remote treatment of panic disorder by Carlbring, Bohman et al. (2006), it was concluded that Internet-distributed treatment for panic disorder, supplemented with short weekly telephone support, was clinically effective.

Tillfors et al. (2008) conducted an investigation on the efficacy of an Internet-based self-help program for university students suffering from social phobia and public speaking fears. A self-help manual was modified based on an existing empirically supported self-help manual (Andersson et al., 2006) and adapted for use via the World Wide Web (Andersson et al., 2006; Carlbring et al., 2006, 2007). The self-help manual was based on CBT principles, tailored to a university population, and targeted on social phobia. The self-help manual and minimal therapist contact via email comprised one of the treatment conditions, the other treatment condition added five sessions of live group exposure sessions to be delivered in conjunction with the manual and therapist email contact. Therapist contact was primarily in the form of support and guidance and homework assignments were reviewed to gauge progress and guide therapist feedback. The time spent with each participant was, on average, 35 min per week. Participants were also encouraged to take part in an online discussion group—each treatment condition had its own group. In short, both treatment conditions were found to be effective in the treatment of university students suffering from social phobia. Moreover, the addition of live group exposure sessions did not produce a significant improvement on outcome measures. It was concluded that the Internet-based self-help program, on its own, was efficient and effective in treating university students with social phobia (Tillfors et al., 2008).

Litz, Williams, Wang, Bryant, and Engle (2004) described the delivery of a therapist-assisted Internet self-help program for PTSD. More specifically, the intervention employed a modified form of stress inoculation training in combination with supportive homework completed with therapist guidance and feedback. The treatment program utilized fewer therapist resources than traditional face-to-face therapy; however, only 14 participants had been randomized and outcome data with respect to program efficacy were unanalyzed at the time of publication. Although none of the 14 participants randomized to SIT had dropped out at publication, it appears that it is premature to provide any substantive comments on the program at hand. In a similar study, Litz, Engel, Bryant, and Papa (2007) employed an 8-week RCT of a therapists-assisted, Internet-based, self-help CBT program versus an Internet-based supportive counseling for PTSD. Overall, results favored the therapist-assisted CBT self-help program. For example, participants in the self-management CBT condition experienced a statistically significant and sharper decline in mean total PTSD symptom severity and a greater reduction in depressive spectrum symptomology when compared to those in the supportive condition. For treatment completers at 6-month follow-up, patients in the self-management CBT condition had significantly lower depression, anxiety, and total PTSD symptoms when compared to those in the supportive condition. Additionally, a greater percentage of participants in the CBT self-management condition no longer met criteria for PTSD—these findings were replicated in an intent-to-treat analysis, that is, a greater percentage of self-management CBT cases no longer met criteria for PTSD when compared to those in the supportive condition at post-treatment. High endstate functioning as assessed by the Beck Depression Inventory-II (BDI-II, Beck, Steer, & Brown, 1996), Beck Anxiety Inventory (BAI, Beck et al., 1996), and PTSD Symptom Scale (Foa & Tolin, 2000) all favored the self-management CBT condition at post-treatment and at 6-month follow-up. Litz et al. (2007) conclude that a self-management CBT program may be of clinical utility for military personnel who often do not receive effective treatment.

One Internet-based treatment program for agoraphobia and panic is *FearFighter*. *FearFighter* is a therapist-assisted computer treatment program consisting of nine treatment steps. The program employs a variety of materials to assist the user in the development and implementation of a personalized program of self-exposure

(Proudfoot, 2004). In both, an uncontrolled study and an RCT investigation, *FearFighter* was as effective as therapist-administered CBT and it achieved this level of effectiveness with a 73% savings in therapist time (Marks et al., 2004). Another Internet-based treatment program, the *Balance system*, has been developed for generalized anxiety. Both programs have received empirical support (Marks, 2004). A computer-aided CBT program developed for the treatment of OCD, *BTSteps*, has demonstrated that it is cost-effective and clinically effective (Proudfoot, 2004).

Internet Support for Depression

Meyer (2007) examined the efficacy of a comprehensive self-help website designed specifically for students. The website (www.studentdepression.org) has close to 100 pages of information and a variety of self-help resources with accompanying personal narratives. Formal therapist involvement is not included in this self-help web-based resource; however, a broad-band in-depth account of depression, empowering perspectives and strategies, and challenges to perceived or actual barriers to help-seeking are provided. With respect to utility, the website was reported to be helpful by a representative group of users and valid by a panel of professional experts (Meyer, 2007). The site has been popular receiving over 50,000 actual visits in the initial year subsequent to its launch—visits more than doubled in the site's second year.

Similar to the foregoing, *MoodGYM* (www.moodgym.anu.edu.au), a cognitive-behavioral therapy/psychoeducation-based Internet site has received a body of supportive research literature indicating the effectiveness of this site in reducing depressive spectrum symptomology and the social stigma related to depression (Christensen & Griffiths, 2002; Christensen, Griffiths, & Jorn, 2004; Griffiths & Christensen, 2007). Another computer-based CBT program for depression, *Beating the Blues*, has amassed an impressive body of literature supporting its clinical effectiveness (Griffiths & Christensen, 2007; Learmonth, Trosh, Rai, Sewell, & Cavanagh, 2008; Proudfoot et al., 2003; Van den Berg, Shapiro, Bickerstaffe, & Cavanagh, 2004) and cost-effectiveness (Proudfoot, 2004). *Beating the Blues* is an interactive multimedia program that also has application in the treatment of anxiety and mixed anxiety/depression. *Beating the Blues* has been recommended as a part of a stepped care program for the treatment of depression (NICE, 2004; as cited in Meyer, 2007).

Griffiths and Christensen (2007) indicate that *MoodGYM* was a cost-effective treatment method; however, it may not be suitable for all users and offer some caveats. More specifically, it was suggested that *MoodGYM* may not be appropriate for individuals with low literacy levels and the CBT-focused learning style may not be experienced as comfortable for those residing in rural communities. Another website (http://bluepages.anu.edu.au) is written at a reading level much lower than *MoodGYM* and it employs a "smiley-face" rating system. *BluePages* is a depression information system similar to the aforementioned student depression website. *BluePages* provides almost 50 different medical, psychological, and alternative interventions for depression (Griffiths & Christensen, 2007). Also available are interactive online screening tests for depression and anxiety, a list of self-help resources, and a relaxation tape that the consumer may download. Finally, *BluePages* provides a search function to search within *BluePages* and internationally for other depression websites.

In a randomized controlled trial with Internet-based self-help for depression, Andersson et al. (2005) found that a self-help CBT with minimal therapist contact and a discussion group produced greater reductions in depressive spectrum symptomology than a discussion group only condition. Treatment gains were generally well maintained at 6-month follow-up. Andersson et al. concluded that Internet-delivered CBT should be considered as a complementary treatment or a treatment alternative for individuals suffering from mild to moderate depression. Another CBT-based computer-assisted program developed for the treatment of depression, *Good Days Ahead: The Multimedia Program for Cognitive Therapy*, has received empirical support (Proudfoot, 2004). More specifically, the CBT computer program produced gains that were equivalent to face-to-face standard CBT and treatment gains were maintained at 3- and 6-month follow-up.

At present, de Graaf et al. (2008) are investigating the cost-effectiveness of a computerized CBT for depression in primary care. An RCT design is being employed to compare a computerized CBT program to TAU by a general practitioner coupled with the computerized CBT program. Results of this investigation are forthcoming.

Internet Support for Depression, Anxiety, and Work-Related Stress

A web-based intervention was developed to provide self-help resources with the intention of reducing symptoms of depression, anxiety, and work-related stress (burnout). The web-based intervention was developed as a course to be completed over a period of 4 weeks. Investigators (van Straten, Cuijpers, & Smits, 2008) employed an intent to treat analysis in an RCT design to determine if the web-based intervention was effective.

The course consisted of weekly automated email messages that explained the contents and exercises for the coming week. All information and exercise forms could be downloaded or completed online. Master's level psychology students were trained to provide feedback on completed exercises—feedback was targeted on mastering the proposed problem-solving strategies and was not intended to be therapeutic. Among course completers, students spent an average of 45 min total per participant.

In general, statistical and clinically significant change was demonstrated for research participants suffering from symptoms of depression and anxiety. Further, among participants with more severe depression and anxiety at baseline, symptom change was more pronounced. A similar finding also held for individuals who completed the course, that is, there appeared to be a dose-response effect associated with the web-based program.

Internet Support for Problem Drinking

According to Riper et al. (2007), self-help interventions have been effective in the treatment of adult problem drinkers; however, their efficacy via Internet delivery has not been well-established. In the Riper et al. investigation, participants were randomized to an experimental drinking less (DL) condition or an online psychoeducational brochure on alcohol use (PBA). The DL condition was a multi-component, interactive, self-help program based on cognitive-behavioral and self-control principles and was delivered via the Internet without therapist assistance. The recommended length of treatment for the DL condition was 6 weeks. In general, the DL intervention received support as an effective program for the reduction of problem drinking. More specifically, those in the DL condition reduced drinking significantly more than those in the control condition and more than three times as many participants in the DL condition fell within the guideline norms for low-risk drinking compared to those in the PBA condition (Riper et al., 2007).

The DL intervention (http://www.minderdrinken.nl) is a free-access web-based self-help treatment program that does not include therapist involvement. Riper et al. recommends this program for problem drinkers who want to reduce their alcohol intake to a level that may be characterized as low-risk drinking. There are four stages in the DL self-help program: (1) preparing for action, (2) goal setting, (3) behavioral change, and (4) maintenance of gains and relapse prevention. Additionally, the program has chat-room capability for peer-support. Based on the findings of the study, the researchers concluded that the DL program appears to be a viable option for community use and a feasible component of an online stepped care treatment model for adult problem-drinkers.

A preliminary investigation of an Internet-based intervention for problem drinkers (Cunningham, Humphreys, Koski-Jannes, & Cordingly, 2005) employed an RCT design and randomly assigned participants to an Internet only condition or an intern plus self-help book condition. The investigators found minimal support for the Internet intervention alone; however, those who received the self-help book reported lower levels of alcohol consumption and fewer alcohol-related consequences of drinking at 3-month follow-up. Cunningham et al. concluded that the self-help book appeared to produce an additive treatment effect and indicated that self-help materials are relatively well-received by individuals suffering from problem drinking.

Internet Support for Miscellaneous Mental Health and Medical Issues

A number of popular Internet-based support groups for cancer patients exist; Seale, Zieband, and Charteris-Black (2006) investigated two of these and found that web forums are generally experienced as safe in terms of privacy and the exchange of intimate information (Seale et al., 2006). Cuijpers et al. (2008) conducted a review of investigations into Internet-administered CBT for a variety of health problems. Patient populations consisted of individuals suffering from pain, headache, and six other health problems. For the interventions targeted on pain and headache, effects obtained from Internet-administered CBT were comparable to those obtained in face-to-face treatments. For the remaining conditions, effects were not as strong for the other conditions under investigation. At present, van Bastelaar et al. (2008) are conducting an investigation on a web-based CBT for diabetes employing an RCT design—results are forthcoming. Prasad and Owens (2001) provided a description of Internet sites that disseminate information and help to those who engage in self-harm behaviors. These investigators utilized an Internet meta-search engine to find resources for their population of interest. Based on their findings, these investigators concluded that most of the support offered came in the form of information and most of the information was focused on suicide, self-injury, and psychological issues. These authors called for more published research about self-harm and the Internet. Haker, Lauber, and Rössler (2005) investigated Internet forums for individuals suffering from schizophrenia. These investigators found that Internet forums are utilized by individuals diagnosed with schizophrenia in the same general fashion as those suffering with other psychiatric disorders and those unaffected by mental health problems. It was concluded that Internet forums can help individuals who are suffering from schizophrenia learn to cope with alienation and isolation.

An Innovative Use of Online Technology in Mental Health

Systematic Treatment (ST) and Systematic Treatment Selection (STS)

The underpinnings of an innovative online and patient-driven resource are the result of three decades of focused psychotherapy research that began in the late 1970s. More specifically, the findings from patient–treatment matching research have been integrated into an Internet-distributed application of ST that is a collection of multi-level and multi-dimensional psychosocial treatment elements. STS (Beutler & Clarkin, 1990; Beutler et al., 2003; Beutler, Clarkin, & Bongar, 2000; Beutler & Harwood, 2000) was the first integrative iteration of patient–treatment matching research findings and technology. Both STS and the newer, more advanced, interactive, and patient-friendly version, ST (aka, InnerLife, www.InnerLife.com), employ empirically derived principles to inform the planning of individualized treatments for psychiatric disorders; most of these treatment planning principles have received recognition and endorsement from Division 29 and/or Division 12 of the APA (Harwood & Beutler, 2008).

All of the ST principles of change have received a substantial amount of empirical support over the years (e.g., Beutler et al., 2003; Beutler & Harwood, 2000; Beutler et al., 2000; Beutler & Clarkin, 1990; Harwood & Beutler, 2008). Unfortunately, the parameters of this chapter preclude a useful description of the 18 STS or ST principles of change; therefore, we will simply list the six empirically supported patient–treatment matching dimensions and provide a description of the information and services provided by the Internet-distributed application of ST. The interested reader is directed to Beutler et al., 2003; Beutler et al., 2000; Beutler & Harwood, 2000; Harwood & Beutler, 2008 for in-depth descriptions of the patient–treatment matching dimensions and specific studies and/or task force endorsements of STS and ST principles of change. Briefly, the six ST patient–treatment matching dimensions are (1) Coping Style (CS, externalizing or internalizing); (2) Functional Impairment (FI, an estimate of the degree that planful behavior is compromised by the patient's problems); (3) Reactance Level (RL, aka resistance, is an index of the patient's level of resistance to therapist-delivered interventions); (4) Social Support (SS, a prognostic indicator utilized in ST treatment planning); (5) Problem Complexity/Chronicity (PCC, related to Functional Impairment—PCC is a prognostic indicator, an indicator of treatment intensity, and suggests the need for multi-person treatment); and (6) Subjective Distress (SD, level of emotional arousal experienced by the patient).

The remainder of this section will provide a brief overview of how technology and research findings have been integrated to produce a treatment program formulated for both patient and clinician access and application. Systematic Treatment (ST, Beutler, Williams, & Norcross, 2009) is an advanced version of the basic idea represented by STS. One major advance is that ST has been developed to be primarily patient-driven rather than clinician-dependent, thus, addressing one of the major criticisms voiced by practitioners utilizing the earlier version. When a patient engages with the ST program, via Internet and completes the ST assessment, they are provided with an informative ST Intake Narrative Report. The ST narrative report includes important treatment-relevant information specific to seven areas with each area representing greater levels of specificity. A brief description of these seven areas follows:

1. *Potential Areas of Concern*: Identifies concerns and provides information specific to the nature of the problem that a patient is experiencing. A determination of the necessity level for formal professional help is provided at this level. Additionally, the problems and difficulties that require attention are identified and the severity of each problem is quantified. Relatedly, the overall severity represented by the patient's unique constellation of problems is also identified and an individually tailored narrative informs the patient about the degree to which these problems warrant attention and the success rates of various forms of psychosocial treatment. More specifically, four major and 14 secondary problem clusters are identified and ranked according to treatment needs.
2. *Treatments to Consider*: Provides a more detailed analysis of the nature of the treatment that research suggests will provide the most help for this particular patient and presenting problem. For example, at this level, ST considers how well the patient's personality (i.e., coping style, trait resistance level) will interact therapeutically with various empirically supported treatments and strategies. Specific brand-name therapies, deemed most helpful, are provided so the patient can discuss these with potential therapists.

3. *Treatments to Avoid*: ST identifies treatments considered ineffective for the patient's specific area(s) of concern. Treatments considered to be discredited for mental health or addictions are also identified.
4. *Compatible Therapist Styles*: Describes how the most compatible therapists, based on information gathered with respect to personality styles and demographics, are likely to interact with each particular patient. The information provided here may be best characterized as suggestions about the type of therapist who has the greatest probability of helping the patient with their presenting problem(s).
5. *Picking Your Psychotherapist*: Provides information on how to locate the therapist best suited to the patient and how to determine if the therapist is employing an empirically supported treatment. Compatibility of personal styles is addressed here as well. Additionally, level of therapist experience with the patient's presenting problem(s) is assessed (PCC, FI, SD, and presenting problem are some of the patient factors used in this assessment), and a list of pertinent questions that the patient may ask potential therapists is provided in order to further help determine the level of patient–therapist compatibility.
6. *Self-Help Resources*: Provides the patient with a list of self-help books, movies, Internet sites, and support groups tailored to their presenting problem and personal preferences.
7. *Online Support Communities*: Offers patients opportunities to receive ideas, support, and skills from people with similar concerns.

ST is a resource readily available to the public and able to provide patients with a wealth of information and various empirically supported and tailored psychotherapeutic elements sans clinician involvement. As already stated, severity of distress and problem complexity are considered important treatment indicators and a careful assessment of these dimensions provides the data needed to determine if a clinician's expertise is necessary or if psychosocial treatment is warranted. If a clinician and treatment are deemed necessary, ST provides information to the patient about those clinicians best suited to treat the patient and their unique problem; i.e., at this point treatment is tailored to the patient at the level of the therapist. Once a clinician's expertise is deemed necessary, various treatments, psychotherapeutic principles, and strategies are identified—at this point, psychotherapy is tailored to the patient at the level of clinical intervention. Not only does ST identify the best clinicians and the best forms of treatment for each patients' unique needs, it also identifies the types of treatments a patient should avoid; that is, some treatments have been found to be unhelpful for certain patients or problems and, in some cases, research has demonstrated that these treatments may be harmful to specific types of patients or to those suffering from the same presenting problem.

For some presenting problems, individuals may be able to obtain the necessary treatment via resources that do not require clinician involvement. Indeed, research on the topic confirms that most individuals with problems seek to handle the issues themselves, resorting to professional help only when all else fails (Norcross, 2006). Patient data and the ST database allow for the identification of self-help manuals, workbooks, or computer-based Internet distributed sources of support that are specifically designed to meet the needs of the patient and their presenting problem. For those patients not suffering from severe or complex psychiatric disorders, these bibliotherapeutic elements may be enough to address their concerns and restore functioning. For others, the addition of various Internet-based resources, self-help groups or other supportive resources (e.g., 12-step groups) may be called for. Any or all forms of psychotherapeutic treatment may be combined in a recipe (i.e., prescription) for success depending on the unique needs of each patient.

ST represents the integration of cutting-edge technology and quality psychotherapy research. An ever-expanding database provides increasingly more accurate treatment relevant information specific to the needs of the patient. Self-help information, focused and tailored treatment recommendations, prognostic information, change trajectories, and outcomes assessment are only some of the features that the ST program can provide. Whether the patient requires all of the resources of ST or only the self-help portion, ST will increase the likelihood and magnitude of change with a savings in time, cost, and personnel—both the patient and the profession of psychology benefit from this blending of technology and empiricism. The interested reader is directed to www.InnerLife.com for more detailed information on this innovative, patient-driven, psychosocial treatment resource.

Quality Assurance

As with any type of information resource that is Internet-based, some of the sites available on the Internet are substandard and others may even provide disinformation or discredited sham treatments (Proudfoot, 2004; Rehm, 2008; Zuckerman, 2003). Clinicians, patients, and consumers should be aware of the guidelines for evaluating sites and be able to access resources where information may be checked for accuracy. Zuckerman provides several websites to help clinicians and others evaluate the quality of Internet resources or to find other useful information on mental health issues:

1. http://helping.apa.org/dotcomsense/, this website offers a downloadable brochure titled *dotcomsense*, which provides information on privacy and quality evaluation.
2. www.webMD.com
3. www.mayoclinic.org/healthinfo/, these last two sites provide accurate informational materials on mental health issues.
4. John Grohol's Psych Central (http://psychcentral.com/) is a meta-site providing a wealth of self-help information and guide to additional resources.
5. Mental Health Net (www.mentalhelp.net) provides an index to at least 10,000 resources for clients and professionals.
6. Mental Health Sourcebook online (http://mentalhelp.net/selfhelp/) provides a list for finding any kind of support group anywhere.
7. Psychologists USA Directory (www.psychologistsusa.com/) provides links to psychologists' websites nationwide.

8. Dr. Wallin's Psychologist's Internet Guide (www.drwallin.com/Internetguide. html), an excellent guide to the Internet with helpful search tips.
9. The International Society for Mental Health Online (ISMHO, www.ismho.org or info@ismho.org) provides operating principles for patients/consumers and the clinicians who provide online mental health services.
10. The American Association for Technology in Psychiatry (formerly the Psychiatric Society for Informatics (http://www.techpsych.org) provides additional information and resources for online psychiatric services (not as comprehensive as the ISMHO website).

Conclusions

Psychotherapy and self-help programs delivered over the Internet are becoming increasing popular among lay persons and clinicians. This raises a number of practical issues that have yet to be addressed sufficiently on a national or international basis. Issues surrounding patient safety and ethical issues are most salient. More specifically, emergency procedures that safeguard patients are relatively easy to establish and implement should the need arise. Proudfoot (2004) discusses crisis procedures that involve recall/reminder systems and clinician report—computer programs can compile important information to be stored automatically and systematically relayed to patient and clinician should the situation warrant such action.

In a similar sense, ethical concerns also present themselves with computer-delivered therapeutic systems. The International Society for Mental Health Online (ISMHO) and the Psychiatric Society for Informatics (PSI; now known as the American Association for Technology in Psychiatry, AATP) have worked together to establish guiding operating principles for clinicians who provide online therapy and for patients or consumers who receive these services (Proudfoot, 2004). Informed consent, potential risks and benefits to treatment and mode of delivery, clinician profiles/credentials, the existence of safeguards and alternative treatments, and legal issues such as confidentiality are examples of the foci for the guiding operating principles established by ISMHO and PSI (Proudfoot, 2004). Even with the foregoing quality assurance and patient-centered organizations, the enforcement of guidelines developed for online mental health services is exceedingly complex, especially when they are delivered across state lines or internationally (Rehm, 2008).

Although safety and ethical concerns still exist, Internet-based and other technology-based self-help interventions have generally been demonstrated to be safe and effective in reducing symptoms of depression and anxiety. Emmelkamp (2005), in his critical review of computer technology and the Internet in mental health care, concluded that computer-driven assessment and intervention has many advantages and few disadvantages. Research support for a variety of other mental health problems such as problem drinking and eating disorders has also been demonstrated; however, more empirical support is required before one can have an acceptable level of confidence about recommendations with respect to these Internet resources. As such, recommendations for these less empirically supported resources should be made with some caution and any reservations about safety, effectiveness, or other issues should be communicated to patients. Clinicians may find online resources, even those with less empirical support, to be useful as adjunctive treatments or helpful as treatments employed in a stepped-care model. Additionally, the reduction in relapse rates associated with many online therapy and self-help resources may also warrant their utilization across a range of mental health issues.

The delivery of psychotherapy and self-help via the Internet or telephone has a number of advantages. For example, patients may access treatment or other resources on a 24/7 basis. Additionally, individuals who might not otherwise access mental health services (e.g., rural residents, those concerned about privacy, socially phobic individuals, individuals who are financially constrained, individuals with problematic work schedules, and those without a reliable means of transportation) may find Internet-delivered or telephone-administered treatments more appealing.

One significant problem with the extant self-help research is that except for a small number of studies on the efficacy of online therapy or self-help, the severity of mental health problems that were treated has generally been on the mild to moderate end of the severity dimension. Presently, it is not clear how many of these Internet-based self-help programs would function among those suffering from complex, chronic, and more debilitating forms of the disorders under study. As such, clinicians tend to correctly view self-help programs and materials as adjunctive treatments or part of a stepped-care model in the treatment of complex/chronic mental health problems. Utilized in this manner, patients may require fewer services, experience enhanced response rates, require less intensive treatment, reduce the frequency or severity of relapse, and allow therapists to focus on those who are in greatest need. Relatedly, many of these programs involve various levels of therapist contact or student-delivered feedback; when problem severity warrants, clinician contact can be increased. Indeed, very few online therapy programs are intended as independent, stand-alone treatment interventions. For the lion's share of online resources, research and refinements are ongoing (e.g., ST, Beutler et al., 2009).

With respect to those with mild or sub-clinical forms of disorders, these technology-based services appear to make sense. As stated in the foregoing, through the use of online resources, psychiatric services may become more available for those most in need. Relatedly, with the use of online resources, the prevention of a progression to clinical mental health problems is realistic for at least some of those suffering from sub-clinical forms of psychiatric disorders.

Finally, as stated above, consumers and clinicians should be aware that Internet self-help resources come in varying levels of excellence. As such, clinicians should be familiar with the quality and effectiveness of web-based interventions before recommending them to their patients. Likewise, consumers seeking self-help without clinician guidance should be aware of the Internet sites and organizations that provide information on the quality and excellence of available resources.

Various Web-Based Self-Help and Informational Resources

Much of the information contained in the following list of resources comes from Gottlieb (2008), a volume dedicated to the dissemination of information and resources for mental health professionals, physicians, and consumers.

Resources for Alcoholism, Problem Drinking, and Substance Abuse and Dependence

1. www.Ncadi.Samhsa.Gov, an informational site about prevention and addiction treatment.
2. www.aa.org, an Alcoholics Anonymous site dedicated to the sharing of information and support.
3. www.aca-usa.org, a referral resource for treatment and DUI classes.
4. www.adictionresourceguide.com, a site providing the description of in-patient and out-patient treatment programs.
5. www.adultchildren.org, a site dedicated to adults raised in families troubled by alcoholism and other dysfunctional behaviors.
6. www.al-anon.alateen.org, a site for relatives and friends of alcoholics or problem drinkers.
7. www.alcoholism.about.com/library provides links appropriate for elders to alcohol-related and drug-related sites.
8. www.doitnow.org/pages/pubhub.html provides brochures on smoking, drugs, and alcohol—has information relevant to younger abusers.
9. www.jacsweb.org, a site dedicated to the issues of denial and misinformation.
10. www.mentalhealth.com, an online encyclopedia—provides a wealth of information on treatments and diagnoses. Received the Top Site Award and the NetPsych Cutting Edge Site Award.
11. www.naadac.org, an educational site on addictions for professionals.
12. www.nida.nih.gov, a wealth of publications, research reports, and information on treatments.
13. www.nida.nih.gov/drugpages provides names of commonly abused drugs, means of detection, and medical uses.
14. www.nofas.org provides information on prevention and education relevant to fetal alcohol syndrome.
15. www.psychcentral.com, a meta-site for support and resources.
16. www.unhooked.com, a non-religious support group resource.
17. www.well.com provides reliable sources with factual information on addictions.

Resources for Anxiety Disorders

1. www.adaa.org, a site dedicated to the prevention and treatment of anxiety disorders.

2. www.aim-hq.org provides a support group focused on recovery from anxiety disorders.
3. www.algy.com/anxiety/files/barlow.html provides an overview of anxiety disorders by recognized experts in the field.
4. www.cyberpsych.org, a wealth of information on a variety of mental health issues and diagnoses.
5. www.distress.com/guided.htm provides information on stress management and methods for maximizing health, wellness, and productivity.
6. www.factsforhealth.org provides a wide range of information on a variety of psychiatric disorders including social anxiety disorder and PTSD.
7. www.freedomfromfear.org provides resources and guidance to patients and families suffering from anxiety and depressive spectrum symptoms.
8. www.healthanxiety.org provides information on treatment groups for individuals suffering from phobias.
9. www.healthyminds.org, an American Psychiatric Association resource.
10. www.jobstresshelp.com, a site dedicated to alleviating workplace stressors.
11. www.lexington-on-line.com provides information on the development and treatment of panic disorder.
12. www.interlog.com/~calex/ocd provides a list of links relevant to OCD.
13. www.nimh.nih.gov/anxiety/anxiety/ocd provides information on anxiety disorders and OCD.
14. www.nimh.nih.gov/publicat/ocdmenu.cfm provides a good introduction to OCD and treatment recommendations.
15. www.npadnews.com, a site dedicated to the dissemination of information from individuals who have recovered from anxiety disorders.
16. www.panicattacks.com.au provides information, resources, and support.
17. www.psychcentral.com, a meta-site for mental health issues.
18. www.ncptsd.org, a site dedicated to the care of Veterans through research, education, and training on PTSD and other stress-related disorders.
19. www.sni.net/trips/links.html provides links to meta-sites and other PTSD resources.
20. www.ptsdalliance.org, the PTDS alliance website.

Resources for Bipolar Disorders

1. www.bpso.org, a supportive website for individuals who interact with those who suffer from Bipolar disorder.
2. www.bpso.org/nomania.htm, an educational site providing information on causes of episodes and how to avoid Bipolar episodes.
3. www.dbsalliance.org provides mental health news updates and local support information for individuals suffering from Bipolar disorder and depression.
4. www.geocities.com/enchantedforest/1068, a meta-site for children suffering from Bipolar disorder.

5. www.manicdepressive.org provides information supported by clinical research and dedicated to educating professionals, the community, and patients.
6. www.med.yale.edu, a research center focused on mood disorders.
7. www.mentalhealth.Samhsa.Gov provides a wealth of information on resources and other aspects of mental health.
8. www.miminc.org, a site dedicated to information on medications in the mood stabilizer category other than lithium.
9. www.moodswing.org/bdfaq.html, a good resource for those recently diagnosed with Bipolar disorder—provides information on symptoms, treatments, and etiology.
10. www.planetpsych.com, a good resource for patient or therapist—provides information on a wide range of psychiatric disorders.
11. www.psychcentral.com, a meta-site providing a wealth of resources.

Resources for Cognitive Disorders

1. www.Nia.Nih.Gov/Alzheimers, a good informational site for evaluation, referral, and treatment.
2. www.aan.com, a site for professionals and laypersons, covers a wide rage of neurological disorders including Alzheimer's, Parkinson's, and stroke.
3. www.agelessdesign.com provides information on Alzheimer's Disease and other age-related diseases.
4. www.ahaf.org/alzdis/about/adabout.htm, a resource for Alzheimer's patients and their caregivers.
5. www.alz.co.uk, a meta-site dedicated to the support of dementia patients.
6. www.alzforum.org provides information intended for the layman.
7. www.mayohealth.org/mayo/common/htm/, an informational site focused on Alzheimer's Disease.
8. www.ohioalzcenter.org/facts.html provides an Alzheimer's Disease fact page.
9. www.psychcentral.com, a meta-site for numerous mental health issues.
10. www.zarcrom.com/users/alzheimers, a site that provides detailed, practical information on Alzheimer's Disease.

Resources for Depression

1. www.Depressedteens.Com, a site focused on informing teenagers, parents, and educators about teenage depression. Resources are provided.
2. www.befrienders.org, a site providing support, help-lines, and advice.
3. www.cyberpsych.org, a site dedicated to a variety of mental health issues.
4. www.nimh.nih.gov/publist/964033.htm, a good resource on late-life depression.

5. www.planetpsych.com offers information on treatments, symptoms, and other psychiatric issues for a wide array of mental health topics.
6. www.psychcentral.com, a meta-site with many resources.
7. www.psychologyinfo.com/depression provides useful information on diagnosis, psychosocial treatments, and pharmacological treatments for depression.
8. www.psycom.net/depression.central.html, a site dedicated to the pharmacological treatment of depression.
9. www.queendom.com/selfhelp/depression/depression/html provides articles on depression, information on pharmacological treatments, and contacts for support groups.

Resources for Eating Disorders

1. www.alt.support.eating.disord provides information on alternative treatments for eating disorders.
2. www.anred.com provides materials on anorexia and related eating disorders.
3. www.closetoyou.org/eatingdisorders, an informational site covering the range of eating disorders.
4. www.cyberpsych.org, a site dedicated to a variety of mental health issues.
5. www.edap.org provides educational materials focused on awareness and prevention of eating disorders. A good site for educators.
6. www.gurze.com provides listing of more than 100 books on eating disorders.
7. www.kidsource.com/nedo/ provides educational materials and treatment options.
8. www.mirror-mirror.org/eatdis.htm, a site dedicated to the prevention of relapse.
9. www.planetpsych.com offers information on treatments, symptoms, and other psychiatric issues for a wide array of mental health topics.
10. www.psychcentral.com, a meta-site with many resources.

Resources for Personality Disorders

1. www.mhsanctuary.com/borderline provides education, support, and resources on Borderline PD.
2. www.planetpsych.com offers information on treatments, symptoms, and other psychiatric issues for a wide array of mental health topics.
3. www.psychcentral.com, a meta-site with many resources.
4. www.nimh.nih.gov/publicat/bpdmenu.cfm provides treatment recommendations.

Resources for Schizophrenia

1. www.health-center.com/mentalhealth/schizophrenia/default.htm, a good site for the provision of basic information on schizophrenia.

2. www.members.aol.com/leonardjk/USA.htm provides links and information on Schizophrenia support organizations.
3. www.mentalhelp.net/guide/schizo.htm provides articles and links.
4. www.mhsource.com/advocacy/narsad/narsadfaqs.html provides answers to medical questions.
5. www.mhsource.com/advocacy/narsad/studyops.html provides information from research studies on schizophrenia.
6. www.nimh.nih.gov/publicat/schizoph.htm provides NIMH information on schizophrenia.
7. www.planetpsych.com offers information on treatments, symptoms, and other psychiatric issues for a wide array of mental health topics.
8. www.psychcentral.com, a meta-site with many resources.
9. www.schizophrenia.com/discuss/Schizophrenia provides online support for both patients and families dealing with schizophrenia.
10. www.schizophrenia.com/newsletter, a psychoeducational website dedicated to disseminating information on schizophrenia.

Resources for Suicide

1. www.lollie.com/about/suicide.html, a site providing comprehensive information on the prevention of suicide.
2. www.members.aol.com/dswgriff/suicide.html, a survival guide for individuals contemplating suicide.
3. www.members.tripod.com/~suicideprevention/index provides assistance for coping with suicidal thoughts and friends contemplating suicide.
4. www.metanoia.org/suicide/ provides good suggestions, information and links for those contemplating suicide.
5. www.psychcentral.com, a meta-site with many resources.
6. www.psycom.net/depression.central.suicide.html provides myriad links to information on suicide.
7. www.save.org, a site dedicated to suicide prevention through public education and support.
8. www.vcc.mit.edu/comm/samaritans/brochure.html provides guidelines for families dealing with suicide.
9. www.vcc.mit.edu/comm/samaritans/warning.html provides the warning signs of suicide risk.
10. www.nineline.org provides information on a nationwide crisis and suicide hotline.

Chapter 6
Manuals for Practitioners

The application of randomized clinical trial (RCT) research to psychotherapy, involving head-to-head comparisons of treatments for specified conditions, led to a proliferation of published and empirically supported treatment manuals. The large-scale NIMH Treatment of Depression Collaborative Treatment Program (TCRCP; Elkin et al., 1989) introduced the methodological innovation of treatment manuals as a way to make treatment comparisons (Beutler, Clarkin, & Bongar, 2000; Beutler et al., 2004; Lambert & Ogles, 2004). Manualized treatments are tools that investigators may utilize to aid in the identification of the signal or active ingredients within treatments and separate these specific treatment elements from the general therapeutic qualities of the therapists delivering the treatment. Unfortunately, the relatively small cadre of therapists used in the TCRCP did not allow investigators to confidently disentangle therapist effects from treatment effects. Generally speaking, therapists are not randomly assigned to treatment conditions within RCTs—participants are the individuals who are randomized and therapists are assigned to their particular treatment of choice. This selective assignment of therapists produces a confound with respect to the effects of therapists versus the effects of treatments. The best methodology to reduce therapist effects is to train a relatively large number of therapists in each of the treatments to be delivered and investigated. In this way, therapists can treat equal numbers of patients in each treatment condition according to the tenets of the specific treatment being applied (Beutler et al., 2000).

The introduction of treatment manuals was heralded by many as a revolution in psychotherapy process research (Luborsky & DeRubeis, 1984; p. 5; as cited in Beutler et al., 2000). The TDRCP promoted a proliferation of treatment manuals and helped to create a variety of applications. For example, manuals are employed in treatment delivery, training, supervision, and for the determination of third party payment for services (Chambless et al., 1996; Lambert & Ogles, 1988; Neufeldt, Iversen, & Juntenen, 1995). Today, granting agencies almost universally require that investigators adopt or develop manualized treatments in an effort to increase treatment fidelity, reduce therapist effects, and ensure the competent delivery of contrasting therapies. The ultimate aim of treatment manuals is to help practitioners improve upon outcome. We will limit our discussion to manuals that have received empirical support, although treatment manuals frequently are published based on

T.M. Harwood, L. L'Abate, *Self-Help in Mental Health*,
DOI 10.1007/978-1-4419-1099-8_6, © Springer Science+Business Media, LLC 2010

theory alone and await scientific scrutiny. Similarly, the array of treatment manuals, even those with empirical support, is vast (Beutler et al., 2004; Chambless & Ollendick, 2001). For example, at least 145 manuals have been identified; therefore, we shall provide a brief, representative sample of the extant empirically supported treatment manuals.

Brief Description of Selected Empirically Supported Treatment Manuals

Couple Therapy for Alcoholism. This is a manualized treatment for problem drinking or alcoholism delivered within a couple format. It was developed for use in a large-scale NIAAA head-to-head RCT comparison against a manualized form of family systems therapy for alcoholism or problem drinking. Couple therapy for alcoholism was published in 1996 by Wakefield, Williams, Yost, and Patterson. The empirical support for this manual comes from the original RCT investigation. The underlying premise for this cognitive-behavioral based form of treatment is that problem drinking or alcoholism is the problematic, destructive, and destabilizing force behind the couple or marital conflict. On the other hand, the family systems treatment conceptualizes alcoholism or problem drinking as symptomatic of a dysfunctional relationship.

Therapist's guide for the mastery of your anxiety and panic II & agoraphobia supplement (Map II) Program series was first published in 1994 by authors Michelle G. Craske, David H. Barlow, and Elizabeth Meadows. The series has updated versions available including the *Mastery of your anxiety and panic: Workbook*, 2006, by Craske and Barlow; *Mastery of your anxiety and panic: Therapist guide* (2006) by Craske and Barlow; *Mastery of your anxiety and panic: Workbook for primary care settings* (2007) by Craske and Barlow; and *Mastery of your anxiety and worry: Workbook* by Craske and Barlow (2006). These treatment resources offer an empirically supported, well-organized, step-by-step, primarily cognitive-behavioral approach to a variety of anxiety spectrum disorders.

The FRIENDS programme. FRIENDS is an empirically supported prevention program for childhood emotional disorders, particularly *anxiety and depression.* FRIENDS was crafted to be developmentally tailored *for children and youth.* It involves a family and peer-group CBT-based protocol and represents a modified form of Kendall, Kane, Howard, and Sigueland (1990; Kendall , 1994) CBT for anxious children. Two manuals are available: *Friends for life! For children. Participant workbook and leader's manual* (Barrett, 2004) and *Friends for life! For youth. Participant workbook and leader's manual* (Barrett, 2005).

Attention-Deficit Hyperactivity Disorder: A handbook for diagnosis and treatment. Barkley published the third edition of this empirically supported treatment manual in 2005. It is appropriate for the *treatment and management of ADHD in children*, adolescents, and adults. A companion workbook (Barkley & Benton,

1998) is available providing questionnaires and useful handouts. Interested clinicians may contact Dr. Barkley directly at DrBarkley@russellbarkley.org for additional information.

Cognitive-Behavioral treatment of borderline personality disorder. This is an empirically supported treatment manual developed by Dr. Marsha Linehan (1993a). The manual reflects an innovative method of treatment, Dialectical Behavior Therapy (DBT), for individuals diagnosed with Borderline Personality disorder or for those showing features of this disorder—these individuals have been described by clinicians as notoriously difficult to treat and some clinicians refuse to accept patients with this diagnosis.

Skills training manual for treating borderline personality disorder. This is the skills training companion manual for the treatment manual described in the foregoing (Linehan, 1993b). The skills training component of treatment is generally carried out in a group context; Dialectical Behavior Therapy is delivered by therapists in an individual format. The skills training manual is well organized into skill modules and skill groups subsumed under the foregoing. Therapists support, in the form of consultation groups, is a major component of treatment.

Parent-Child Interaction Therapy (PCIT). Originally conceptualized and developed by Sheila Eyberg, PCIT integrated elements of behavior therapy, play therapy, family systems theory, and social learning theory. PCIT was ultimately manualized by Hembree-Kigin and McNeil in 1995 and is empirically supported for the treatment of *conduct disorder*. The PCIT manual is a step-by-step guide that has a variety of supplementary materials available (e.g., videotapes, a PCIT manual adapted for group format and use with older children, and resources to help ensure fidelity of treatment delivery). For additional information: Chsbs.cmich.edu/PCIT, pcittraining.tv, http://www.ucdmc.ucdavis.edu/caare/mentalhealthservices/pcit.html

Cognitive Therapy of depression: A treatment manual. Beck, Rush, Shaw, and Emery, crafted this treatment manual in 1979. It was based on empirical findings in the treatment of depression and since then, it has garnered a great deal of additional empirical support. The manual is comprehensive—among other areas of strength, it covers the cognitive theory of depression and provides the clinician with the information and resources necessary to approach the treatment of depression from a cognitive perspective.

Interpersonal Psychotherapy of Depression. Klerman, Weissman, Rounsaville, and Chevron (1984) originally developed IPT as a treatment manual for the New Haven-Boston Collaborative Depression Research Project. It was subsequently described in a textbook for the purpose of training clinicians (Cornes, 1990). Since its inception, IPT has been employed in numerous investigations and it has been demonstrated to be efficacious for the treatment of depression. Following modifications, IPT has also demonstrated efficacy in the treatment of substance abuse, dysthymia, and bulimia. IPT is generally employed as a short-term treatment

Mindfulness-based cognitive therapy for depression: A new approach to preventing relapse. Published by Segal, Williams, and Teasdale (2002), this therapist manual is a good resource for clinicians treating patients who suffer from *multiple recurring major depressive episodes*. A companion manual for patient use, *The mindful way through depression: Freeing yourself from chronic unhappiness*, was published by Williams, Teasdale, Segal, and Kabat-Zinn in 2007.

Defiant Children: A Clinician's Manual for Assessment and Parent Training, Second Edition. Barkley's (1997) manual is based on Behavioral parent training (BPT), an empirically supported treatment program. According to Antshel and Barkley (2008), BPT employs operant conditioning techniques including contingent application of positive reinforcement (e.g., praise, privileges, and tokens) or punishment such as the imposition of time-out, absence of praise and loss of privileges or tokens. A related manual developed by Barkley (2005) is titled *Attention-Deficit Hyperactivity Disorder, Third Edition: A Handbook for Diagnosis and Treatment*. The handbook has a companion workbook with permission to copy a variety of forms, questionnaires and handouts. Barkley's (2005) handbook is based on scientific findings.

Focused Expressive Psychotherapy (FEP). FEP was manualized by Daldrup, Beutler, Engle, & Greenberg and published in 1988. Empirical support for FEP is strong and FEP has been applied to a variety of problems that are symptomatic of or partially due to blocked affect. For example, marital issues, drug and rehabilitation treatment, victims of violence, individuals suffering from mood and anxiety disorders are all possible candidates for FEP *if constricted emotional expression is a salient factor* in the recovery or maintenance of their particular problem. It should be noted that some experiential or expressive treatments have been found to be harmful (Lilienfeld, 2007); however, the Daldrup et al. (1988) FEP manual has not been identified as a harmful treatment.

Negotiating the therapeutic alliance: A relational treatment guide. This treatment manual was published in 2000 and authored by Jeremy D. Safran and J. Christopher Muran. This manual may be most effective for therapists who work with difficult patient populations such as those with character pathology. This manual is a valuable resource and it may be most useful when there are ruptures in the therapeutic alliance or when the development of a healthy therapeutic alliance is problematic. This manual is a valuable resource for anyone who wishes to engage in productive therapy.

Cognitive-Behavioral therapy for OCD. Published in 2004 and authored by David A. Clark, this manualized form of treatment has been found to be efficacious for individuals suffering from OCD. As the title indicates, the manual blends elements of cognitive therapy with previously established behavioral therapy in an effort to eliminate the symptoms and distress associated with OCD. The manual is well-organized and complete with a variety of helpful forms for both the patient and therapist. For example, therapists have case conceptualization forms for OCD and patients have various behavioral and cognitive rating scales.

Parent Management Training: Treatment for oppositional, aggressive, and antisocial behavior in children and adolescents. Published 2005, Kazdin's Parent Management Training (PMT) manual is an excellent guide for clinicians who work within a family context involving some of the more common forms of pathology among children and adolescents. The manual has a sound empirical base, is well-organized, and relatively comprehensive (One review, Allan & Workman, 2006, called for more in-depth discussion of problem-solving skills training, an important component of PMT). In 2008, *The Kazdin method for parenting the defiant child with no pills, no therapy, no contest of wills* was published—this manual for parents is a useful companion to Kazdin's 2005 PMT manual.

Personal therapy for schizophrenia and related disorders: A guide to individualized treatment. This manual was published in 2002 and authored by Gerald Hogarty. The personal therapy approach described in this manual is meant to afford flexibility in application. More specifically, the components of this therapeutic modality may be tailored to the patient's unique needs, strengths, and stage of recovery. The manual incorporates aspects of supportive therapy and the result, personal therapy, has demonstrated efficacy in patient stabilization, improved functioning, and reductions in relapse rates.

Behavioral Treatment for Substance Abuse in People with Serious and Persistent Mental Illness: A Handbook for Mental Health Professionals. This treatment manual, published in 2006 and authored by Alan S. Bellack, Melanie E. Bennett and Jean S. Gearon, is an extension of a previously developed treatment protocol specifically geared toward substance abuse among patients suffering from schizophrenia. This new version has been manualized and broadened to include an array of serious and persistent mental illness including schizophrenia, depression, and bipolar disorders.

Cognitive Therapy of Substance Abuse. Published in 1993 by Beck, Wright, Newman, and Liese, this treatment manual provides a comprehensive conceptualization of substance abuse. A large body of quality research supports the efficacy of this manualized treatment. Additionally, the manual provides the clinician with myriad useful resources including a variety of homework assignments, problem-solving strategies for non-compliant for difficult patients, and rating forms for patients to help foster awareness and gauge progress.

Prescriptive Psychotherapy (PT). This manual, authored by Beutler and Harwood (2000), is a flexible, evidence-based practices approach to *patient-treatment matching*. Clinicians are guided in the selection of specific interventions based on overarching empirically supported principles and strategies of change. Maximal flexibility is afforded because a wide range of effective interventions are subsumed under each guiding principle or strategy. The PT principles of change have received empirical support in the treatment of depressive-spectrum disorders, alcohol abuse, stimulant abuse, poly-substance abuse, and anxiety disorders. Additionally, these principles have been employed through individual, couple, and group therapy.

Supportive Expressive Psychotherapy (SE). The Original SE treatment manual was published in 1984 and authored by Dr. Luborsky. Since then, SE has been manualized and tested for efficacy within a variety of populations including participants suffering from *personality disorders, depression, generalized anxiety disorder, opiate drug dependence, and cocaine dependence*. SE has a large body of research literature supporting its application with the foregoing problems. In general, SE is a short-term psychodynamic therapy; the primary goal of treatment is to foster insight, specifically focused on current conflicted relationships based on previously cathected interpersonal themes. Signal techniques include the development of a healthy therapeutic alliance and the timely use of interpretation to facilitate insight.

Stress Inoculation Training (SIT). A variety of publications (e.g., Meichenbaum, 1996, 1994, 1985) describing this method of treatment for individuals are available from Meichenbaum, the originator of SIT. This method of treatment helps train individuals to cope with a variety of stressors including upcoming stressful events (a preventative "inoculation" measure) and coping strategies in the aftermath of exposure to stressful events. The method may be applied to individuals, couples and groups. It may constitute a very brief intervention (20 min in the preparation for surgery) or treatment may extend to 40 sessions. SIT has been applied for *problems related to military combat, athletic performance, surgery/medical concerns, the stress involved in police work, the treatment of PTSD, and anger management.*

Cognitive Therapy for inpatients with Schizophrenia. This may be a manual that is available in the near future.

Additional Manuals for Empirically Supported Treatments

Woody and Sanderson (1998) independently published a listing of the empirically supported treatment manuals that were considered well-established or probably efficacious by the Division 12 Task Force on Psychological Interventions. The following represents a sample of treatment manuals specific to several diagnostic categories included in the 1998 update and not included in the foregoing. Additional information on empirically supported treatments may be obtained from Chambless et al. (1998). An update on empirically supported treatment manuals has not been published in the last ten years (Chambless, personal communication, 12.28.2008).

Bulimia
Fairburn, C. G., Marcus, M. D., & Wilson, G. T. (1993). Cognitive-behavioral therapy for binge eating and bulimia nervosa. In C. G. Fairburn & G. T. Wilson (Eds.) *Binge eating: Nature, assessment, and treatment.* New York: Guilford Press.

Chronic Headache
Blanchard, E. B., & Andrasik, F. (1985). *Management of chronic headache: A psychological approach.* Elmsford, NY: Pergamon Press.

Depression
Lewinsohn, P. M., Antonuccio, D., Steinmetz, J., & Teri, L. (1984). *The coping with depression course: A Psychoeducational intervention for unipolar depression.* Eugene, OR: Castalia.

Treatment of Pain Associated with Rheumatic Disease
Keefe, F. J., Beaupre, P. M., & Gil, K. M. (1997). Group therapy for patients with chronic pain. In R. J. Gatchel & D. C. Turk (Eds.) *Psychological treatments for pain: A practitioner's handbook.* New York: Guilford Press.

Couple Therapy
Baucom, D. H., & Epstein, N. (1990). *Cognitive-behavioral marital therapy.* New York: Brunner/Mazel.

Generalized Anxiety Disorder
Brown, T., O'Leary, T., & Barlow, D. H. (1994). Generalized anxiety disorder. In D. H. Barlow (Ed.), *Clinical handbook of psychological disorders*. New York: Guilford Press.

Obsessive-Compulsive Disorder
Steketee, G. (1993). *Treatment of obsessive compulsive disorder*. New York: Guilford Press.
Riggs, D. S. & Foa, E. B. (1993). Obsessive compulsive disorder. In D. H. Barlow (Ed.), *Clinical handbook of psychological disorders* (2nd ed., pp. 180–239). New York:Guilford.

Panic Disorder
Barlow, D. H., & Cerny, J. A. (1988). *Psychological treatment of panic*. New York: Guilford Press.
Clark, D. M. (1989). Anxiety states: Panic and generalized anxiety. In K. Hawton, P. Salkovskis, J. Kirk, & D. M. Clark (Eds.), *Cognitive behavior therapy for psychiatric problems*. Oxford University Press.

Social Phobia
Turner, S .M., Beidel, D. C., & Cooley, M. (1997). *Social effectiveness therapy: A program for overcoming social anxiety and phobia*. Toronto: Multi-Health Systems.

Specific Phobia
Craske, M. G., Antony, M. M., & Barlow, D. H. (1997). *Mastery of your specific phobia, therapist guide*. San Antonio, TX: The Psychological Corporation.

The Argument for and Against Treatment Manuals

Manuals are Useful Clinical Tools

A number of practitioners and investigators have argued for the dominance of clinical impressions in the development of individualized treatment plans (Davison & Lazarus, 1995; Malatesta, 1995; Persons, 1991; as cited in Beutler et al., 2000); however, "Meehl's (1960)...conclusion that diagnostic accuracy and behavioral predictions based on simple statistical formula are more accurate than even the most complex clinical judgment has never been refuted empirically (Dawes, Faust, & Meehl, 1989)" (Beutler et al., 2000, p. 316). As Beutler and colleagues go on to state, faith in the accuracy of clinicians' perceptions and opinions is outweighed by the objective accuracy of these opinions and viewpoints (Houts & Graham, 1986). Further, clinicians are frequently persuaded by illusory correlations (Chapman & Chapman, 1969) and often influenced by relatively irrelevant events and personal biases (Houts & Graham, 1986; Nisbett & Ross, 1980). Clinical experience appears to increase the likelihood that illusory correlations will be accepted as factual and clinicians are prone to believe firmly in the validity of their own clinical judgment even though their formulations are inaccurate and their ability to predict behavior is no better than chance (Beutler et al., 2000).

At present, there are more than 400 brand-name therapies and they continue to proliferate at an alarming rate. This proliferation suggests that no single-theory formulation is adequate for all individuals or all presenting problems. Moreover, many treatments are developed within complex permutations of abstract theories of patient pathology rather than theories of patient change. Other theories are no more than vague representations of loosely structured clinical opinions and lore. Treatments that rely upon complex theory frequently lack sound empirical support. Treatments that rely upon impression and lore frequently lack a detailed method of application (Beutler et al., 2000).

Evidence is mounting that specialized and structured training in manualized forms of psychotherapy has the potential to enhance treatment effectiveness (Burns & Noel-Hoeksema, 1992; Henry, Schacht, Strupp, Butler, & Binder, 1993; Schulte, Kunzel, Pepping, & Schulte-Bahrenberg, 1992). Additionally, effectiveness of treatment appears to be correspondent with the level of treatment compliance, regardless of the type of treatment manual employed (Dobson & Shaw, 1988; Shaw, 1983) and treatment manuals appear to increase therapist consistency (Crits-Christoph et al., 1991). Additionally, training in manualized treatments may be most useful for therapists who know the least (Beutler & Harwood 2004). In a similar vein, although using a highly structured, inflexible treatment manual may be problematic from some perspectives, some evidence suggests that adherence to such a manual is more effective than allowing the therapist to unsystematically modify and adapt the manual to individual patients and needs (Emmelkamp, Bouman, & Blaaw, 1994; Schulte et al., 1992). Further, there is evidence that the demonstrated efficacy of manualized treatments in randomized clinical trials (RCTs) can be transported in the form of effectiveness to clinical settings (Tuschen-Caffier, Pook, & Frank, 2001; Wade, Treat, & Stuart, 1998). Finally, in a study by Schulte et al. (1992) the fallibility of clinical judgment was illustrated by the tendency for clinicians to misidentify which manualized treatments were most effective in spite of clear empirical evidence to the contrary (Beutler et al., 2003) .

Manuals are Problematic and Limiting

There are a number of problems associated with treatment manuals. For example, head-to-head comparisons of manualized treatments have generally failed to find meaningful differences between them. Some researchers interpret these findings as proof that common factors are the meaningful mechanisms of change (Lambert & Bergin, 1994). Conversely, the failure to find consistent differences between manualized treatments has been interpreted by others to represent a failure in methodology. More specifically, most investigations that have compared manualized treatments do not disaggregate patients based upon individual predispositions to different psychotherapeutic interventions—they group patients by diagnosis failing to recognize treatment-relevant variability that exists among patients within a diagnostic category (Beutler et al., 2000). The potentially fruitful aptitude-by-treatment interactions available for investigation number in the millions (Beutler, 1991).

A second problem arises within the area of psychodynamic therapies—investigations from Strupp and his group at Vanderbilt found that the therapists with the best treatment compliance were the least empathic and most angry (Beutler et al., 2000). Apparently, within psychodynamic treatments, manualization attenuated the important human, common elements that are beneficial to outcome (Henry, Schacht, et al., 1993; Henry, Strupp, Butler, Schact, & Binder, 1993). Perhaps the structure inherent in treatment manuals has an attenuating effect on those common variables that may ultimately prove to be more important to the change process than unique theory-specific elements.

A third problem centers on the issue of competence/skill. More specifically, therapists may learn a particular form of manualized treatment; however, this does not necessarily mean that these same therapists will competently deliver the treatment (Bein et al., 2000; Castonguay, Goldfried, Wiser, & Raue 1996; Lambert & Ogles, 2004). The findings reported by the foregoing investigators suggest that it may be valuable to differentiate between specific competence and general competence. The former refers to compliance or adherence to a manualized form of treatment while the later refers to the skill level of the therapist in the administration of the treatment (Beutler et al., 2004). In a similar vein, there is evidence suggesting that the ability of a therapist to learn a manualized form of treatment is negatively correlated with that therapist's interpersonal skills (Henry, Schacht et al., 1993; Henry, Strupp, et al., 1993). Relatedly, strict adherence to manualized treatment may interfere with the development of a healthy working relationship (Henry, Strupp, et al., 1993) and attenuate the likelihood or magnitude of positive outcome (Castonguay,et al., 1996). Additionally, there is wide variability in the manner in which a given manual is applied—as such, therapy effects have been detected within manuals. That is, the setting and nature of the treatment population appears to influence how a given manual is delivered (Malik, Beutler, Alimohamed, Galagher-Thompson, & Thompson 2003).

Another potential problem is that treatment manuals vary among a number of important dimensions. For example, some manuals suffer because they adhere strictly to a single theory, as such, they provide guidance; however, they limit the range of interventions available and allow for little in the way of flexibility or creativity (e.g., Beutler, 2000; Strupp & Anderson, 1997). More specifically, these types of manuals are single-theory specific, proscribe certain interventions, strategies, or principles of change while at the same time prescribing a set of relatively narrow and theory specific interventions—each patient is treated as if they are the same. In the more extreme examples of these types of manuals, each treatment session is scripted and specific objectives and tasks are assigned (e.g., Wakefield et al., 1996). The primary criticism of unitheoretical and scripted manuals is that they are overly restrictive, inflexible, and they tend to treat each individual as if they will respond equally to the interventions allowed regardless of the patient's unique presentation, context, and predilections or distaste for certain interventions (Beutler et al., 2000; Beutler & Harwood, 2000; Beutler et al., 2003; Norcross & Prochaska, 1982, 1988).

Managed care systems may utilize treatment manuals in an effort to help contain treatment costs. These systems typically attempt to maintain costs at a level that does not fall below "the bottom line", sometimes irrespective of patient need. To this end, manuals are employed to control costs by restricting, standardizing, and limiting coverage and the number of treatment sessions allocated for chronic conditions that require more broadband, intensive, and lengthy treatments (Beutler et al., 2000).

Another shortcoming alluded to in the above, centers on the tendency for manuals, due in the main to their inflexibility, to ignore the artistry of psychotherapeutic practice. We have already cited evidence to support the notion that the technical consistency manuals provide is often helpful; however, inflexibility may offset the gains provided by conformity. This is a salient criticism because Anderson and Strupp (1996) demonstrated that the most effective psychotherapists occasionally found it necessary to depart from manualized guidelines. In other words, manuals generally limit clinicians to a truncated array of interventions or strategies and prevent them from creatively or systematically adapting treatments to the unique needs, nondiagnostic states, and predispositions of individuals (Beutler et al., 2000). Relatedly, manuals have been criticized for being inadequate for application with patients suffering from complex and chronic co-morbid problems—the type of patients that often seek help for their problems through psychotherapy (Beutler, Kim, Davison, Karno, & Fisher, 1996; Silverman, 1996; Wilson, 1996).

The Present Status of Manualized Treatments

It is generally accepted that manualized treatments are productive within research settings because they allow investigators to train therapists, more accurately assess the effects of training, examine the effects of adherence, measure the degree of differences between the delivered therapies, and allow investigators to extract detected therapy factors from the noise generated by therapist and patient factors (Beutler et al., 2004; Lambert & Ogles, 2004). On the other hand, there is scant evidence to support the notion that manuals improve upon treatment effects—in fact, the collective evidence suggests that there are few mean differences in outcomes between manualized treatments and TAU in clinically relevant samples (Beutler et al., 2004; Beutler, 2009).

Given the available research on this topic, it appears that the general effectiveness of treatment manuals is still highly questionable and a great deal of ongoing research in this area is needed. For example, a meta-analysis of 90 studies indicated that naturalistically applied psychotherapy was just as effective as manualized treatments (Shadish, Matt, Navarro, & Phillips, 2000). Additionally, a mega-analysis that included more than 300 meta-analyses and involved a variety of psychotherapies revealed that structured treatments performed similarly to treatment as usual (TAU) within naturalistic settings (Lipsey & Wilson, 1993). On the other hand, manuals may prove fruitful in clinical settings and training programs by improving the effectiveness of those who are in need of training in the treatment of specific disorders.

Methodological weaknesses and poorly formulated treatment manuals may explain the absence of differential outcomes across manuals and between manuals and TAU. For example, many studies do not randomly assign therapists to manualized treatments—instead, therapists often select the form of manualized treatment they wish to deliver making selection bias a potential confound in these investigations. Additionally, manuals that fail to clearly distinguish important patient attributes and methodology that fails to provide distinguishing characteristics between manuals results in overly simplistic designs that are unable to investigate potentially fruitful aptitude-by-treatment interactions (ATIs). Future investigations involving treatment manuals should not neglect ATIs and more rigorous designs should be required for any future research in this area.

A Uniquely Formulated Treatment Manual

The failure to find consistent and meaningful differences between manualized treatments in RCTs may simply be a reflection of unsophisticated methodologies and statistical procedures. For instance, it is traditional for RCT designs to consider patient groups as homogenous simply because they have earned a specific diagnosis. These designs fail to recognize that myriad non-diagnostic treatment-relevant variables may be important considerations in the determination of treatment effectiveness. What we are referring to is research that incorporates specific aptitude-by-treatment interactions that are selected for investigation because prior research has supported their contribution to differential treatment response.

A manual based upon the foregoing would essentially allow investigators to disaggregate patients according to a set of distinguishing characteristics or patient qualities that result in differential treatment responses to specific therapist delivered interventions. Diagnosis would no longer be the single or dominant guiding criterion for treatment application—instead, clinicians would select principles and strategies of change that house families of interventions; treatment decisions involving the selection of specific interventions would be informed by each patient's unique pattern of interpersonal style and emotional response states.

Effective manuals would guide clinicians in the selection of empirically supported principles of change, identify specific strategies, and highlight an array of interventions that are most appropriate for application. In a systematic manner, the manual would target the principles, strategies, and interventions that have the highest likelihood of producing positive change and are also most likely to generate the greatest magnitude of change.

At the positive end of the flexibility dimension are manuals that do not prescribe specific single-theory formulations. Instead, these manuals place their emphasis on flexibility, patient non-diagnostic dimensions, and an inclusiveness of the array of empirically supported interventions, strategies and principles of change (Beutler, Moleiro, Malik, Harwood, Romanelli et al., 2000; Beutler & Harwood, 2000; Beutler et al., 2003; Housley & Beutler, 2006). In fact, these manuals are relatively consistent with the two major premises underlying the psychotherapy integration movement: (1) a variety of ingredients from different psychotherapies may be combined to create a unique and more effective treatment, and (2) various ingredients from the many therapies may be combined to produce a unique treatment for each specific individual. The manuals developed by Beutler and Harwood (2000) and by Housley and Beutler (2006) are examples of the later premise and promotes psychotherapy integration at the level of principles, strategies, and interventions tailored to meet the needs of each patient and proclivities of each therapist.

Prescriptive Psychotherapy (PT)

Systematic Treatment Selection (STS; Beutler & Clarkin, 1990) is a model of patient–treatment matching that incorporates the ideal qualities for a treatment manual briefly described in the foregoing section. This model has undergone a number of changes over the years incorporating additional patient predisposing variables and identifying a number of prognostic indicators for treatment modification and success. The most recent manualized rendition of STS is Prescriptive Psychotherapy (PT; Beutler & Harwood, 2000)—this manual represents a prescriptive approach to intervention that cuts across theoretical frameworks (Beutler et al., 2000).

The principles of change embodied in PT are empirically supported and independent of any particular theoretical framework. PT is first and foremost a manual directed toward treatment planning—as such, PT guides the clinician in the selection of principles of change, informed by the various patient qualities that produce differential treatment responses, thereby increasing the likelihood and magnitude of positive treatment outcome. More specifically, this multi-component method of intervention involves targeted assessment, the identification of treatment-relevant patient dimensions, and a guiding systematic patient–treatment matching model that informs clinicians in the selection of specific interventions. The primary patient dimensions employed by the STS model are: (1) Coping Style, (2) Functional Impairment, (3) Reactance Level, (4) Subject Distress, (5) Social Support, and (6) Problem Complexity/Chronicity. We will provide a brief discussion of these dimensions and their empirical support in the following paragraphs. The interested reader is directed to Harwood and Beutler (2008) for more detailed information on STS and a newly reformulated version, Systematic Treatment (ST, aka InnerLife, www.InnerLife.com).

Patient Coping Style: This dimension may be determined via a variety of methods, the most efficient method employs a patient-driven computerized ST system (discussed in the chapter, Online Therapy, this volume) that identifies a patient's dominant coping style. A ratio of several clinical scales (Beutler & Harwood, 2000) derived from the MMPI-2 (Butcher, 2000) may also be employed to determine a patients dominant style of coping. The STS principle that corresponds to coping style is dependent upon the patient's identified status as an externalizer or internalizer. For patients identified as externalizers, the corresponding STS principle suggests that these extroverted or externalizing and impulsive patients will benefit from treatments designed to employ interventions that directly alter symptomatic behavior and enhance skills. On the other hand, the introverted, internalizing, and restricted patient will benefit from treatments that employ interventions specifically designed to directly affect insight and awareness. Recently, the Division 29 Task Force identified coping style as a participant factor meaning that this STS principle should be considered an empirically supported principle based on "a preponderance of the available evidence" (Castonguay & Beutler, 2006a, p. 634; Harwood & Beutler, 2008).

Functional Impairment: Is an estimate of the degree to which a patient's planful behavior has been compromised by their presenting problem. The newly formulated ST system provides the most efficient and accurate assessment of this patient dimension. The STS principle that corresponds to Functional impairment (FI) states that "benefit corresponds with treatment intensity among high functionally impaired patients" (Beutler & Harwood, 2000, p. 149; Harwood & Beutler, 2008). In other words, as FI increases, so should the number of treatment sessions attended per week, or the length of treatment sessions, or therapy may take on a multi-person treatment (including group, family, couple, or pharmacotherapy). FI was recently identified by the Division 29 Task Force as a participant factor (Castonguay & Beutler, 2006a; Beutler, Castonguay, & Follette, 2006; Harwood & Beutler 2008). Relatedly, FI was recently identified by the Dysphoria Work Group of the Task Force on Empirically Based Principles of therapeutic Change (Castonguay & Beutler, 2006c; Harwood & Beutler, 2008).

Reactance Level: Reactance is sometimes referred to as "resistance" in the treatment literature. Reactance is defined as the patient's perception of efforts on the part of the therapist to control her or his behavior—a patient's tendency toward reactance may become activated when ". . .a patient's sense of freedom, image of self, safety, or psychological integrity, or power is threatened" (Beutler & Harwood, 2000, p. 115). The STS principles that correspond to reactance are: (1) Therapeutic change is most likely when procedures do not evoke patient resistance and, (2) therapeutic change is greatest when the directiveness of interventions is either inversely related to the patient's current level of reactance or the therapist authoritatively prescribes a continuation of the symptomatic behavior (Beutler & Harwood, 2000). Empirical support for these principles have been found in more than 30 different investigations with a combined sample size of more than 8,000 inpatient and outpatient samples (Beutler et al., 2000; Harwood & Beutler, 2008).

Subjective Distress: The STS principles for managing distress are: (1) The likelihood of therapeutic change is greatest when the patient's level of emotional distress is moderate and, (2) therapeutic change is greatest when a patient is stimulated to emotional arousal in a safe environment until problematic responses diminish or extinguish (Beutler & Harwood, 2000). Empirical support for these principles have been found in at least eleven investigations with a combined sample size of both inpatients and outpatients totaling more than 1,250 (Beutler et al., 2000; Harwood & Beutler, 2008).

Social Support: Social support has been identified and employed as a positive prognostic indicator, and as an inverse correlate of functional impairment, in the STS model (Beutler et al., 2000; Beutler & Harwood, 2000; Beutler et al., 2003; Harwood & Beutler 2008). At least 37 investigations with a combined sample of more than 7,700 inpatients and outpatients have provided empirical support for this patient dimension (Harwood & Beutler, 2008). Further, the Dysphoria Work Group of the Task Force on Empirically Based Principles of Therapeutic Change recently identified social support as a patient prognostic indicator (Castonguay & Beutler, 2006b; Harwood & Beutler, 2008). The ST principle that corresponds with this dimension calls for the establishment or enhancement of social support whenever it is nonexistent or weak.

Problem Complexity/Chronicity: Like social support, this patient dimension is related to FI; however, a subset of patients is able to function adequately, in various aspects of their lives, even when saddled with complex/chronic problems (Beutler, Brookman, Harwood, Alimohamed, & Malik, 2002). Problem Complexity/Chronicity (PCC) is a highly informative patient dimension. More specifically, PCC is a prognostic indicator, an indicator of treatment intensity, and PCC suggests the need for multi-person treatment (Beutler et al., 2000; Beutler & Harwood, 2000). Patients suffering from highly complex and chronic problems respond best to intensive broad-band treatments; within the domain of psychotherapy, systemic and dynamic treatments should perform better than symptom-focused treatments. Among medical treatments, ECT or ECT in combination with pharmacotherapy would generally be favored over pharmacotherapy alone (Beutler et al., 2000; Gaw & Beutler, 1995). Facilitating social support increases the likelihood of positive change among patients with complex/chronic problems (Harwood & Williams, 2003) and prognosis is attenuated by PCC and by the absence of patient distress (Beutler et al., 2000; Harwood & Beutler, 2008). The STS treatment matching dimension that corresponds to PCC has received empirical support in at least 23 investigations with a combined sample size of nearly 2,000 inpatients and outpatients (Harwood & Beutler, 2008).

Concluding Remarks

The parameters of this chapter prevented comprehensive coverage of the empirically supported treatment manuals available today; however, we hope we have provided a fairly representative cross-section. Manuals continue to be developed at a rapid pace. For example, it was recently reported (DeAngelis, 2008) that Barlow has proposed the development of a new manualized treatment that shares some of the features of Prescriptive Psychotherapy. More specifically, the manual functions at the level of principles of change, is flexible, and research suggests that it is efficacious (DeAngelis, 2008). Barlow claims that his proposed manual may be applied across mental disorders, thus, therapists will only need one manual to treat all diagnoses. This approach to mental health treatment makes sense. Indeed, the principles embedded in Prescriptive Psychotherapy (Beutler & Harwood, 2000) have already been applied across patient populations and they have received empirical support among various diagnostic groups. Although PT is likely to be efficacious across additional untested groups of patients (e.g., Harwood, Fraga, & Beutler, 2001), it claims to have efficacy with only those populations in which empirical support has been obtained already. Irrespective of the type of manual a practitioner may select for a particular patient or condition, the manual serves as a method of self-help for the treating clinician.

Unfortunately, the research on the effectiveness of manualized treatments is mixed. Collectively, the empirical support for treatment manuals is outweighed by a number of negative findings and meta- or mega-analyses that cast doubt on their importance or clinical utility. Of course, psychotherapy process and outcome research has benefited from the use of treatment manuals. Additionally, fledgling therapists and therapists who need additional training with a specific disorder or population of patients, and the patients they treat, may reap the greatest benefit from manualized forms of treatment. In a similar vein, many treatment manuals have companion workbooks that extend treatment beyond the confines of the therapist's office—a resource and practice that is likely to enhance treatment outcomes.

The effectiveness of a treatment manual appears to depend on a variety of elements such as therapist skill, competency, creativity, and the willingness to depart from the manual when deemed clinically necessary. A manual that guides individualized treatment planning, encourages creativity, and promotes seamless adjustments in empirically supported principles of change, strategies, and techniques (e.g., Beutler & Harwood, 2000; Housley & Beutler, 2006; DeAngelis, 2008) appears to hold the most promise for clinical utility across a wide range of patients. An additional element, signal to a potentially effective manualized treatment, is the ability of a clinician to skillfully apply empirically based practices.

Therapists must be able to effectively utilize empirically supported principles of change in the treatment planning stage; however, they must also be able to make skillful in-session adjustments based on patient cues and the introduction of clinically relevant information. There is some evidence to suggest that seasoned clinicians may find it most difficult to learn new and complex manualized treatment models. This evidence prompted Beutler and Harwood to hypothesize that effective and transferable training in Systematic Treatment Selection (e.g., Beutler & Clarkin, 1990; Beutler & Harwood, 2000; Housley & Beutler, 2006) models may require specialized instruction for fledgling therapists. To this end, virtual reality (VR) technology may serve training programs, trainees, and patients quite well (Beutler & Harwood, 2004). Virtual reality training methods, geared toward instruction in treatment models such as Prescriptive Psychotherapy, can circumvent the dangers that patients suffering from complex and chronic disorders may face when being treated by a fledgling therapist. More specifically, virtual patients suffering from difficult to treat complex conditions may be developed and may serve as an effective and safe method for the initial and on-going training in patient–treatment matching models.

Cucciare, Weingardt, and Villafranca (2008) discuss the use of blended learning, to implement evidence-based psychotherapies. Blended learning is defined as the "...systematic integration of several complementary informational delivery mechanisms in an effort to optimize learning and skill acquisition" (Singh, 2003, as cited in Cucciare et al., 2008, p. 299). Chu (2008) expands upon the foregoing by discussing the who, what, and how of blended learning. Empirically based manualized psychotherapies, especially those that function at the level of principle and strategy, may demonstrate significant improvements over TAUs if VR technology is one of the elements integrated in blended learning. Indeed, through comprehensive blended learning, we may finally observe incremental improvements in training and ultimately realize the promise of significant improvements in the clinical utility of treatment manuals that employ empirically based principles of change.

At present, the debate over the general clinical utility of treatment manuals remains vigorous. A clear consensus has not been reached; however, refinements in research design are likely to provide some clarification on this topic of great importance to researchers and practitioners alike. The interested reader is directed to the following for more in-depth coverage of treatment manuals and their efficacy and effectiveness.

Part III
Self-Help and Self-Change Approaches for Specific Conditions: Initiated, Administered, Guided, Maintained, and Monitored by Professionals

Up to this section, SH methods were reviewed as they apply to a variety of non-clinical and clinical conditions. In this Section, SH is paired with self-change (SC) methods for specific clinical conditions, where a variety of SH methods have been used to help individuals and their intimates improve their behavior to reach higher levels of functioning. As discussed in Chapter 1 of this volume, where Mark Sobell's (2007) model was presented and expanded, SH within this context means more than changing by approaching and adding new behaviors, it means also SC, avoiding past undesirable behaviors and initiating new ones, a much more difficult level obtainable by many people who do need to be guided, monitored, and followed-up over time, perhaps for a lifetime. We start with what at first blush may seem a relatively mild condition i.e., shyness, and social phobia. However, in spite of this perception, shyness may be a much more pervasive condition that it may appear in many phobias, fears, and avoidance behaviors. In this Section, we increase the relative severity of disorders concluding with more serious disorders, including medical ones.

Chapter 7
Anxiety Disorders

Anxiety spectrum disorders comprise the most common of psychiatric diagnoses in the U.S. They occur approximately twice as often in women than in men (Gottlieb, 2008). The high prevalence rates for anxiety, increasing demands on mental health treatment providers, and pressure from insurance companies to limit treatment time has created a need for brief, less expensive, but effective psychotherapeutic procedures and resources targeted on the treatment of anxiety spectrum disorders (Newman, Erickson, Przeworski, & Dzus, 2003).

As with most psychiatric disorders, many individuals suffer needlessly because they resist entering treatment for a variety of reasons—economic, limited treatment access, social stigma, and time constraints are just a few of the problems people face in seeking mental health treatment from a professional. In a different vein, many suffer from what may be best characterized as sub-clinical anxiety—they may not yet meet diagnostic criteria for any of the anxiety disorders; however, they may eventually earn the diagnosis if they continue living with their anxiety without seeking some form of intervention.

Fortunately, a variety of SH workbooks for a wide range of anxiety disorders are available to the general public. Therapists are typically well aware of their clinical utility as an adjunctive treatment for anxiety; however, individuals who have not entered treatment are often unaware of the existence of these treatment workbooks unless they are informed by someone "in-the-know". The availability of these materials via the Internet and SH section of their local bookstores provides easy access for the motivated and informed consumer.

Self-Administered Treatments for Anxiety

Ethical concerns centered on the proliferation of SA treatments have prompted debate, especially for treatments that have yet to receive empirical support (Rosen, 1987). More recently, Newman (2000) has questioned the clinical utility of SH materials for all individuals suffering from anxiety spectrum disorders and has called for more investigation and prescriptive practices based on empirically supported predictors of positive treatment response. It is still unclear if limited therapist

T.M. Harwood, L. L'Abate, *Self-Help in Mental Health*,
DOI 10.1007/978-1-4419-1099-8_7, © Springer Science+Business Media, LLC 2010

contact, or no therapist contact, endangers the individual suffering from anxiety or other psychiatric disorders. A good portion of the likely signal elements in the treatment of anxiety disorders are considered by some to be technique (e.g., Lambert, 1992); therefore, an investigation on the contribution of therapist contact in the treatment of anxiety was conducted by Newman et al. (2003).

The foregoing researchers provide solid empirical support for undertaking such an investigation. For example, meta-analyses have demonstrated the effectiveness of SH materials for fear reduction and anxiety (Gould & Clum, 1993; Mars, 1995). As pointed out by Newman et al., 2003, effect sizes derived from meta-analyses on the efficacy of these SH materials are comparable to those achieved from therapist-delivered treatments (i.e., $d=0.74$). Relatedly, treatment gains from these SH materials were relatively durable with effect sizes remaining stable between end of treatment and follow-up (Newman et al., 2003). When individuals were provided with SH media, such as audiotapes, to supplement their bibliotherapy, effect sizes approximately doubled (Gould & Clum, 1993; Newman et al., 2003).

The foregoing findings suggest that, at least for some, SH materials targeted on the treatment of anxiety may be valuable as stand-alone, self-administered treatments; however, treatment studies rarely employ a methodology that does not involve some type of therapist contact with varying degrees of time spent in therapist contact. For example, investigations often employ several or all of the following: (1) regularly scheduled check-ins with their therapists, (2) a pre-assessment, (3) a rationale for the SH treatment typically delivered by the therapist, (4) introduction to the SH materials, (5) clinic appointments to engage in the SH treatment (Newman et al., 2003). Based on the variety of therapist contacts involved in studies on anxiety and SH, Newman et al. (2003) chose to investigate if minimal structure and therapist contact was sufficient for positive treatment outcome. Five different anxiety spectrum disorders were included in their analysis of the literature. More specifically, Newman et al. (2003) covered SH for phobias, panic disorder, obsessive-compulsive disorder (OCD), generalized anxiety disorder (GAD), and social phobia.

In general, the review of the literature by Newman et al. (2003) indicated that significant benefits from SA treatments were achieved with only a few exceptions. Additionally, SA treatments were as effective as those involving greater amounts of therapist contact. Further, predominantly SH (PSH) and minimal-contact (MC) therapy were just as effective as SA desensitization via audiotape and booklet on phobic anxiety. Relatedly, computerized vicarious exposure was as effective as MC therapist-led exposure and educational reading about snakes was as effective as therapist-directed education about snakes. One caveat with respect to the foregoing findings is that several of the studies involved interventions administered in a laboratory setting (Newman et al., 2003), that is, Hellstrom & Öst (1995) found that the location of exposure (lab versus home) explained differences in percentage of change across settings (i.e., 63% of laboratory self-exposure individuals improved versus 10% of home-delivered self-exposure individuals).

In a systematic review of the literature on the efficacy of SH manuals for anxiety disorders in primary care settings, van Boeijen et al. (2005) found that, in general, SH manuals have clinical utility and can be regarded as an effective treatment possibility for primary care participants suffering from anxiety. More specifically, although some of the investigations included in the review failed to support the inclusion of a SH manual in the treatment of anxiety, most of the investigations produced positive findings in favor of the SH manuals. Most of the effect sizes (Cohen's *d*) from the studies reviewed were in the moderate to large range. Additionally, van Boeijen and colleagues reported that a SH manual was effective in ameliorating anxiety in a sample of participants with a duration of anxiety complaints greater than 1 year. In the White (1995) study, treatment gains were maintained at 12-month and even at 3-year follow-up. It is noteworthy that only six studies were included in the review; however, all six involved RCT designs strengthening the conclusions reached by the authors in the review. Further, there was a positive association between therapist contact or guidance on the use of the manual and accrual of therapeutic benefit.

Depression is typically co-morbid with anxiety; therefore, studies that examine the utility of self-therapy for these often co-existing disorders are of interest. One such investigation was carried out by Stant, Ten Vergert, den Boer, and Wiersma (2008). In this RCT, 151 participants were assigned to cognitive self-therapy (CST) or treatment as usual (TAU). The findings suggested that CST was a cost-effective and useful treatment with the effectiveness of CST at least comparable with that of TAU—on some treatment relevant indices, CST outperformed TAU. For example, CST appeared to be more cost-effective and it had the potential to relive the burden of an already over-burdened mental health care system. The authors suggest wider implementation of CST may improve the health care system and provide help to persons who might otherwise not be served.

Shyness

Although the prevalence of shyness (aka social anxiety) is high, there is a paucity of appropriate resources for this problem available to the consumer and clinician. When available, resources generally take the form of workbooks and are typically subjected to limited scientific scrutiny. In spite of the paucity of empirical support for these resources, the availability of resources, such as interactive workbooks, may represent a positive step, especially if these resources can be adapted to the Internet and given the scrutiny they require.

Workbooks

The second author published a Shyness workbook for shyness in children (L'Abate, 1992e, pp. 228–231) patterned after a paradoxical approach (Weeks & L'Abate, 1982) that consisted of three computerized practice exercises for parents or caregivers about (1) a *description* of the disorder, especially in children, according to their frequency, duration, intensity, origin, consequences for participants, and previous attempts to deal with this problem; (2) *explanation*, in which 12 *positive* explanations (reframing) for this behavior were given, asking parents to rank-order those explanations according to how they applied to the individual participant. If none of the explanations applied to the child, parents were asked to come up with a more likely explanation for this behavior in their child with possible suggestions on how this behavior could be decreased; and (3) *prescription*, in which parents were asked to provoke and replicate this behavior in the child at prescribed spaces and times, keeping notes of what happened whenever they instituted this paradoxical prescription of the symptom. Unfortunately, this program was never administered to anyone due to the second author's retirement from teaching and private practice.

The most helpful SH book/manual in this area is Carducci's (1999) classic, which is not only extremely readable but also replete with programmed, self-administered SH materials involving therapeutic writing exercises. Writing requires thoughtful reflection and internal locus of control from participants. For instance: (1) a shy-life survey (pp. 22–29), (2) incorrect assumptions of an unhappy shy person (p. 49) versus positive assumptions of a successful shy person (pp. 50–51), with (3) the beginning of a shy life journal, (4) instructions on how to work on such a journal (pp. 76–77, 99), (5) Shyness Attributional Questionnaire (pp. 114–1150, and (6) the real-self/ideal-self quiz (pp. 138–140). Additionally, Carducci covers shyness at various stages of the lifecycle, including different stigma that occur at those different stages. Throughout these stages there are penetrating questions that need to be answered in writing.

Even more importantly, Carducci has followed up with research (2000) that analyzed the written responses of shy individuals to investigate the nature of the self-selected strategies they used to deal with their shyness. A content analysis of written responses of 158 shy individuals indicated that 91% of the individuals utilized at least one self-selected strategy to deal with their shyness while 40% tried two strategies and 15% tried as many as three strategies. The classification, along with the frequency of their use, of the self-selected strategies by four raters identified 10 separate categories, with the top five labeled forced extraversion (65%), self-induced cognitive extraversion (26%), educational extraversion (15.2%), sought professional help (14.6%), and liquid extra-version (12.7%). An evaluation of the self-selected strategies indicated that they were associated with characteristic features that were incomplete, self-defeating, and/or potentially dangerous (e.g., self-medication). Suggestions as to how shy individuals might improve the effectiveness of these self-selected strategies for dealing with their shyness and the therapeutic implications associated with seeking professional assistance for shyness are presented, along with a discussion of the value of employing qualitative research methodology in the study of shyness.

A shyness workbook for teens (Carducci & Fields, 2007) covers this topic with systematic practice exercises that are extremely relevant at this age, including an initial assessment (pp. 5–6) and comments (voices) by teenagers who have completed these assignments. A shyness workbook for adults developed by Carducci (2005) contains a list of self-contained written homework assignments contained in Table 7.1 not requiring any interaction with a helper, a departure from the interactive practice exercises presented in Chapter 3 of this volume. It would be valuable to examine what outcome would be produced by administration of this workbook

Table 7.1 List of homework practice exercises for shyness

1. Defining shyness: What shyness really is
2. Born shy?
3. Shyness is not all in your head: Putting it into perspective
4. Understanding approach-avoidance conflict: The sources of the conflict
5. The slow-to-warm-up tendency: Time to adjust
6. Understanding the comfort zone: The role of routine
7. Shyness and self-esteem: It's not what you think
8. Assessing your shyness: What makes you shy?
9. Becoming successfully shy: Taking control of your shyness
10. Making the right decisions: The key to your success
11. Defining shyness of the mind: The most critical component
12. Understanding the role of anxiety: A misunderstood emotion
13. Strategies for controlling your anxiety: The anxiety advantage
14. Narcissism and selective attention deficit: The problem of excessive
15. Self-consciousness
16. Controlling excessive self-consciousness: Promoting realistic self-evaluations
17. Explaining attributional process: Playing the blame game
18. Common attributional errors: Losing the blame game.
19. Controlling attributional errors: Playing the blame game fairly
20. Common social comparison errors: When uncertainty promotes unfairness
21. Controlling unfair social comparisons: Promoting self-confidence with fair comparisons
22. Expanding your comfort zone: Gently widening your range of experiences
23. Performing social reconnaissance: Planning and preparing for your social success
24. Taking advantage of the warm-up process: Actively responding to the passage of time
25. Preventing social medication: Avoiding the trap of liquid extroversion
26. Practicing quick talk: Setting the stage for conversational contacts
27. Taking advantage of rejection: Finding useful information
28. Focusing on your social successes: Creating opportunities for personal enhancement
29. Helping other shy individuals: Becoming a host to humanity
30. Becoming a volunteer: Helping yourself by helping others
31. Living the successfully shy life: A day-to-day adventure

*From Carducci (2005).

on a spaced rather than massed administration with or without feedback. The basic issue with all these materials is outcome. What immediate and long-term results have been produced by this workbook?

Another workbook about shyness and social anxiety was developed by Antony and Swinson (2000) that deals with topics such as appearing, acting, or talking in front of an audience at one end of a continuum of avoidance to complete withdrawal from social events and contacts at the other end. Each chapter in this workbook is coupled with homework assignments about conquering one's fears, feeling confident about new relationships, and living without being controlled by fear and anxiety. It would be important to evaluate how this workbook compares with Carducci & Field (2007) workbook and what difference interactive feedback or no feedback would have on outcome.

Treating Social Phobia at a Distance

Titov and his collaborators (Titov, Gavin, Schwencke, Probny, & Einstein, 2008; Titov, Gavin, and Schwencke, 2008) performed a very important series of studies that supports highly the use of distance writing and Internet interventions for disorders of this kind. In the first study a clinician-assisted computerized CBT program was administered to 105 participants high on social phobia divided into an experimental and a waiting list control group. After evaluation of social phobia with two different paper-and-pencil self-report tests, experimental participants entered into a treatment program composed of four components: (1) six online "lessons," (2) homework assignments, (3) participation in an online discussion forum, and (4) regular e-mail contact with a therapist.

Outcome was assessed by how many participants completed this program (78%) and effect sizes comparing social phobia measures with those of non-participants controls were $d=1.15$ and $d=0.95$ respectively. The important aspect of this study lies in its results comparing favorably with "exemplary" F2F TB treatment programs. Even more importantly, Titov and two of his collaborators (Titov, Gavin, and Schwencke, 2008) replicated the same study with 85 participants with exactly the same procedures used in the first study. Completion of the program was found in 80% of participants with effect sizes of $d=1.18$ and $d=1.20$. In this study researchers tracked the average amount of time spent between each participant and the therapist, an incredible 127 min of contact time spread over the 10 weeks of treatment with 22 e-mail messages between the two parties. Furthermore, this treatment, without ever seeing the therapist, was found to be very acceptable to participants. Research of this kind should be the gold standard for publication in the mental health field, where replication of results seldom occurs. Another important application to the treatment of social phobia might be virtual reality therapy.

Virtual Reality Therapy

Virtual Reality Therapy (VRT) has been very successful in treating phobias since 1994 (North, North, & Code, 1997). Since that time, a plethora of studies have shown how many phobias can be treated through a technology that exposes participants to feared situations (fear of flying, closed spaces, spiders, snakes, etc.) by repeated exposure and desensitization (North, North, & Burwick, 2008). Fear of public speaking could be conceived as an expression of shyness and social phobia. North et al. (1997) involved 16 participants selected through a two-stage screening process by which they were assigned to an experimental and to a do-nothing control group. The VRT group was subjected to 5 to 10–15 min sessions. Real world follow-up showed a significant reduction in anxiety symptoms, comparable to other studies, in spite of the small sample size. Anderson et al. (2003) reported on two case studies in which VRT was used to treat social phobia according to a mixture of one or two in vivo and at least two VR exposures. Combination of real exposure and VR exposure seemed to produce significant reduction in anxiety levels in both participants.

Harris et al. (2002) discussed the prevalence and impact of public speaking anxiety as a type of social phobia, reviewing also the literature about VRT as an emerging treatments specifically targeted to phobias. In their study (Harris et al., 2002) one group of 8 students completed individual VRT treatment and post-testing while 6 students were in a waiting list control group assessed also on a post-treatment basis. Assessment measures included four self-report, paper-and-pencil inventories, self-report of Subjective Units of Discomfort during exposure to VRT, and physiological measurements of heart rate during speaking tasks. Four weekly individual exposure treatment sessions of approximately 15 min each were conducted by the first author serving as therapist. Results on self-report and physiological measures suggested that the four VRT sessions were effective in reducing public speaking anxiety in university students, corroborating earlier studies of VRT effectiveness as a psychotherapeutic modality. Future research directions should be focused on younger populations where social anxiety may have emerged earlier than in college.

Specific Phobias

Specific phobia is characterized by anxiety generated by exposure to a specific feared object or situation. The major types of specific phobia are animal, natural environment, blood-injection injury, and situational. The ratio of women to men with specific phobia is 2:1; however, ratios differ by type, still favoring women. Community surveys indicate point-prevalence rates of 4–8.8% and lifetime prevalence rates ranging from 7.2 to 11.3%. Onset of specific phobia is generally identified in childhood or early adolescence and it appears to occur earlier in women than in men (DSM-IV-TR, 2000).

Self-Administered Treatments

With respect to specific phobias, exposure has been designated the most successful treatment strategy (Chambless, 1990). Self-administered exposure has been found to be particularly efficacious prompting some to suggest that therapist involvement in exposure for social phobia is relatively redundant (Marks, 1991). Self-administered (SA) treatments for specific phobias have been employed for snake phobia (Barrera & Rosen, 1977; Clark, 1973; Cotler, 1970; Girodo & Henry, 1976; Hogan & Kirchner, 1968; Rosen, Glasgow, & Barrera, 1976) and spider phobia (Gilroy, Kirkby, Daniels, Menzies, & Montgomery, 2000; Hellstrom & Öst, 1995; Öst, Salkovskis, & Hellstrom, 1991; Öst, Stridh, & Wolf, 1998; Smith, Kirkby, Montgomery, & Daniels, 1997). The foregoing studies ranged in their method of treatment delivery from home application to self-administration in a laboratory setting and most utilized objective forms of outcome assessment (Newman et al., 2003). Additionally, attrition rates were generally within expectations.

Newman et al. (2003) suggest that some people may respond better if individual contact with a therapist is part of the treatment protocol. In a comparison of MC therapist-directed SA treatment and home self-directed treatment, positive responses were found for 71% versus 6% respectively. Similar findings were reported in subsequent studies. For example, 100% of individual MC treatment participants responded with positive clinical change compared to 68% of group MC individuals and 27% of home-based SA treatment individuals. In a separate study, three hours of therapist-directed exposure produced positive change in 88% of individuals compared to only 63% improvement among individuals who engaged in clinic self-exposure. Finally, a single session of therapist-delivered exposure outperformed one hour of SA-exposure performed in a lab. Based on the foregoing, Newman et al. (2003) suggest that more therapist contact than is typically provided with SH materials or self-administered treatments may be a necessary component of change for some individuals.

Newman et al. (2003) provide some evidence of predictors of differential optimum treatment response for self-administered treatments for specific phobias. For example, an investigation by Smith et al. (1997) provided evidence that self-administered vicarious exposure was effective for both phobic relevant and phobic irrelevant targets. Additionally, in an investigation by Öst et al. (1998), bibliotherapy produced greater positive change than did video therapy. Moreover, Gilroy et al. (2000) found that self-administered vicarious exposure produced a better therapeutic response than did an audiotape delivery of a relaxation technique. Further, Hellstrom & Öst (1995) found that a detailed SH manual was better than a general and briefer manual. Finally, Öst et al. (1998) found that positive treatment outcome predictors included a respected treatment manual and motivation for psychosocial treatment. Newman et al. (2003) conclude, based on the foregoing, that the treatment of specific phobias has a higher likelihood of positive therapeutic response if a treatment manual has credibility, motivation for change is adequate, therapists impose an acceptable level of externally imposed structure or contact, and the principle of exposure is part of the treatment strategy.

Predominantly SH

PSH treatments are described by Newman et al. (2003) as those SH treatments where, "therapist contact beyond assessment is for periodic check-ins, teaching participants how to use the SH tool, and/or for providing the initial therapeutic rationale" (p. 253). Only three PSH treatments had been tested by the time of the Newman et al. (2003) review, one for spider, one for snake, and one for mixed phobias. Unfortunately, the findings from these three investigations are mixed. For example, a 20-min therapist-delivered rationale combined with self-desensitization delivered in-home produced effects similar to those derived from a 65-min therapist-delivered rationale and hierarchy construction coupled with phone check-ins on a weekly basis. In this investigation, both active treatment conditions produced effects that were significantly more effective than a control condition (Phillips, Johnson, & Geyer, 1972). Similarly, 30 min of role-play coupled with bibliotherapy self-desensitization developed for lab delivery by a friend or stranger resulted in the same effect as a therapist-delivered desensitization (Moss & Arend, 1977). A study that produced differential treatment response was conducted by Öst, Ferebee, and Furmark (1997). In this investigation, the findings indicated that PSH videotape-administered vicarious exposure and live vicarious exposure were less effective than a therapist-led, group-administered in-vivo exposure.

Minimal Contact Treatments

MC treatments have been defined as those that include "active involvement of a therapist, though to a lesser degree than traditional therapy for this disorder, includes any treatment in which the therapist helps with initial hierarchy construction" (Newman et al., 2003, p. 253). As Newman et al. (2003) report, MC treatments have been applied to phobias for spiders (Arntz & Lavy, 1993; Öst, 1996), snakes (Lang, Malamed, & Hart, 1970; O'Brien & Kelly, 1980), injections (Öst, Hellstrom, & Kaver, 1992), blood/injury (Hellstrom, Fellenius, & Öst, 1996), flying (Öst, Brandberg, & Alm, 1997), heights (Baker, Cohen, & Saunders, 1973), and dental situations (de Jongh, Muris, ter Horst, G., & van Zuuren, 1995). Exposure is the guiding treatment principle for each of these MC treatments with specific treatment strategies or interventions varied across investigations. Many of these investigations combined other treatments or elements of treatments such as Cognitive Therapy, modeling, muscle tension techniques, and relaxation training.

Although the amount and duration of MC sessions varied, each of the treatment interventions were effective at reducing phobias. Moreover, treatment gains were maintained in at least one, three, and predominantly at 12 months follow-up. The addition of Cognitive Therapy proved superior to the addition of information for dental anxiety (de Jongh et al., 1995) and most of the foregoing studies employed objective outcome measures (Newman et al., 2003). When MC treatments were compared to therapies with greater therapist contact, the MC interventions fared as well or better, especially at follow-up (e.g., Baker et al., 1973). As Newman et al. (2003) suggest, the foregoing indicates that, at least some participants may be better served by MC treatments than more traditional treatments requiring greater therapist contact and greater expense.

Some indicators of MC treatment efficacy that were identified include (1) better outcomes were observed when groups were kept to a minimum (i.e., three or four members) compared to groups of seven or eight participants (Öst, 1996), (2) therapist-guided exposure of as little as 30 min was more effective than non-therapist guided exposure (O'Brien & Kelly, 1980), (3) education was positively associated with treatment response, and (4) greater anxiety and avoidance at pretest were prognostic indicators for successful treatment response (Baker et al., 1973). Collectively, these findings suggest that externally imposed structure and/or some contract with a clinician may result in a more effective treatment, among a wider array of participants, for specific phobias (Newman et al., 2003).

Panic Disorder

The key feature of panic disorder is unexpected panic attacks coupled with severe concern over their recurrence. Lifetime prevalence rates have been reported as high as 3.5%. Panic disorder without agoraphobia is diagnosed twice as often in women than men. Panic disorder with agoraphobia is diagnosed three times as often in women than in men. Co-morbidity with other anxiety disorders is common with prevalence rates varying for specific disorders. Additionally, co-morbidity with major depressive disorder has widely varying prevalence rates depending on source ranging from 10 to 65% (DSM-IV-TR, 2000).

Self-administered treatments may be useful for those suffering from Agoraphobia because of the difficulty these individuals experience when it is necessary to leave the house for treatment or other purposes. A SA treatment may produce the changes necessary for an individual to leave their home and engage in psychosocial treatment or pharmacotherapy. SA treatments may also be useful for those suffering from Panic Disorder without Agoraphobia. As pointed out by Newman et al. (2003), some investigators have suggested that therapist contact may lead panic disordered persons to become dependent on their therapist while increasing rates of relapse (Jannoun, Murphy, Catalan, & Gelder, 1980; Mathews, Teasdale, Munby, Johnston, & Sahw, 1977). Indeed, longer term treatment may be counterproductive for individuals suffering from panic disorder related problems and limited therapist contact may be indicated (Newman et al., 2003).

In an effort to find predictors of positive treatment response to SH for panic attacks, Baillie and Rapee (2004) developed a prognostic scale to identify who will likely recover from panic attacks with minimal help and who will likely require more intensive forms of treatment. In their investigation, 117 participants experiencing panic attacks participated in a 9-month trial of a psychoeducational booklet, a SH workbook, and brief group CBT. In sum, baseline social anxiety and poorer general mental health were prognostic indicators of less successful outcome on a scale of panic disorder and agoraphobia (PDA) symptoms. More specifically, a positive screen for problem drinking, high baseline neuroticism scores, earlier onset of first panic attack, and severity of PDA was associated with poorer general mental health at baseline and this was subsequently associated with poorer outcome. It was concluded that, among people presenting with panic attacks, a score of four or less on the prognostic scale may be provided with psychoeducation and SH along with regular monitoring. For those scoring five or greater on the prognostic scale, recovery from psychoeducation and SH is less likely and face-to-face therapy is indicated.

SA Treatment for Panic Disorder

There is limited available research on SA treatments for Panic Disorder. Among extant investigations, one uncontrolled study (Harcourt, Kirkby, Daniels, & Montgomery, 1998) and two controlled studies (Parry & Killick, 1998; Febbraro, Clum, Roodman, & Wright, 1999) provide evidence for the efficacy of SA treatments for panic disorder. More specifically, in the Harcourt et al. study, self-reported panic attack symptoms were reduced immediately and at 18-month follow-up following a computer-administered vicarious exposure. The Parry investigation found that, in a RCT head-to-head comparison of cognitive-behavioral bibliotherapy versus video therapy prior to therapist assignment, both forms of SA treatment were effective at reducing panic symptoms; however, participants who experienced the video found it more encouraging than did those who utilized the manual. In the Febbraro study, therapist contact was not utilized—instead, cognitive-behavioral bibliotherapy, bibliotherapy plus self-monitoring, self-monitoring, and wait-list conditions were compared on the dimension of panic symptoms. All active-treatment groups showed improvement; however, no differences were detected between any groups at end of treatment. Newman et al. (2003) suggest that some therapist involvement may be necessary to increase the efficacy for SA treatments for panic disorder.

PSH Treatments for Panic Disorder

Among the more methodologically rigorous studies involving comparison conditions, bibliotherapy was consistently more effective than wait-list control (Gould & Clum, 1995; Gould, Clum, & Shapiro, 1993; Lidren et al., 1994). Moreover, home-administered bibliotherapy and lab-administered computerized treatments were equally effective as their therapist-delivered versions (Ghosh & Marks, 1987; Gould et al., 1993; Lindren et al., 1994; Wright, Clum, Roodman, & Febbraro, 2000) and no difference on clinically significant change was detected between PSH and therapist versions at follow-up (Lindren et al., 1994). Additionally, few differences were detected on dimensions of homework compliance, treatment satisfaction, or attrition rates between PSH and therapist delivered treatments (Newman et al., 2003).

MC Treatments for Panic Disorder

According to Newman et al. (2003), SH approaches such as cognitive therapy, exposure-based interventions, problem solving strategies, multi-component CBT, bibliotherapy, and palmtop computer-administered treatment, employed as an adjunct to minimal therapist contact, all produced significant reductions in panic symptoms. Further, in several of the studies reviewed by Newman and colleagues, positive change was maintained or increased at 6-month follow-up. Finally, 67–90% of participants in some investigations were designated panic-free at follow up (Newman et al., 2003).

When optimal conditions for MC treatments for panic disorder were examined, exposure-based interventions were found superior to problem solving techniques. Additionally, the inclusion of a spouse as co-therapist did not result in a statistically significant improvement over treatment alone (Newman et al., 2003). When MC and a standard-length treatment were compared, no differences were identified on the patient dimension of panic. More specifically, a four session computer-assisted version of cognitive-behavioral therapy was as effective as twelve sessions of CBT without computer assistance. Finally, when severely agoraphobic participants were treated with a MC treatment, they failed to respond favorably until therapists implemented exposure-based interventions (Newman et al., 2003). As Newman and colleagues point out, these findings suggest that MC therapy is often sufficient for panic disorder treatment; however, for those suffering from severe agoraphobia, additional therapist involvement may be required for treatment benefits to accrue. Additionally, the efficacy of SA treatments for panic disorder is questionable, MC and PSH appears to be a more reliable form of treatment for most participants suffering from panic attacks.

Obsessive-Compulsive Disorder

OCD typically begins in adolescence or early adulthood; however, childhood onset is not uncommon. Males generally experience an earlier age of onset than females—between the ages of six and fifteen for males and 20 and 29 for females. Prevalence rates are ultimately equal across sexes (Gottlieb, 2008). Several forms of SH interventions have been employed in the treatment of OCD including, computer programs, SH manuals, voice-activated phone messages in combination with a SH manual, and self-exposure homework. In all of the studies reviewed by Newman et al. (2003), a variety of exposure and response prevention (ERP) techniques were examined.

SA treatments for OCD

An interactive computer program was developed as a SA vicarious treatment for dirt ERP for hand washing (Clark, Kirkby, Daniels, & Marks, 1998). A significant reduction in self-reported symptoms and a decreased urge to vicariously ritualize within therapy sessions was observed; however, the change was modest and not clinically significant—Newman et al. (2003) indicates that the findings may be characterized by some as a failure from a clinical standpoint. It was suggested that the computer program might be more effective as an adjunct to more traditional therapy or used in a MC treatment (Newman et al., 2003).

PSH Treatments for OCD

Two uncontrolled investigations were conducted on a program (BT Steps) that employed a self-guided treatment manual and an interactive voice response (IVR) system compatible with any touch-tone telephone (Bachofen et al., 1999; Marks et al., 1998). The BTSteps program includes self-assessment and self-treatment elements (Newman et al., 2003). Any use of the IVR system resulted in a computer-generated report containing summary information, positive feedback, and homework reminders that was mailed to the participant. As Newman and colleagues summarize, the BTSteps program was helpful for about half of the participants. A strong indicator of negative outcome was program non-compliance, severity of OCD symptoms, low levels of motivation for change at baseline, and higher levels of symptom-based functional impairment (Newman et al., 2003). In a follow up RCT of BTSteps, Kenwright, Marks, Graham, Franses, and Mataix-Cols (2005), it was found that proactive phone support from treatment staff significantly enhanced OCD patient's compliance and improvement with the computer-assisted SH program when compared to study participants who were left on their own to request phone support.

MC Treatments for OCD

Newman et al. (2003) reviews four MC investigations for OCD. Therapist contact varied across studies from three and one half hours to five hours. The findings from the investigations included in the Newman review indicate that MC produced significant positive change in clinician-rated and self-rated measures of OCD symptoms. Additionally, gains were maintained at one month follow-up in one study and active treatment participants fared better than those in delayed-treatment in a separate investigation. Still, as the Newman review points out, the investigation that obtained clinically significant improvement did so for only 33% of the study participants. Moreover, one investigation obtained relapse rates that were high on measures of depression and OCD symptoms with 79% of participants seeking additional treatment post follow-up. The MC treatments investigated in the Newman literature review do not appear adequate in the treatment of OCD.

PTA Treatments for OCD

Only two case studies on PTA treatments were identified by the Newman et al. (2003) review—we will not cover these investigations because we consider them of limited clinical utility, especially due to the relative failure of these treatments to reduce OCD symptoms. Newman and colleagues (2003) summarize the PTA, PSH, MC, and SA treatments along the following lines: (1) all SH treatments produce some reduction in OCD spectrum symptomology, (2) vicarious ERP proved insufficient as a stand-alone treatment, (3) an interactive home-accessed PSH program was relatively effective for motivated, compliant participants and those with moderate OCD and with moderate functional impairment, and (4) MC treatments were helpful for approximately 33% of participants.

Generalized Anxiety Disorder

Among individuals diagnosed with GAD, many report feeling anxious all their lives. GAD is reported to have a 1-year prevalence rate of approximately 3% and a lifetime prevalence of 5%. It is diagnosed more often in women with epidemiological studies on GAD indicating that approximately 66% are female. Often, GAD is a co-morbid diagnosis seen among individuals seeking treatment from a clinic specializing in anxiety disorders (DSM-IV-TR, 2000).

Few studies on SA treatments for GAD were identified in the Newman et al. (2003) review. Some PSH and MC treatment designs have been tested; however, not enough investigations have been conducted to make more than tentative conclusions. In general, PSH and MC treatments show enough promise to encourage further investigation.

Social Phobia

The hallmark of Social Phobia is debilitating anxiety provoked by social or performance situations. The lifetime prevalence for Social Phobia ranges from 3 to 13%, based on epidemiological and community-based studies. Social Phobia is reported to be more common in women than in men but clinical samples appear to have equal representation across sexes. Onset typically occurs in the mid-teens and duration of the disorder may be lifelong in some cases (DSM-IV-TR, 2000).

SH studies for social phobia are relatively rare and typically employ CT and exposure techniques within an MC format. Newman and colleagues (2003) identified two such investigations where group treatment and bibliotherapy were components of these studies. Results have been primarily supportive of MC treatments; however, the addition of bibliotherapy did not improve upon the group treatment and a palmtop computer-assisted eight session treatment regimen was equivalent to twelve sessions of therapy at six month follow-up (Newman et al., 2003).

Post-Traumatic Stress Disorder

PTSD is characterized by the involuntary re-experiencing of a traumatic event that produces symptoms of increased arousal, hyper vigilance, and avoidance behaviors (DSM-IV-TR, 2000). The lifetime prevalence rate for PTSD is estimated at 8% of the adult U.S. population. In the general population, females are over-represented in this diagnostic category; however, among those in at-risk groups (e.g., combat veterans, survivors of rape), the rate is generally highest.

Despite the suggestion by some that men and women respond similarly to traumatic events (e.g., Housely & Beutler, 2006), the preponderance of research on the topic indicates otherwise. For example, Bryant and Harvey (2002) conclude that, "[p]eritraumatic dissociation and acute stress disorder is a more accurate predictor of PTSD in females than males. This gender difference may be explained in terms of response bias or biological differences in trauma response between males and females (pp. 226)." Additionally, Holbrook and Hoyt (2004) conclude that women are at greater risk of early psychiatric morbidity and poorer quality of life outcomes following major trauma than men. These findings are independent of mechanism and injury severity and are consistent with findings from Holbrook, Hoyt, Stein, & Steiber (2002). Further, Breslau and Anthony (2007) analyzed data from a representative sample of 1,698 young adults and found that women's risk for PTSD was greater than men's risk following assaultive violence. "When assaultive violence preceded a later nonassaultive trauma in women, there was an increased risk (relative risk = 4.9) for PTSD, which was not observed in men (pp. 607)." Finally, Stein, Walker, and Forde (2000) concluded that "women were found to be at significantly increased risk for PTSD following exposure to serious trauma (odds ratio ~5), even when sexual trauma-which predominates in women-was excluded (odd ratio ~3). Adjusting for gender differences in the number of lifetime traumata, or in the likelihood of the trauma being associated with particular reactions to or consequences of the event (i.e., thinking that one would be killed or seriously injured; sustaining a serious physical injury; seeing someone else seriously injured or killed) did not result in lessening of the PTSD risk in women (pp. 619)"

Focused Expressive Writing (FEW) involves writing one's deepest thoughts and feelings about the most stressful or traumatic event of their life. Smyth and Helm (2003) found that FEW improved coping with stress in healthy populations. Moreover, these investigators found that FEW was effective in reducing PTSD symptoms in women. In a separate study, Busuttil (2004) found that social support and SH outpatient groups were useful because traumatized individuals were able to disclose trauma-related information in a controlled and supportive environment.

Some PTSD SH information books were found to be unhelpful or possibly detrimental, sensitizing people and disrupting the natural recovery process (Ehlers et al., 2003; Turpin, Downs, & Mason, 2005). Still, some individuals have found these books to be helpful; however, they should be used with caution. For example, the Responses to Traumatic Injury booklet offered advice on facing trauma and seeking help (Turpin et al., 2005); however, the booklet titled Understanding Your Reactions To Trauma did not lead to better outcome than untreated participants or those who participated in repeated assessments (Ehlers et al., 2003). In sum, the investigation failed to support the efficacy of an informational booklet offered in an effort to attenuate symptoms of PTSD.

An Internet-based SH program for traumatic event related consequences was found to decrease some PTSD symptoms and increase coping skills. The 8-week CBT program consisted of relaxation training techniques, cognitive restructuring, and exposure modules. The program provided some promising results; however, more empirical support is needed before definitive comments can be made (Hirai & Clum, 2005). In a similar vein, Litz, Williams, Wang, Bryant, & Engel (2004) describe a therapist-assisted Internet SH program for traumatic stress. It begins with a face-to-face intake/assessment session—the rest of the eight weeks are spent over the Internet with guided exercises and homework. The program was developed to be tailored to the unique needs of the individual. The SH intervention is based on stress inoculation training (SIT) and the program requires empirical support.

At present, both the NIMH and Housely and Beutler (2006)—suggest that individuals who have experienced trauma seek help and comfort from their own social support networks and give the natural recovery process a chance to work. If the trauma-related stress is particularly debilitating or if the stress does not become increasingly more manageable in a period of one to two weeks, then it may be more appropriate to seek professional counseling in addition to SH via one's social support network.

A Naturalistic Design Investigation

Finch, Lambert, and George (2000) conducted an investigation involving a naturalistic design to examine the effectiveness of a multimedia SH program (Attacking Anxiety) specifically developed for the self-administered treatment of anxiety. These investigators found that 61% of their participants were classified as improved or recovered and only one individual self-reported deteriorating. On the other hand, the group mean on the outcome measure (OQ-45) fell well within the dysfunctional range and approximately 40% of the participants failed to show a significant change in the positive direction.

Some interesting group comparisons revealed that among younger individuals with less education, the Attacking Anxiety SH program appeared to perform best. Conversely, among individuals who were older and with more education, the Attacking Anxiety program was less successful. Finch and Lambert suggested that greater academic achievement and a more chronic anxiety disorder (associated with age) may attenuate the effectiveness of this SH program.

Several weaknesses in the methodology of the foregoing investigation render the findings of questionable clinical utility. For example, a naturalistic design prevents randomized assignment, the use of a control or other comparison group, the evaluation of treatment compliance, and causal inference. Additionally, as the authors point out, the participants in this investigation self-selected. There may have been differences between those who chose to purchase Attacking Anxiety compared to those who did not purchase the program. Relatedly, a high attrition rate, approximately 66%, weakened the findings further because it is impossible to know if the participants who completed the study were different from those who dropped out on important variables. Finally, only one self-report outcome measure was employed to investigate change and this measure is not designed to render a diagnosis; therefore, the diagnoses that were characteristic of this sample are unknown.

Conclusion

Findings on SA treatments for anxiety disorders are mixed. In general, some benefit is achieved through the use of these SH materials and treatment benefits accrue with greater therapist involvement. Prognostic indicators include motivation level, severity of the disorder, functional impairment, and compliance. More specifically, prognosis is good if the participant is highly motivated to engage in SH treatment. Moreover, the likelihood of positive outcome is enhanced if the disorder is not severe. If severity is high, greater therapist involvement is indicated. Additionally, high levels of functional impairment do not augur well for treatment success—therapist intervention directed at stabilizing the participant and reducing the frequency of, or eliminating, problematic symptoms/ behavior may be necessary before SH materials can be of clinical utility. Finally, for SH materials to be of maximal benefit for the participant, compliance with the use of the materials is an obvious necessity.

Even with the mixed findings and paucity of rigorous RCT research on SH materials, SA treatments do appear useful for a significant number of individuals. Finding the materials that are best suited to the unique needs of each person presenting with anxiety involves a little effort on the part of the consumer. If a manual, workbook, or other commercially produced resource has empirical support, the marketer of those materials is likely to make sure the consumer is aware of the science behind the product. In other cases, some manuals developed for practitioner use, but still of use to a subset of consumers, may not have advertising that touts the scientific support of the resource. Consumers are their own best advocates and it makes good sense to see what information is available on the resource in consideration via Internet (e.g., google) searches. There are literally hundreds of resources available for the SH treatment of anxiety, far too many to do justice in a chapter devoted to this topic. As a way to facilitate the access to information, we provide some resources to the interested/motivated consumer below.

Available Resources

Associations and Agencies and Web Sites

1. Anxiety Disorders Association of America: www.adaa.org
2. Center for Mental Health Services Knowledge: www.mentalhealth.org
3. Agoraphobics in Motion: www.aim-hq.org
4. Freedom from Fear: www.freedomfromfear.org
5. Anxiety Disorders: www.healthyminds.org
6. Meditation, Guided Fantasies, and Other Stress Reducers:
   www.selfhelpmagazine.com/articles/stress

Books

1. 100 Q&A About Panic Disorder: www.www.jbpub.com
2. Anxiety & Phobia Workbook: www.newharbinger.com
3. Anxiety Cure: Eight Step-Program for Getting Well: www.wiley.com
4. Anxiety, Phobias, and Panic: www.www.hachettebookgroupusa.com
5. Anxiety, Phobias, and Panic: A Step-By-Step Program for Regaining Control of Your Life: www.twbookmark.com
6. Coping with Social Anxiety: The Definitive Guide to Effective Treatment Options: www.henryholt.com
7. Coping with Trauma: A Guide to Self Understanding: www.adaa.org
8. Dying of Embarrassment: Help for Social Anxiety and Social Phobia: www.newharbinger.com
9. Flying without Fear: www.newharbinger.com
10. Free from Fears: New Help for Anxiety, Panic, and Agoraphobia: www.adaa.org
11. Freeing your Child from Anxiety: Powerful, Practical Solutions to Overcome your Child's Fears, Worries, and Phobias: www.www.randomhouse.com
12. Master your Panic and Take Back Your Life: www.adaa.org
13. Master of Your Anxiety and Panic: Workbook: www.www.oup.com/us

Support Groups and Hotlines

1. Agoraphobics Building Independent Lives: www.www.mhav.org
2. Pass-Group: 716-689-4399
   (This group offers a 3-month counseling program via telephone for panic/agoraphobia sufferers—also includes "The Panic Attack Recovery Book")
3. Phobics Anonymous: 760-322-2673

Chapter 8
Mood Disorders

Introduction

Depression is the prototypical mood disorder with approximately 17 million Americans suffering from some sort of depressive illness each year (Gottlieb, 2008). Among the major psychiatric disorders in North America, depression is the most prevalent and most costly with respect to both personal functioning and work productivity (Beutler, Clarkin, & Bongar, 2000). Depression can affect anyone at any age and women tend to earn the diagnosis at least twice as often as men (Beutler et al., 2000; Gottlieb, 2008). Some have promoted social theories (e.g., socialization, inequality) to explain the sex differences in depression rates; however, evidence does not support this notion. More specifically, there is strong evidence that biological/hormonal stresses experienced by women are a strong contributor to higher depression rates—the fact that, following menopause, female depression rates fall to a rate that is almost equal that for males supports a biological etiology. According to Areán, McQuaid, and Muñoz (1997), if another diagnostic category such as premenstrual dysphoric disorder was used to diagnose dysphoric women, the rates of depression would be approximately equal between men and women. Another potential explanation for differential rates of depression between men and women may be due to the fact that women and men respond differently to personal stress (Areán et al., 1997). Additionally, the fact that the 2:1 ratio is seen world wide across cultures and nations does not support a cultural/social effect—women are treated very differently across cultures with great variability in rights and opportunities; however, we do not see any changes in depression rates.

Prevalence rates for depression vary widely. For example, the NIMH epidemiological catchment area (ECA) study estimated a point-prevalence for depression at 5% of the U.S. population; however, the National Co-morbidity Survey (NCS) provided evidence that the prevalence rate for recent or current depression was 10%. The lifetime prevalence rate for depression from the ECA was estimated to be 7%; however, the NCS survey revealed a lifetime-prevalence for depression at 19%. When examined by sex, the lifetime prevalence of depression in women ranged from 7 to 21% and between 4 and 8% for dysthymia. For men, lifetime prevalence rates of depression range between 3 and 13%—for dysthymia, the range is 2–5%.

T.M. Harwood, L. L'Abate, *Self-Help in Mental Health*,
DOI 10.1007/978-1-4419-1099-8_8, © Springer Science+Business Media, LLC 2010

The above rates have been documented throughout the world and appear to reflect true sex differences (Areán et al., 1997)

In an effort to resolve the discrepant findings from the ECA and NCS studies, Eaton, Dryman, Sorenson, and McCutcheon (1989) reanalyzed data from the ECA utilizing statistical procedures to compensate for symptom interdependence and measurement intercorrelation effects—their findings indicated a lifetime-prevalence rate for depression of 14%. Based on the prevalence rates from depression literature, Beutler et al. (2000) concluded that the prevalence rate for major depression is something over 10%. When these authors utilized probability samples to derive an estimate for the prevalence of minor and transitory (life adjustment) depression, figures ranged from 15 to 25%. The rates of double depression may be present among 20% of the population at any given time and almost 33% of the U.S. population may experience clinically significant, impairing, but transient dysfunction from depression sometime in their lives (Beutler et al., 2000). Recent evidence suggests that prevalence rates for depression are increasing and the average age of onset for the first episode of depression is becoming lower with each succeeding generation.

Among the elderly, depression is often a missed diagnosis or depressive spectrum symptomology may be mistaken for "normal" aging; however, a recent study suggests that depression among the elderly ranges anywhere from 6.5 to 9.0%. General medicine practitioners have demonstrated that they are reluctant to address depression among elders and elders present with more somatic than affective symptomology (Mellor, Davison, McCabe, George, Moore, & Ski, 2006). The elderly comprise a population that tends to utilize mental health services at a lower rate than younger cohorts; therefore, it is perhaps most important to identify effective self-help resources available to this population.

Because depression is a psychiatric disorder, it does not dissipate through the use of behaviors or activities that people typically use to cheer us, or others, up. Additionally, depression is often a recurring disorder—about 50% of patients who experience one episode of depression will experience another episode later. The bad news is that this rate of recurrence increases with each additional episode. On the other hand, depression is one of the most treatable of psychiatric disorders and response rates are high for psychotherapy, pharmacotherapy, and electroconvulsive therapy. Response rates would likely improve through the use of self-help materials and relapse rates would likely drop for patients, clients, or individuals not yet receiving treatment if self-help methods were willingly employed.

Depression is a costly mental illness and much of the burden shouldered by individuals and society is attributable to subclinical depression. In an already overburdened health care system, the dissemination of evidence-based self-help options is one practical solution to the treatment of depression (Jorm & Griffiths, 2006). Ease of access and application coupled with the savings in time and financial resources make self-help resources acceptable to many. Acceptability and effectiveness coupled with the potential to avert the development of clinical depression make self-help materials all the more attractive and useful (Jorm & Griffiths, 2006).

Self-Help for Depression

Self-Administered Treatments for Depression

Menchola, Arkowitz, and Burke, (2007) conducted a meta-analysis on self-administered treatments (SAT) for depression and anxiety. The investigators employed strict criteria in the selection of outcome studies. For example, these investigations had to be randomized clinical trials with head-to-head comparisons between SATs, a control group (placebo or no treatment), or a therapist-administered treatment (TAT). Additionally, the SATs had to be designed to be administered by the depressed individual sans regular therapist contact and it had to be the primary method of treatment, not an adjunctive treatment. If meetings or phone contacts were part of any investigation, these contacts could not be greater than 15 min per week and they had to be for the sole purpose of monitoring change or compliance with the SAT. Finally, the investigations selected involved individuals with depressive spectrum symptomology severe enough to meet clinical criteria for depression and only adolescent or adult samples were included. This investigation appears to be the only extant meta-analysis involving individuals who warrant a clinical diagnosis of depression.

The primary findings from the foregoing meta-analysis indicated that SATs were more effective than no-treatment controls; however, the improvement produced by SATs was significantly lower than those produced by therapist-delivered treatments. The authors also concluded that preliminary evidence for the efficacy of SATs appeared better than placebo; however, there was no such effect identified when compared to therapist-administered group treatments. Additionally, TATs were found to be significantly more effective than SATs among individuals suffering from clinical levels of depression. Menchola et al. (2007) concluded that although a body of literature suggests that SATs appear to be efficacious for individuals suffering from mild forms of depression, SATs may be less effective as stand-alone treatments for more serious presentations of depression—for these individuals, therapist involvement seems indicated.

Stant, Ten Vergert, den Boer, and Wiersma (2008) conducted an investigation on the cost-effectiveness of cognitive self-therapy (CST) for patients with depression and anxiety disorders (not necessarily co-morbid). Patients were randomly assigned to CST or treatment as usual (TAU). Treatment as usual was characterized as 10–20 contacts with a psychologist, psychiatric nurse, or social worker—no specific treatment protocol was followed and therapy consisted primarily of problem-solving and coping strategies. The CST condition involved the use of a manual (Contact & Relationship, Den Boer, & Raes, 1997) comprised of three components: (1) self-therapy theory manual, (2) manual for practicing cognitive self-therapy, and (3) manual for self-assessment of the treatment process. Additionally, CST involved a preparatory, orientation, basic course, and self-therapy phase. The preparatory phase consisted of one to three 45-min informational meetings that also assessed the patient's willingness and ability to participate. The orientation phase involved three morning meetings within a week's time. The basic course, running for 5 days in a week's period, helped patients learn how to manage a CST session. Finally, self-therapy meetings were conducted once a week, led by peers and in accordance with manual guidelines. Self-therapy patients could attend any weekly meeting they liked—attendance was entirely voluntary during the course of the investigation.

Costs were assessed both within and outside the healthcare system (e.g., medical costs, direct non-medical costs such as cost related to travel and time, and indirect non-medical costs; i.e., productivity losses). The primary outcome measure was the Symptom Checklist-90 (SCL-90; McKinnon & Yodofsky, 1986). Other symptom measures included the Beck Depression Inventory (BDI; Beck & Steer, 1993), State-Trait Anxiety Inventory (STAI; Spielberger, Gorsuch, & Lushene, 1970), Groningen Social Disabilities Schedule (Wiersma, De Jong, & Ormel, 1988), and the Quality of Life Assessment-BREF (World Health Organization, 1998). Results indicated that not only was the CST cost-effective, it was also found to be at least as effective, with respect to clinical utility, as treatment as usual. The investigators call for the implementation of CST in an effort to allocate health care resources most efficiently.

With respect to the Stant et al. (2008) study, the investigators recommended that future studies of this type employ a non-inferiority design instead of a superiority design because the former design allows to compare interventions on dimensions other than effectiveness. For example, a non-inferiority design allows for the investigation of lower health care costs associated with interventions such as self-help treatments.

In a recent study, primarily qualitative employing interviews and focus-groups to gather retrospective data, Wisdom and Baker (2006) found that depressed teens voluntarily employ self-help interventions to relieve depressive symptoms. In many cases, these teenagers ($n = 14$) had never received formal instruction in self-help for depression and many had never entered psychotherapy for depression. More specifically, a total of 142 interventions, many empirically supported, were reported by the fourteen adolescent participants. The number of interventions employed ranged from 2 to 24 with a mean of 9.6 interventions. The activities or interventions, many cognitive-behavioral in nature, were categorized by Wisdom and Baker as (1) Behavioral Activation, (2) Cognitive Restructuring, (3) Problem Solving, (4) Counseling, (5) Social, (6) Emotional Expression, (7) Risky Activities, and (8) Non-productive.

As might be expected, in the Wisdom and Baker investigation, it was found that teens who had been in psychotherapy reported more attempted interventions in an effort to reduce depressive spectrum symptomology. Further, there were no remarkable differences in the amount of interventions reported by gender. Somewhat surprisingly, participants did not mention the use of Internet or bibliotherapy to learn about depression treatment. The investigators suggest that, for many teens, recovery from depression may not be spontaneous, but rather recovery from depression is often the result of concerted efforts to engage in activities and employ interventions that are effective.

A study, the Women and Depression Project (WPD), conducted by Laitinen, Ettorre, and Sutton (2006) employed professionally guided self-help groups as a therapeutic intervention in mental health. Technically, this was a professionally guided psychoeducation group; members learned interventions that they eventually employed individually in their everyday lives. More specifically, the group members learned, through a series of thirty self-help exercises, women-focused, self-help techniques including consciousness raising, assertiveness training, diary work, and straight talking. The authors adhered to what they considered an essential tenet of self-help: one's own personal growth was the guide for what members learned; i.e., members learn for themselves.

Results for the Laitinen et al. (2006) investigation revealed statistically significant improvement on eleven dimensions of individual feelings (i.e., feelings directed towards oneself) and statistically significant change was detected on 10 dimensions of social feelings (i.e., feeling having an external impact). In general, the majority of the treatment gains were maintained at 12-month follow-up. According to the investigators, women made constructive changes in their lives immediately subsequent to end of treatment.

Bibliotherapy as Self-Help Treatment for Depression

A survey indicated that between 60 and 97% of psychologists prescribed bibliotherapy as an adjunct to depression treatment (Mains & Scogin, 2003). A meta-analysis of bibliotherapy for populations of depressed adolescents through older adults produced an effect size of 0.83 (Cuijpers, 1997), large enough to indicate that bibliotherapy is efficacious and comparable to the 0.73 effect size generated in the literature review on psychotherapies for depression conducted by Robinson, Berman, and Neimeyer (1990). Bibliotherapy has been suggested as an effective component of a stepped-care treatment model for depression (Scogin, Hanson, & Welsh, 2003). More specifically, bibliotherapy may be an effective initial intervention for mild to moderate depression. Patients suffering from severe depression should initially receive psychotherapy and/or pharmacotherapy (Scogin et al., 2003). In a proposed stepped-care model, the first step would involve assessment of depression severity—if appropriate, treatment would then begin with bibliotherapy. If necessary, the next step would be a combination of bibliotherapy and pharmacotherapy (Scogin, Hason & Welsh suggest that psychotherapy included at step 2 would be most consistent with the research literature on depression; however, they recognize that this does not appear to be a frequent practice). If a third step is required, psychotherapy would be combined with pharmacotherapy and the final step, if necessary, would involve psychiatric referral (Scogin et al., 2003).

If a stepped-care model is to be employed, patients should be monitored on a regular basis. For example, Scogin et al. (2003) recommend assessment within 1 month or less, following the initiation of bibliotherapy, depending upon patient presentation and unique life circumstances at baseline assessment. Telephone monitoring, self-report measures (e.g., BDI-II), or clinical interview (e.g., Hamilton Rating Scale for Depression) are acceptable forms of follow-up assessment to determine if subsequent steps in care are indicated.

Among patients suffering from mild to moderate depression, bibliotherapy has been found to be an effective treatment alternative and superior to an attention control and delayed treatment control condition (Scogin, Hamblin, & Beutler, 1987; Scogin, Jamison, & Gochneaur, 1989). Additionally, bibliotherapy may also be an acceptable and credible treatment approach for depression among older respondents (Landreville, Landry, Baillargeon, Guerette, & Matteau, 2001), middle-aged adults (Jamison & Scogin, 1995), and adolescents (Ackerson, Scogin, Lyman, & Smith, 1998).

Bibliotherapy offers several potential advantages including (1) the ability for patients to work, with varying levels of independence, and at their own pace in their own home; (2) a treatment method that can reach a larger population of individuals suffering from depression; (3) a cost-effective approach for individuals who may not have the financial resources to utilize psychotherapy or pharmacotherapy; and (4) the provision of coping skills targeted on the management and treatment of depression that remain at their fingertips after treatment has ended.

An investigation of the efficacy of bibliotherapy among older adults is relatively rare. According to Floyd et al. (2006), only four studies on the clinical utility of bibliotherapy among older adults have been conducted to date. Findings indicate that behavioral bibliotherapies are as effective as cognitive therapy and both treatments are more effective than wait-list controls (Scogin et al., 1989). Another investigation of this type indicated that cognitive bibliotherapy was as effective as individual cognitive therapy with treatment gains maintained in both conditions at 3-month follow-up (Floyd, Scogin, McKendree-Smith, Floyd, & Rokke, 2004). At 2-year follow-up, Floyd et al. (2006) found that individual treatment gains were generally well-maintained across conditions; however, those participants in the bibliotherapy condition had a higher rate of relapse than those in the individual cognitive therapy condition. The foregoing suggests that, at least among the elderly, some individuals may require more in the way of treatment for depression than bibliotherapy alone. When investigations are examined in the collective, bibliotherapy for the elderly has clinical utility and this form of therapy should be considered a viable treatment option.

Of the four studies described by Floyd et al. (2006), Burns (1980) *Feeling Good* was the book chosen for bibliotherapy. There are a number of other texts or manuals available for use as bibliotherapy for depression. For example, *Mind Over Mood* (Greenberger & Padesky, 1995) is a cognitive restructuring manual specifically designed for the treatment of elders suffering from depression. *Control Your Depression* (Lewinsohn, Munoz, Youngren, & Zeiss, 1986) is a behavioral-therapy self-help book for depression. As with all bibliotherapies, *Feeling Good*, *Mind Over Mood*, and *Control Your Depression* may be employed as an adjunct to individual, group, or family therapy, or it may be used as a stand-alone form of treatment. *Mind Over Mood* is a user-friendly manual, designed as a self-help resource; however, empirical support for the utility of this manual still needs to be established. Empirical support for *Feeling Good* and *Control Your Depression* already exists (Mains & Scogin, 2003; Scogin et al., 2003).

More recently, Bilich, Deane, Phipps, Barisic, and Gould (2008) examined the effectiveness of bibliotherapy self-help for depression with varying levels of telephone helpline support. Employing a sample of 84 mildly to moderately depressed adults, change in depression spectrum symptomology was assessed for participants who were randomly assigned to one of three groups: (1) a control group, (2) a self-help with minimal contact (MC) group, and (3) telephone assistance self-help (AS) group. The self-help manual utilized in this investigation was *The Good Mood Guide* (GMG; Phipps et al., 2003). Based on Cognitive-Behavior therapy, this manual employs a variety of CBT techniques designed to be self-administered. The CBT techniques are divided into eight separate modules containing selected readings and activities. Each module is designed to be completed in a week; therefore, the entire program may be completed in an 8-week period.

Depressive symptoms were measured with the Beck Depression Inventory-II (BDI-II, Beck, Steer, & Brown, 1996). Additional outcome measures included the Depression, Anxiety, and Stress Scale (DASS-21; Lovibond & Lovibond, 1995), and the Kessler Psychological Distress Scale (K10; Andrews & Slade, 2001).

Eighty-five percent of participants in the treatment conditions reported reading the entire GMG. Both the minimal contact and telephone assistance treatments obtained clinically significant reductions in depression compared to the control group. One month follow-up assessment indicated that treatment gains were maintained. Although both active treatment groups received assistance, the AS group received more assistance than the MC group and the magnitude of treatment gains was related to amount of assistance received. The control group was eventually provided with the GMG sans assistance (Bibliotheraphy Only; BO group). The BO group experienced some reduction in depressive spectrum symptomology; however, the reduction was not statistically significant. The investigators suggest that for self-help bibliotherapy to be most effective, some level of assistance, even minimal contact, is necessary for adults suffering from mild to moderate depression.

In a study comparing cognitive bibliotherapy to self-examination therapy and a wait-list control, the bibliotherapy and self-examination therapy conditions produced greater reductions in depression spectrum symptoms than the wait-list control group (Bowman, Scogin, & Lyrene, 1995). Another study examined a self-administered treatment for depression, COPE, which combines bibliotherapy booklets, a video, and 11 periodic phone calls over the course of treatment. In the foregoing study, time spent on the phone by participants correlated with treatment gains (Osgood-Hynes et al., 1998).

An investigation comparing a cognitive therapy-based bibliotherapy and a behavioral therapy-based bibliotherapy found that both self-help treatments outperformed a control group; however, no differences between therapies were detected (Scogin et al., 1989). When bibliotherapy was compared to psychotherapy, findings indicated that psychotherapy produced greater post-treatment improvement than did bibliotherapy (Floyd, Scogin, McKendree-Smith, Floyd, & Rokke, 2004).

In a meta-analysis, Den Boer, Wiersma, and Van Den Bosch (2004) concluded that self-help materials for significant emotional disorders were more effective than no treatment or wait list control conditions. The meta-analysis was conducted on 14 investigations where participants met clinical criteria—the bulk of the investigations (13) employed bibliotherapy as their self-help intervention. When bibliotherapy was compared to short-term psychiatric treatment, no group differences were found.

These authors concluded that bibliotherapy was an effective treatment for emotional disorders such as depression and anxiety.

Another meta-analysis involving 29 investigations on cognitive forms of bibliotherapy for depression yielded effect sizes that were comparable to those obtained from individual psychotherapy (Gregory, Canning, Lee, & Wise, 2004). More specifically, when the 17 most rigorous studies were separated and analyzed, an effect size of 0.77 was obtained—when all studies were considered, the analysis yielded an overall weighted effect size of 0.99. The authors suggest that the effect size yielded from the 17 between-group investigations is the best estimate of bibliotherapy effect size from the study at hand.

An interesting finding from the Gregory et al. (2004) investigation revealed an age effect. More specifically, five studies involving teenagers yielded an average effect size of 1.32. When the 15 studies involving adults were examined, the average effect size obtained was 1.18. Finally, among the nine studies with older adults, an average effect size of 0.57 was obtained. The older adult sample effect size significantly differed from the effect sizes obtained on the teenage and adult samples; however, the teenage and adult sample effects sizes did not differ significantly from each other. The authors conclude that the differences in effect sizes across groups may be due to different baselines for the various groups. That is, the older adults were substantially less depressed than their adult and teenage counterparts—they simply did not have as much room to improve when compared to the other groups. Although meta-analyses indicate that bibliotherapy is clearly an effective form of self-help treatment, Gregory and colleagues suggest that bibliotherapy may be most appropriate for less severe forms of depression.

Computer-Administered Treatments for Depression

An investigation comparing the efficacy of content-identical cognitive-behavioral therapist-led treatment and cognitive-behavioral computer-administered treatments, no differences were found between the two treatments (Selmi, Klein, Greist, Sorrell, & Erdman (1990). McKendree-Smith, Floyd, and Scogin (2003) indicate that the foregoing study provides preliminary evidence that cognitive-behavioral interventions can be successfully administered through a computer format.

In an investigation on another computer-administered cognitive-behavioral treatment program titled Overcoming Depression (Colby, 1995), three conditions were tested: (1) treatment as usual, (2) treatment as usual with therapist-delivered cognitive-behavioral therapy, and (3) treatment as usual with the computer-administered Overcoming Depression program. Treatment as usual with therapist-delivered cognitive-behavioral therapy outperformed the computer-assisted treatment at post-treatment rendering significantly lower BDI and HRSD scores; however, neither group differed significantly from treatment as usual at post-treatment. McKendree-Smith et al. (2003) point out that the small sample size in the Colby investigation makes interpretation of the interesting findings difficult.

   In a study on computer-administered treatments for depression delivered in a hospital setting, four different conditions were compared: (1) standard hospital treatment (SHT), (2) SHT with a computer-placebo control, (3) SHT with the Overcoming Depression program (Colby, 1995), and (4) SHT with the program developed by Selmi et al. (1990). The only significant between-group difference indicated that the Selmi et al.'s program outperformed the SHT group on post-treatment scores—positive patient change as measured by the BDI was evident in all conditions (McKendree-Smith et al., 2003). Although patient improvement was noted in all conditions, the investigators concluded that this treatment format may not be appropriate for individuals suffering from severe forms of depression requiring hospitalization and stabilization (Stutzke, Aitken, & Stout, 1997).

Bipolar Disorder

Self-help materials or resources and research are sparse for bipolar disorder. This paucity of resources may be due to the complexity involved in the treatment of bipolar disorder combined with the potential for risky behavior. One resource available for self-help with bipolar disorder is a workbook titled *The Bipolar Workbook: Tools for Controlling your Mood Swings* (Basco, 2006). This workbook allows the user to individualize their treatment and supplies the consumer with guidelines and worksheets to help reduce the recurrence and severity of symptoms. Another related resource is *The Cyclothymia Workbook: Learn How to Manage your Mood Swings and Live a Balanced Life* (Price, 2004). Neither of these resources has received the empirical support necessary to provide a strong recommendation or prescription.
   A study by Rivas-Vasquez (2002) involved bipolar patients who were taught to identify early symptoms of relapse. The participants developed personalized treatment seeking plans, had them laminated, and carried them in their wallets. When compared to routine care, these participants showed improvement in social functioning, employment, and they had significantly longer intervals between relapses at 18-month follow-up.

Medical Co-morbidity

Schultz (2007) acknowledges the relationship between medical co-morbidity and depression. Kamholz and Unützer (2007) report on the relationship between hip fracture and depression. More specifically, the incidence of depression following hip fracture ranges from 9 to 47%. Relatedly, depression is associated with greater risk of falls among the elderly. In a similar vein, depression is negatively associated with proper hygiene, adequate diet, regular exercise, and social support. On the other hand, depression and hip fractures account for a significant amount of morbidity and mortality among the elderly.

As the foregoing suggests, it isn't clear if diet or other factors associated with depression and falls are causal or consequence; however, proper diet, regular exercise, good hygiene, and social support are all recognized as having an attenuating effect on the severity of mood states. Moreover, falls and fractures are likely to be reduced if one is engaged in good physical and social health activities. With respect to self-help resources, the aforementioned activities/behaviors are within the behavioral repertoire of most individuals, elderly or not. Many of the bibliotherapy resources for self-help for depression recommend these activities; however, maintaining these activities before depression develops would be one way to reduce its rate of occurrence or relapse.

Collaboration between one's primary care physician and one's psychotherapist may be a useful way to motivate individuals to incorporate self-help-related behaviors into a multifaceted (self-help) treatment regimen. Indeed, this type of collaboration may reduce the frequency of physician and psychotherapist visits by providing an optimal form of treatment among elders and younger adults.

Discussion

The findings on self-help treatments for depression are somewhat inconsistent. The meta-analyses offer the best evaluative information for clinicians and these generally favor the use of self-help treatments for depression; however, even when meta-analyses are used as the guide for self-help treatments, some caveats are in order. First, few meta-analyses include investigations on selected severely depressed individuals. In general, participants in self-help studies are suffering from sub-clinical, mild, or moderate levels of depression. Relatedly, these investigations involve some form of supportive contact with mental health professionals. Therefore, it is premature to suggest that self-help materials are adequate as stand alone treatments for all individuals—none of the investigators involved in this review are suggesting anything of this kind and it is important to underscore this caveat.

Second, a stepped-care model of treatment would seem to be the most clinically prudent mode of intervention. At the very least, for individuals suffering from sub-clinical or mild forms of depression, minimal contact with a therapist would make good clinical sense. More specifically, some individuals may present with sub-clinical or milder forms of depression; however, this does not preclude a progression to more serious forms of depression. Minimal contact with a mental health professional, to provide initial assessment and periodic re-assessment, is a reasonably convenient and cost-effective way to track individual treatment trajectories. Moreover, early intervention and minimal contact may serve as a preventative measure and it would free up needed resources that are better directed to those suffering from more debilitating and chronic forms of depression.

Taken together, the investigations reviewed herein clearly indicate that self-help treatments are efficacious for many individuals—in some cases the effect sizes associated with self-help materials are not remarkably different from those found in studies involving individual, professional treatment of depressed patients. Still, among those diagnosed with more severe forms of depression, self-help materials may be best viewed as an adjunctive treatment complementary with professional care. Further, it is recommended that individuals suffering from symptoms of depression seek initial consultation with a mental health professional and consider periodic monitoring of functioning and mood state.

Conclusion

The general consensus from investigators is that self-help materials for depression serve an important function in the treatment of depression irrespective of severity. For sub-clinical depression, self-help materials may prevent a progression to more severe forms of depression and may improve mood. Mild and moderate depression may be treated, to varying degrees, with self-help materials—in some cases, depression may remit. In all cases of depressive spectrum symptomology, ranging from sub-clinical depression to severe forms of depression, therapist contact ranging from minimal to intensive is clinically indicated, respectively.

Self-help interventions may be more important than originally thought—their contribution to the reduction of case load, potentially preventive role, cost-effectiveness, therapeutic effectiveness, and likelihood that treatment will be enhanced if self-help materials are included as adjunctive treatment all augur well for their proliferation and increased use in both clinical and non-clinical settings.

Self-Help Resources for Mood Disorders

Associations and Agencies

1. Depression and Bi-Polar Support Alliance: www.dbsalliance.org
2. Depression and Related Affective Disorders Association: www.drada.org
3. Depression after Delivery: www.depressionafterdelivery.com
4. Emotions Anonymous International Service: www.EmotionsAnonymous.org
5. National Alliance on Mental Illness: www.nami.org
6. National Institute of Mental Health: www.nimh.nih.gov
7. Postpartum Support International: www.postpartum.net
8. SAMHSA'S National Mental Health Info Center: www.mentalhealth. samhra.gov

Books

1. Against Depression: www.us.penguingroup.com
2. Breaking the Patterns of Depression: www.randomhouse.com

3. Clinical Guide to Depression in Children and Adolescents: www.appi.org
4. Depression Workbook: A Guide for Living with Depression: www.newharbinger.com
5. Drug Therapy and Postpartum Disorders: www.masoncrest.com6. Encyclopedia of Depression: www.factsonfile.com
7. Growing Up Sad: Childhood Depression and Its Treatment: www.wwnorton.com/psych8. Manic-Depressive Illness: Bipolar Disorders and Recurrent Depression: www.oup.com/us/
9. The Cognitive Behavioral Workbook for Depression: A Step-By-Step Program: www.newharbinger.com
10. Treatment Plans and Interventions for Depression and Anxiety Disorders: www.guilford.com
11. Winter Blues: www.guilford.com

Support Groups and Hotlines

1. Depressed Anonymous: www.depressedanon.com
2. Recovery: www.recovery-inc.com

Video and Audio

1. Bundle of Blues: www.fanlight.com
2. Day for Night: Recognizing Teenage Depression: www.drada.org
3. Depression and Manic Depression: www.fanlight.com
4. Why Isn't My Child Happy? Video Guide: www.addwarehouse.com
5. Women and Depression: www.fanlight.com

Web Sites

1. www.depressedteens.com
2. www.ifred.org3. www.nimh.nih.gov/publicat/depressionmenu.cfm4 www.planetpsych.com5. www.psychcentral.com6. www.queendom.com/selfhelp/depression/depression.html

Chapter 9
Eating Disorders: Anorexia, Bulimia, and Obesity

Eating disorders are often times included among addictive behaviors (Klingemann & Sobell, 2007; L'Abate, Farrar, & Settitella, 1992) where they rightly belong because of their single-minded concentration on unique patterns of behavior, exclusion of other alternatives, and their repetitive and compulsive nature. On the other hand, the SH and SC literature on these disorders is so vast that they deserve separate coverage (Buchanan, 1992; Buchanan and Buchanan, 1992; Williams, 2003). There is a high rate of mortality for anorexia nervosa (AN) with less than one-half of those who survive recovering fully from the disorder. There may be a natural progression from anorexia nervosa to bulimia nervosa (BN) (Polivy, 2007, p. 119; DSM-IV-TR, 2000). Within 5 years of manifesting the restricting subtype of AN, a significant number of these individuals will experience a change in diagnosis first developing the binge eating/purging subtype of AN—among these patients, many will eventually earn the diagnosis of bulimia nervosa, "...patients treated for bulimia nervosa are more likely to recover fully from the disorder" (Polivy, 2007, p. 122). Not all types of the eating disorders respond better to treatment than no treatment. We need to specify which eating disorder is most responsive to self-help treatments, face-to-face verbal treatments, or online treatments. "The three most commonly mentioned factors [responsible for recovery] were supportive relationships outside the family, therapy, and maturation" (Polivy, 2007, p. 122).

Both anorexia nervosa and bulima nervosa are related to how we control our weight and how we can prevent weight loss or weight gain. For instance, the National Weight Control Registry, initiated over a decade ago, received more than 5,000 enrollees in the program who reported having lost weight successfully and maintaining the loss for at least a year (Polivy, 2007, f. 123; Latner & Wilson, 2007). The issue here is how many of these enrollees used self-help resources and how many were diagnosed with either anorexia nervosa or BN. We cannot reliably determine the composition of the sample because self-diagnosis, the method employed by the Registry, is unreliable. It is possible that a small percentage of spontaneous recoveries occurred among those in the Registry; however, this possibility should not mean that eating disorders should be left untreated.

The most important issue to keep in mind about eating disorders refers to gender differences, especially in anorexia nervosa and bulimia nervosa. By a ratio of 10

T.M. Harwood, L. L'Abate, *Self-Help in Mental Health*, DOI 10.1007/978-1-4419-1099-8_9, © Springer Science+Business Media, LLC 2010 to 1, more women develop these two disorders than men (Bekker & Spoor, 2008). Although eating disorders are serious and potentially life threatening, the lifetime prevalence rate for anorexia nervosa among females is only 0.5% (DSM-IV-TR, 2000). The lifetime prevalence rate for BN among women is approximately 1–3% (DSM-IV-TR, 2000). Perhaps the second most important issue about these disorders refers to a lack of awareness and the ability to admit and eventually share hurt feelings with loved ones (Bekker & Spoor, 2008). This inability has serious health implications to the extent that when those feelings, inaccurately called "negative emotions" or "distress" in the literature, are suppressed, the individual's immune system is compromised (L'Abate, 2009b). This issue will be discussed further in Chapter 14 of this volume in regard to a model of relational competence theory related to hurt feelings and how their non-admittance, expression, and sharing with loved ones may be a major source of psychopathology.

Genetic factors in eating disorders are typically ignored by social scientists in favor of social factors. Although social factors and psychosocial treatments may be relevant to addressing the problem of eating disorders, genes may play a greater role in the development of eating disorders than social elements or expectations. For example, Novotney (2009) recognizes the important contribution that many genetic and biological risk factors play in the development of eating disorders. Klump (2007) conducted a series of twin studies and found that "...the heritability of eating disorder symptoms increases during puberty, from zero before puberty to 50% or greater after puberty" (cited in Novotney, 2009). Stice (unpublished fMRI brain-imaging work) has suggested that bulimia may be "hard wired" in some females and Marsh has demonstrated that the brains of women with bulimia appear to react with greater impulsivity compared to women without an eating disorder (as cited in Novotney, 2009).

In a study (Miotto, de Coppi, Frezza, & Preti 2003) of a mixed male–female sample of 1,000 adolescents of age 15–19 years in northeastern Italy, the relationship between eating disorders and suicidal tendencies was investigated. Investigators employed the Eating Attitudes Test (EAT), the Bulimic Investigatory Test of Edinburgh (BITE), the Body Attitudes Test (BAT), and the SCL-90-R psychiatric symptom inventory. Findings indicated that more females reported abnormal eating patterns than their male counterparts. More specifically, 100 females (15.8% of sample) and 8 males (2.8% of sample) scored above the suggested cutoff on the EAT. Additionally, 26 females (4.1%) and 1 male (0.3%) scored above the suggested cutoff on the BITE. Further, 287 females (45.5%) and 24 males (8.6) scored above the suggested cutoff on the BAT. More females than males reported symptoms of hopelessness (44.3% versus 30.5%) and suicidal ideation (30.8% versus 25.3%). Females and males who reported suicidal ideation produced significantly higher scores on the eating disorders inventories, with no independent contribution resulting from age, socioeconomic status, or body mass index. The foregoing suggests that studies on mood disorders and suicidality in youth should consider including measures of eating disorders.

There are a variety of self-help (SH) programs for eating disorders, with bibliotherapy being the most common. Myriad books are available commercially and are presently being used and read by many women with eating disorders (see Chapter 4 of this volume). Support groups, focused on women and Internet-based, are becoming more and more popular with professionals, para-professionals, and peer-leaders functioning as helpers. More structured Internet programs, following a cognitive-behavioral approach, with limited professional guidance are also available (Carrard et al., 2006; Rouget, Carrard, & Archinard, 2005; Winzelberg et al., 2008). Internet programs are especially useful for participants who cannot attend either individual or group meetings during working hours; however, these programs typically require professional monitoring because eating disorders have the potential to be life threatening.

It has been hypothesized that appearance-based comparisons are relevant to eating psychopathology; however, the evidence for this phenomenon is based on samples other than eating-disordered samples. The foregoing illustrates how little we actually know about the genesis and maintenance of eating disorders. It can be hypothesized that greater levels of general socially based comparisons may be associated with eating pathology and that poor self-esteem will account for some of this difference between groups. A study by Morrison et al. (2003) investigated the social comparison hypothesis. More specifically, a sample of 92 female patients, aged 18–63, diagnosed with either anorexia nervosa or bulimia nervosa was recruited to determine (1) if the frequency of general social comparison (focusing on abilities/behaviors and opinions) differs across clinical groups and non-clinical females and (2) if self-esteem level contributes to pathology. Results suggested there is no difference between eating-disordered individuals and non-clinical women in absolute levels of self-esteem and judgment of abilities/behaviors and opinions in comparison with others, despite a relationship between some non-clinical eating characteristics and appearance-based social comparisons.

In spite of a small proportion of self-made changes (Polivy, 2007), drop-out rates are extremely variable depending on the characteristics of the experimental and clinical contexts and settings. Winzelberg et al. (2008, pp. 167–171) include a summary of structured self-help approaches for bulimia nervosa (BN) and binge eating disorder (BED). Anorexia nervosa does not enter into such approaches, supporting Latner (2001) position that this disorder is too lethal to leave it in the hands of non-specialists. As Winzelberg et al. (2008, p. 179) concluded:

> The research to date suggests that self-help approaches for women with eating disorders [not including AN] and those at risk for developing an eating disorder are widely used, feasible to deliver and effective. Studies conduced in Europe, Canada, and the United States contribute to the generalizability of findings.

Latner et al., (2002) classified self-help for eating disorders into five different categories that complement Sobell's (2007) model summarized in Chapter 1 of this volume (Fig. 1.2): (1) independent, unguided self-help that includes self-guided approaches to weight loss (Butryn et al., 2007) and popular and fad diets (Stevens et al., 2007); (2) partially assisted guided self-help that included strategies for promoting and maintaining physical activity (Marcus et al., 2007), guided approaches for binge eating disorder (BED; Grilo, 2007), for BN (Sysko

& Walsh, 2007), and self-help treatments for body-image disorders (Hrabosky & Cash, 2007); (3) computer-assisted SH that includes Internet-based prevention and treatment of obesity and body dysfunction, and BN and BED (Scmidt & Grover, 2007); (4) group SH that includes commercial and organized SH programs (Tsai & Wadden, 2007), guided group support for long-term management of obesity (Milsom et al., 2007), and continuing care and SH for the treatment of obesity (Latner & Wilson, 2007); and (5) practical strategies and considerations that include behavioral treatment of obesity (West et al., 2007), prevention of obesity with young children and families (Dolan & Faith, 2007), treatment of overweight children using practical strategies with their parents (Henderson & Schwartz, 2007), SH for night-eating syndrome(Allison & Stunkard, 2007), appetite-focused CBT for BED (McIntosh et al., 2007), and strategies for coping with the stigma of obesity (Puhl & Brownell, 2007).

All these contributions will be summarized and included in this chapter because all cover the SH literature on eating disorders in more detailed and complete ways than we could have ever accomplished on our own. In their introductory chapter about self-guided approaches to weight loss, for starters, Butryn, Phelan, and Wing (2007) established the National Weight Control Registry (NWCR) to study weight-loss maintenance on a large scale, including registration of self-dieters, prevalence of self-guided dieting, characteristics of self-guided dieters, behaviors during weight loss, behaviors during maintenance, as well as comparisons of experiences of self-guided dieters registered in the NWCR with other dieters. Collection of large data allowed these researchers to evaluate duration and success of self-guided diets as well as the effectiveness of weight-loss programs that provide minimal guidance. They started to define and evaluate the outcome of (1) minimal contact alone, (2) minimal contact plus bibliotherapy, and (3) minimal contact plus meal replacements. Unfortunately, the lack of consensus in defining what constitutes minimal contact makes it difficult to evaluate accurately which individuals tend to profit by which approach, since all three approaches did produce some results; however, no results were replicated involved large numbers of participants because attrition rates are high in weight-loss programs.

The Importance of Diets in Eating Disorders

Diets have become so ubiquitous in the American culture that we are over-whelmed by advertisements about particular commercially available diets. Fortunately, Stevens et al. (2007) developed the following ten criteria consisting of the 10-Cs to evaluate popular SH reducing diets (p. 22): calories, composition, coping with excessive weight problems, continuation of provisions for long-term maintenance, containment of all essential components for sound weight management, consumer friendliness, cost, comparison with dietary guidelines (i.e., the Nutrition Pyramid), common sense test, and customization. These authors also included a list of caloric levels of reducing diets with pros and cons of each diet (p. 24) with serious potential side effects due to misuses of very-low-caloric diets (p. 25). After a detailed consideration of their criteria, caloric levels of carbohydrates, fiber, fat, water/fluids, and protein, these authors proceeded to evaluate the most popular commercial diet programs in the United States, according to their caloric composition (p. 36) and their percentage of micronutrient content. Additionally, popular diets were evaluated according to the contents of different food groups within the USPH Food Pyramid (p. 40). Within these criteria and guidelines, perhaps the most stringent and complete in the extant literature, Stevens et al. examined: OPTIFAST, Slimfast, South Beach, McGraw's Ultimate Weight Solution, Maker's, Atkins for Life, Curves, Body for Life for Women, Abs, and French Women's Don't Get Fat.

Using their evaluative criteria (10-Cs) included in the analysis of quality and effectiveness of ratings for these diets, Stevens et al. (2007) concluded that

> ...nutritional adequacy, safety, and efficacy of popular diets can be evaluated and those wanting separated out. Many of the latest offerings lack one or more of these characteristics. A few popular diets, such as OPTIFAST; some but not all the phases of the South Beach diet; and the actual regimens but not all of the rhetoric of Body for Life for Women diet, the Abs diet, and the SlimFast diet contain some good recommendations. However, until further empirical evidence becomes available, we suggest to those who would use popular diets: *caveat lector*; a page never rejected ink (p. 50).

Potential dieters need to be careful about the hype and seductive claims made by most weight control commercial programs, most diet programs reviewed possessed relevant features; however, none of the diets were substitutes for a careful, measured food intake and exercise. A well-crafted diet is necessary but generally not sufficient, exercise is extremely important for successful weigh reduction. One could follow a sensible diet but if their lifestyle is sedentary it will offset the impact of the diet. If one wants to take care of one's weight, exercise and food intake are characteristics of most weight reduction programs. In one way or another, directly or indirectly, diets force all participants to pay attention to *how*, *when*, and *what* they eat.

The Importance of Exercise in Eating Disorders

There is an indisputable inverse relationship between physical exercise and obesity (Marcus et al., 2007) with no need to rehash here the many undeniable health benefits accruing from physical activity and exercise. The major value of physical activity and exercise are par excellence; the most helpful of all kinds of SH because little if any face-to-face TB contact with a professional is needed. What is laudable in this regard is Marcus et al. (2007, p. 58) insistence on the emphasis of a theoretical basis for successful SH. Their insistence is based on the following grounds: (1) "...programs based on theory may be more likely to be supported by empirical evidence for the various components of the program" than those programs that include diet components *ad hoc* simply because of their seemingly reasonable nature; (2) a theoretical framework specifies how a program's components relate to each other; and (3) theory-derived programs may include reliable and valid assessment instruments to determine whether program components are effective on their own or in combination with other components; components that are not effective or minimally effective can be eliminated.

Marcus et al. (2007) refer to Bandura's social-cognitive theory as, "...the most widely researched framework" (p. 58) to be used as a base for such a desired theoretical background. Another relatively new theoretical framework (L'Abate, 2005; L'Abate & Cusinato, 2007; L'Abate & De Giacomo, 2003) will be condensed in Chapter 14 of this volume to give readers an additional perspective on how self-help and self-change can be viewed in more specific and verifiable way than could be done otherwise.

Cognitive and behavioral processes of change are listed by Marcus et al. (2007, p. 62); they are defined and explained through examples. Whether these processes derive directly from a theoretical or from a practical viewpoint remains to be seen. For instance, Marcus et al. (2007, p. 65) link physical activity promotion to the following five stages of change (Prochaska & DiClemente, 1984; Prochaska, DiClemente, & Norcross, 1992) are apparently easily visible in the process of self-change: pre-contemplation, contemplation, preparation, action, and maintenance and relapse. However, these stages are nowhere to be found in social-cognitive theory. Nonetheless, the insistence for a theoretical framework is echoed by the one presented in Chapter 14 of this volume, where specific interventions are also linked to specific models of the theory through enrichment programs for couples and families in prevention (L'Abate & Weinstein, 1987; L'Abate & Young, 1987), interactive practice exercises (L'Abate, 2010), and prescriptive relational tasks for couples and families in psychotherapy (L'Abate, 2005; L'Abate & Cusinato, 2007; L'Abate & De Giacomo, 2003).

Anorexia Nervosa

The severity and mortality of anorexia nervosa is such that Latner and Wilson (2007b) do not even consider it as part of any self-help approach. They feel that anorexia nervosa should be treated entirely by professionals (p. xii). This conclusion is supported by the latest evidence summarized by Gura (2008). This evidence indicates that anorexia nervosa may represent a profound psychiatric disorder that spawns an addiction to starvation. This seemingly paradoxical conclusion is based on viewing anorexia nervosa as a multi-faceted mental illness whose effects extend beyond appetite. Apparently,

> ...AN may produce cerebral disturbances in the reward circuitry that may render patients unable to feel delight from life's pleasures, such as food, sex, or winning the lottery, [comparable] to drug addiction...[these] biological risk factors appear to exert much of their insidious power at puberty, underscoring the importance of timing in prevention (Gura, 2008, p. 62).

However, in spite of such a frightening conclusion, we cannot help wondering whether any of the four self-help approaches included in Part II of this volume might not be helpful as an adjunctive treatment, especially if nothing is applied in the prevention of this psychiatric diagnosis. Brown (2008, p. 19) reports on ". . . the connection between the pressure to be thin and the perception of being fat. In some women, negative body images [apparently] give rise to extreme attempts to conform to the 'ideal' of female beauty." The dissonance between feeling fat and wanting to be thin has been put to use in the prevention and treatment of AN in young women. Any outcome data on the prevention and treatment of anorexia nervosa in young women needs to be evaluated with caution—a lifetime prevalence rate of 0.5% makes it difficult to evaluate any "prevention" program. Brown's theory must be evaluated for plausibility in light of the fact that obesity is a much greater problem than anorexia nervosa in America and females are more likely to be obese than males. What makes such a small subset of females develop anorexia nervosa, and if the thin "ideal" is signal in the genesis of AN, why does obesity have a much higher prevalence rate? With female obesity on the rise, and at a greater rate than anorexia nervosa, the current social theory of anorexia nervosa is somewhat questionable. Additionally, phenomena identical to anorexia nervosa have been reported in the medical literature for centuries—long before the current standard of thinness for females ever existed. Anorexia nervosa was first officially identified by Morton in 1694—bulimia nervosa was later identified by Osler in 1892 (Kinder, 1997).

A significant aspect of anorexia nervosa is a pathological disturbance in body image—this exists even when the female is already emaciated and has long exceeded the thinness "ideal" that some believe contributes to the development of anorexia nervosa. This severe perceptual disturbance in body image is not an aspect of current mainstream social theories on anorexia nervosa. Moreover, this disturbance in body image cannot be convincingly explained via social mechanisms—emaciated anorexics "feel fat" (Kinder, 1997, pp. 468) and tend to overestimate their body size and body parts to a significant degree. This phenomenon is particularly interesting in light of the finding that undergraduate female college students not only overestimate body size, they also overestimate the size of inanimate objects—this perceptual abnormality may merely be part of a general perceptual disturbance that is inherent in the individual (Kinder, 1997) and represents a vulnerability to the development of anorexia nervosa. An inherent perceptual abnormality would explain the durability of anorexia nervosa and its resistance to treatment.

Evidence from the biological and genetic realm supports the notion of a heritable component leading to anorexia nervosa. More specifically, an increased risk of developing anorexia nervosa has been found in first-degree biological relatives manifesting the disorder (*DSM-IV-TR*, 2000). Relatedly, twin studies on anorexia nervosa find that concordance rates are higher for monozygotic twins than they are for dizygotic twins (DSM-IV-TR, 2000; Nowlin, 1983). Thus, extant treatments may have low success rates because the perceptual disturbances (and perhaps other detected genetic and familial elements) seen among individuals suffering from anorexia nervosa are not central to any mainstream treatment or theory of AN.

Stice et al. (2008) developed two group-counseling interventions that may reduce the risk for eating disorders and obesity. These researchers recruited 481 female high school and college students who felt dissatisfied with their bodies but that did not have an eating disorder and were not obese. Participants were divided into four groups: Group 1 learned how to control their weight by receiving information about metabolism, nutrition, exercise, and thinking more carefully about what they ate. In Group 2, therapists used a script designed to induce cognitive dissonance between participants' attitudes about weight control and how participants actually behaved through group discussion and role-playing (Tavris & Aronson, 2007). Groups 3 and 4 were used as control with activities unrelated to eating disorders. All four groups met for only three 1-h sessions, with follow-up interviews and standard psychological tests at 6 months and then annually for 3 years. Even after 3 years both experimental groups showed striking differences from controls. In Group 1, there was a 61% reduction in the risk of developing an eating disorder and 55% reduction in the risk to develop obesity. In Group 2, there was a 60% reduction in the risk of developing eating disorder.

What is more important about these results lies in their application to sorority houses in various colleges, where students themselves are trained to administer one or both approaches. If both approaches generalize reliably to various college populations through peer training, they could become an important example of cost-effective SH in the field of health promotion and prevention of eating disorders.

A number of concerns remain that bring the conclusions from Stice et al. into question. First, the authors indicate that their sample was self-selected based on an appeal to individuals who felt dissatisfied with their bodies—self-selection may have inflated the findings in an investigation of this type. Second, the reported significant difference between the study sample and a community sample does not address the issue of clinical significance. More specifically, the mean differences between the two groups on the body-dissatisfaction scale and the ideal-body scale was less than one point in each instance—what does a difference of one point mean from the perspective of clinical utility (need to check the foregoing for accuracy)? With a sample size of almost 500, it isn't surprising that statistical significance was achieved. On a different note, it isn't clear from the investigation if all participants were evaluated for the presence of an eating disorder or weight-loss or weight-gain at various assessment points. Another concern centers on the denial aspect of those with an eating disorder—how might social response bias impact on self-report data of this type? Finally, how reliable and valid are the risk factors employed in the analysis and why weren't individuals reliably evaluated for the presence of an eating disorder. It would seem that the impact of the intervention on the development of an eating disorder is paramount to determining if the intervention has any clinical utility.

Unfortunately, the SE_m for the scales used in the investigations at hand are not reported in either of the published studies so the reader does not know if the SE_m is greater than the differences between the two groups. Additionally, the six items on the Ideal-body scale (IBS) contained items that the culturally aware would naturally endorse as typical of the beauty stereotype—a measure that included items that would typically not be endorsed by those who hold a stereotyped view of beauty would be more telling about one's perception and internalization of beauty in general—what Stice et al. may be measuring with the Ideal-body scale is *knowledge* of the typical American stereotype of beauty—the findings do not demonstrate that the respondent has internalized this stereotypical view. Related to the foregoing is that validity data for both measures are not reported in the article and internal consistency is not reported for the samples—internal consistency is sample-dependent and although high based on some earlier investigation, this coefficient may simply be a reflection of redundancy in item content.

One annoying habit from Stice et al. is that these investigators consistently refer the reader to previous studies on the validity of the measure; however, they cite articles that, in turn, cite earlier articles, that again cite earlier articles on validity for this measure and the reader has to devote too much time to find what the original validity study provided—this information should be provided to the reader in each investigation employing the IBS. After accessing at least four articles that were successively cited as sources of validity coefficients for the IBS, I finally gave up looking. In a similar vein, it isn't clear if any validity studies were conducted by independent investigators or if a multi-trait, multi-method matrix approach to establishing validity was employed.

The authors should also provide validity coefficients reflecting the degree of sensitivity and specificity (predictive validity) for the "risk indicators" employed in the study and the methodology used to obtain these data should be included in any article claiming that risk factors were reduced. Relatedly, the apparent reduction in some form of risk does not provide us with overall indicators of health or the actual development of an eating disorder—it would be interesting to determine if differential diagnostic rates and long-term health status are apparent for the participants in the various groups involved in the Stice et al. investigations.

Finally, both of the recent studies by Stice et al. (2005, 2008) on risk factors for eating disorders or obesity used very large samples (near 500) and in each of the foregoing studies, one or more scales were "modified"—this is troubling with respect to the psychometric properties of these measures and sample size brings up the issue of over-powered investigations. At present, the foregoing studies on risk factors should be viewed as preliminary—more rigorous investigation is needed in this potentially fruitful area before these programs are widely adopted.

Binge Eating Behavior

Binge eating behavior (BED) is defined as a repetitive, obsessive overeating followed by a loss of control and vomiting (i.e., purging) to get rid of the food accumulated in the body; however, this disorder is usually coupled with a variety of concerns about food and eating, irregular eating patterns, and distorted cognitions about healthy weight and body size and shape. Depression and a low sense of self-importance and self-esteem are typically co-morbid with this disorder. Obesity is another correlate of this disorder (Grilo, 2007, p. 72). Based on the foregoing disorders, a logical intervention is to employ antidepressant medication—this has been accomplished with rather successful results (Grilo, 2007, p. 75). Psychotropic medication is frequently prescribed in primary care settings by physicians who do not possess the appropriate specialization. Additionally, there is a paucity of skilled psychiatrists in many parts of the country and often not enough physicians and primary care settings to manage large numbers of eating disorder cases. Consequently, guided self-help seems a reasonable alternative and it may be the most cost-effective solution for this disorder because this approach, usually based on CBT, seems to be successful "...in both guided and pure SH formats" (Grilo, 2007, p. 76). Furthermore, it seems possible to produce outcomes comparable to those obtained by professionals by simply employing a widely used manual administered by paraprofessionals (p. 82). Adding Orlistat (trade name Xenical, a medication for the treatment of obesity; it inhibits gastric and pancreatic lipase and prevents absorption of a significant amount of dietary fat) to a specific version of CBT specifically revised for binge eating disorder seems to reduce weight loss in obese participants (p. 83). In spite of these overall results, there is still no general conclusion that can be drawn about how successful and cost-effective guided is self-help for this disorder.

McIntosh et al. (2007, pp. 327–336) introduced a novel way to treat binge eating disorder and BN, emphasizing the role of appetite or awareness of body sensations that in this case are disordered and inadequate. Consequently, a variation of CBT called CBT-A has been devoted to these sensations; McIntosh et al. described a model of appetite-focused CBT for binge eating disorder (p. 331) that includes society, family, and self-risk factors, increased awareness of the consequences of strict dieting, including ignoring appetite and increasing inconsistent overeating and purging followed by feelings of guilt, shame, and anxiety. To help participants in this process, they are given a daily self-monitoring form typical of CBT (p. 333) that allows them to record date and time, food and fluid eaten, the context (i.e., situation) of the eating, description of sensations of hunger and fullness, followed by thoughts and feelings. Through this process, similar to the process guided by Daily Thought Records used in CB treatments for depression, participants would become more aware of their food choices and the volume of a particular food choice consumed. Part of the treatment involves education about satiety-signaling mechanisms, including learning about the dietary functions of proteins, carbohydrates, glycemic load and its effects on physiological processes. From all of the above, McIntosh et al. emphasized the importance of adapting CBT-A to a self-help format, a questionable goal because supportive outcome evidence is non-existent for this interesting variation and adaptation of CBT.

Delinsky, Latner, and Wilson (2006) conducted an investigation of binge eating disorder and weight loss in a self-help behavior modification program. The program used was the Trevose Behavior Modification Program, a self-help group that offers continuing care for obesity. Although bulimic episodes were reported by 41% of the participants, they were not associated with poorer weight-loss outcomes. For treatment completers (12 months of treatment), mean weight loss for this group was almost 19% of initial body weight. For the full sample, employing an intent-to-treat analysis yielded a loss of 10.5% of initial body weight. The authors concluded that a continuing care treatment program produced significant weight loss for individuals experiencing frequent and infrequent binge eating disorder.

A new category of body image disturbance, muscle dysmorphia, appears to contribute to eating disorder pathology and excessive exercise (Chung, 2001; Novotney, 2009). This psychological construct is theorized as existing more commonly in males than females. According to Novotney, this problem often goes unrecognized because the symptoms are less noticeable than the clinically diagnosable eating disorders typically over-represented by women. An excessive desire for muscle development may lead to compulsive exercise, unhealthy eating in the form of over-eating, and insistence on high-protein and low-carbohydrate and low-fat diets. Some individuals are motivated to achieve a certain body shape/size that they may abuse anabolic steroids. According to Klump (2007, as cited in Novotney, 2009), "we now know ... that, just like any other psychiatric condition such as schizophrenia and bipolar disorder, eating disorders have a strong genetic component (pp. 50)."

Body-Image Disturbances

Body-image disturbances (BID) are concomitant with many eating disorders. Unfortunately, BID does not seem to have received the attention it deserves from the research community. Body-image disturbances consist of dissatisfaction and over-concern about body shape and physical appearance (Hrabosky & Cash, 2007) ranging from occasional worry to anxious obsessions about one's negatively perceived looks. Individuals suffering from BID often elect to engage in extreme, sometimes grotesque, if not dangerous surgical corrections. Other functionally impairing features include social avoidance, restrictive diets, and obsessive-compulsive behaviors that may eventually lead to disordered eating. These disturbances of body image are similar to those seen in body dysmorphic disorder—that is, the disturbances are often based on perceptions that have no basis in reality or they may represent a preoccupation with slight imperfections that most individuals would not notice.

Developmentally, body-image disturbance seems to start in adolescence and reach its peak after high school. Hrabosky and Cash (2007, pp. 120–123) developed a specific, structured CBT program consisting of eight steps: (1) assessment and goal-setting, (2) psychoeducation and self-discoveries, (3) relaxation and body-image desensitization, (4) identifying and challenging appearance assumptions, (5) identifying and correcting cognitive errors, (6) changing self-defeating body-image behaviors, (7) enhancing positive body image, and (8) relapse prevention and maintaining body-image changes.

Results obtained from this kind of structured CB treatment indicated the superiority of therapist-lead interventions; however, weekly group therapy sessions, individual face-to-face control visits, and regular telephone check-ins produced equivalent outcomes. There are several major concerns with a structured CBT approach as

a possible self-help form of treatment including (1) the difficulty in identifying participants who may require consistent face-to-face therapist-lead treatment,
(2) participants who may realize significant benefit from guided self-help supplemented with occasional check-ups, and (3) individuals who may improve through
their own efforts with minimal but available contact with a para-professional or
Internet-mediated form of self-help (Hrabosky & Cash, 2007, pp. 129–134).

The number of Americans who are significantly overweight or morbidly obese
has reached epidemic proportions. The problem has grown so quickly that individual
psychosocial treatment is often unavailable to many—paucity of technically trained
personnel or prohibitive costs are the primary barriers to therapy. By the same
token, body dissatisfaction is a risk factor for the development of eating disorders.
The predictive reliability and validity of body dissatisfaction in the developmental
course of an eating disorder remains unanswered. Undoubtedly, most individuals
experience some dissatisfaction with their bodies, some experience high levels of
dissatisfaction, yet these individuals never develop an eating disorder.

Paradoxically, weight-loss programs may "inadvertently increase body-image
dissatisfaction" (Taylor & Jones, 2007, pp. 141–142). Consequently, the Internet
appears as the next frontier in the self-help/self-change mental health movement
based on its potential to reach untold numbers of cases who do not seek help
due to fear of stigma or other intra-psychic avoidance elements. In addition to
what has been presented in Chapter 3 of this volume, Taylor and Jones (2007,
pp. 143–144) discuss in greater detail the various challenges and uses of the
Internet for the treatment of body-image disturbances and obesity. These researchers
reviewed the literature on the Internet crafted for the enhancement of body image
and weight reduction (pp. 144–152) and treatment of obesity (pp. 152–160), including a summary of randomized controlled trials of online weight-control programs
(pp. 154–155) and of online commercial weight-loss programs (p. 156). The
conclusion of these researchers is worth including here:

> The existing research suggests that Internet technology can effectively address the growing
> problem of obesity and body dissatisfaction in the United States and perhaps across the
> globe (p. 162).

Bulimia Nervosa

Of all the eating disorders, BN has received the most attention because of its
widespread nature, especially in the American culture. It consists of binge-eating
and alternative activities, such as eating too many unhealthy foods, irregular eating
patterns with irregularity in when to eat, what to eat, and how to eat. Because of its
widespread nature, BN has received a great deal of attention from the medical and
preventive communities. For instance, there are at least 14 self-help interventions
designed specifically for women with bulimia nervosa and binge eating; however,
their safety and efficacy still needs to be investigated (Garvin et al., 2001). There
seems to be a significant incremental benefit when self-help is used to augment the

treatment of eating disorders. In one investigation of this phenomenon, 78% of a selected group of study participants diagnosed with bulimia nervosa found self-help groups to be useful. It would have been instructive had an anorexia nervosa group been included in the foregoing study's design. Participants who receive a combination of individual therapy and appropriate self-help experience reduced occurrences of BED and BN. At present, more widespread and systematic controlled studies are required before we can provide any definitive conclusions about the efficacy of augmented individual therapy (Stefano et al., 2006).

The demand for the treatment of bulimia nervosa and binge eating disorders is high (Williams, 2003); however, skilled therapists are in short supply. In some cases, self-help and guided self-help programs that employ books and manuals have shown promise as an alternative to full psychotherapy; systematic evaluation of well-defined studies will determine who benefits from this form of treatment and the degree of benefit achieved. The efficacy and effectiveness of SH, for BED and BN, delivered with various forms of face-to-face guidance, led to improvement after four months, with some evidence to support the use of telephone guidance. Compared to self-help alone, participants who received guided self-help demonstrated a lower attrition rate over time. Guided self-help might be an effective treatment alternative or adjunct when delivered in primary care and in other non-specialist settings (Palmer et al., 2002).

Factors perceived to contribute to the efficacy of guided self-help treatment as delivered by general practitioners (GPs) might include (1) improved eating behaviors, body image, and emotional and general well-being, (2) the empathic and practical style of the treatment manual, and (3) specific behavioral change strategies. Factors perceived as contributing to treatment ineffectiveness included lack of changes in eating behaviors and body image, inadequacies of the treatment program and approach, inadequate treatment dose, poor service delivery, and perceptions of low general practitioner competence and professionalism along with a weak therapeutic alliance (Banasiak et al., 2007).

Many potential participants with BN might find it hard to access evidence-based treatment such as cognitive-behavioral therapy (CBT). This difficulty could be alleviated in part by the creation of a novel CD-ROM based on CBT principles for use as a SH intervention. Sixty participants volunteered for an eight-session form of a CD-ROM-based SH sans therapist input; at follow-up, significant reductions in binging and compensatory behaviors (with the greatest reduction in self-induced vomiting) were evident among the 47 participants who completed treatment. This CD-ROM form of self-help holds promise as a first step in the treatment of BN and supports the dissemination of non-specialist-led interventions (Bara-Carril et al., 2004). What needs to be monitored and controlled in such interventions is the degree of patient activity and interactivity associated with programs of this kind. A stepped-care model that employs various self-help programs may prove to be most effective from a cost–benefit ratio. For example, pure SH treatments may be applied first, followed by progressively more intensive and more professionally directed treatments for those who do not respond favorably to treatments applied at a previous step or steps.

Thiels, Schmidt, Treasure, Garthe, & Troop (1998) evaluated the effectiveness of guided self-change for bulimia nervosa. Sixty-two patients with Diagnostic and Statistical Manual of Mental Disorders-III-Revised (DSM-III-R)-defined bulimia nervosa were randomly assigned to (1) use of a self-care manual plus eight fortnightly sessions of cognitive-behavior therapy (guided self-change) or (2) 16 sessions of weekly cognitive behavior therapy. At the end of treatment and at follow-up an average of 43-week post-therapy, substantial improvements had been achieved in both groups on the main outcome measures: eating disorder symptoms according to experts' ratings (Eating Disorder Examination sub-scores on overeating, vomiting, dietary restraint, and shape and weight concerns), self-reports (Bulimic Investigatory Test Edinburgh), and a 5-point severity scale. Also, improvement was seen on the subsidiary outcome measures: the Beck Depression Inventory, the Self-Concept Questionnaire, and knowledge of nutrition, weight, and shape. At follow-up, 71% of the cognitive behavior therapy group had not binged or vomited during the week preceding. In the guided self-change group, 70% had not binged and 61% had not vomited during the week before follow-up.

Mitchell et al. combined fluoxetine with a self-help manual geared toward suppressing bulimic behaviors. The Mitchell investigation involved 91 adult women between 18 and 46 years of age. The duration of treatment was 16 weeks. This combination of antidepressant medication and a self-help manual resulted in significant reductions in the frequency of vomiting episodes and in the rates of vomiting and binge-eating episodes. The placebo-control group did not show the same degree of positive outcome.

The use of manuals (see Chapter 6 in this volume) has been found to be the most cost-effective way to administer guided SH: (1) Getting Better Bit(e) by Bit(e), (2) Bulimia Nervosa: A Guide to Recovery, and (3) Overcoming Binge Eating are examples of some manuals developed specifically for bulimia nervosa. Sisko and Walsh (2007) give detailed chapter outlines for each manual with summaries of empirical studies that have evaluated their effectiveness. Sysko and Walsh conclude their excellent review of these manuals thusly:

> Several well developed SH manuals articulating the principles and implementation of CBT for BN are available. Controlled studies consistently demonstrate that the use of these manuals is associated with greater improvement than assignment to a waiting list. However, the efficacy of SH relative to more established interventions is not clear. Similarly, it is not certain whether SH adds substantially to antidepressant treatment nor how it is best employed in a sequence-care model of treatment. SH books may be more useful in informing potential patients of the nature of BN and the available treatment approaches and in offering a treatment program when no other therapeutic options are available (p. 115).

As these studies demonstrate, manuals seem to constitute a frequent self-help method in the treatment of bulimia nervosa (Bailer et al., 2004), even though their contents, their formats, and the nature and frequency of any interactive processes between participants and helpers are usually not given. The foregoing highlights the importance of evaluating compliance levels in GSC treatment (Thiels et al., 1998, 2000).

There are commercially available computer programs for BN that are reviewed by Schmidt and Grover (2007). Supposedly, from computer use these programs may expand to the Internet: (1) *Overcoming Bulimia* is a multimedia SH package based on cognitive-behavioral approaches, and (2) the *SALUT* project consists of seven sequential steps, including: motivation, self-observation and modification, dietary plans and strategies to avoid binges and automatic thoughts, problem-solving, self-affirmation, conclusion, and relapse prevention. Thus far, participants in these programs have responded positively to their expansion/extension to Internet use (Schmidt & Graver, 2007, p. 169).

Presently, acceptance of computer programs and their expansion to the Internet is viewed with concern by many MH professionals who are still wedded to the face-to-face talk-based personal contact paradigm that was established early in the last century (L'Abate, 2008c). Fortunately, some therapists have remained open-minded and can foresee positive outcomes resulting from technological advances in the delivery of mental health interventions. For example, "... therapists who identified themselves as predominantly cognitive-behavioral in their therapeutic orientation held significantly more positive attitudes toward computerized SH than therapists from other orientations (Schmidt & Grover, 2007, p. 171)." Of course, the computer/Internet approach is still in need of resolving two important problems: (1) patient screening and selection, and (2) delivery of the treatment that matches the referral problem (Schmidt & Grover, 2007, p. 172–173) and is tailored to the patient.

The foregoing constitutes issues that have long been present in the MH field and especially in the area of prevention (L'Abate, 1990). This is why we included experimental information in Chapter 1 and suggest a stepped-care model of SH/SC based on actual performance rather than what participants write on paper (Chapter 14 this volume). Consequently, a word of caution is necessary, as Schmidt and Grover (2007, p. 174) conclude their review: "Thus, in any clinical setting in which computerized treatments are to be used, training of therapists in the package and how to deliver it is vital for a successful implementation of the package."

Obesity

Obesity has received attention in some circles because it has reached what many consider to be an epidemic in the United States; however, anorexia nervosa and bulimia nervosa, disorders with relatively low lifetime prevalence rates, continue to dominate the psychosocial literature on eating disorders. Obesity is more prevalent than all other eating disorders combined—it also claims more lives and represents a greater strain on the economy and medical system than all eating disorders combined. Consequently, a variety of SH, promotional and preventive approaches have been created. For instance, 126 community participants with a mean age of 38.4 years participated in a 10-week weight-reduction program: (1) four groups used a behavioral manual, (2) four groups used an alternate manual under various degrees of therapist guidance, and (3) one group served as a delayed-treatment control.

Results at post-treatment and 3-, 6-, and 16-month follow-ups supported the behavioral manual's effectiveness in producing modest weight loss. The manual could be applied under various degrees of therapist guidance without significant differences in effectiveness, but with increased cost-effectiveness as therapist contact decreased (Pezzot-Pearce et al., 1982).

The cornerstone of any weight management for obesity is lifestyle modification consisting of dietary/nutritional counseling, increased physical activity, and behavior therapy (Tsai & Wadden, 2007, pp. 179–180; Tsai, Thomas, Womble, & Byrne, 2005). These researchers reviewed guidelines for commercially available weight-loss programs applied in a group SH format that included (1) program content, (2) staff qualifications, (3) costs, and (4) program risks (Tsai & Wadden, 2007, pp. 181–182). Non-medical programs that were evaluated included (1) Weight Watchers, Jenny Craig, LA Weight Loss, HMR, OPTIFAST, Medifast/TSFL, (2) Internet-based weight-loss programs such as eDiets.com, and (3) organized SH programs such as Take Off Pounds Sensibly, and Overeaters Anonymous.

Among non-medical programs Weight Watchers seemed relatively more successful than the other programs in this category; however, Weight Watchers is also the most expensive of the programs under consideration. No strong conclusions can be made about the outcome of the other programs at this time. Nevertheless, in spite of their modest evidence and questionable outcome, no SH program should be overlooked. The obesity epidemic is too devastating to rely solely on one approach or a single method and individuals respond differentially to different programs.

Guided group support for the long-term management of obesity must deal with the fact that there are many obese individuals who drop out of each form of treatment. Furthermore, even if the obese are successful in reducing weight, risk of relapse is very high and the result is often a greater weight gain overall. This is the principal reason that obese individuals need long-term guided-group support (Milsom et al., 2007). Oftentimes, management of obesity requires drastic lifestyle changes that typically need to last a lifetime. Milsom et al. (2007) reviewed all of the lifestyle interventions with extended care provided via guided group support during follow-up (pp. 209–211). These group procedures provide a sense of group cohesion necessary to individuals who have experienced isolation and rejection throughout their lives. Long-term intervention with guided support appears to provide clear benefits for those participants who remain in the program (Milsom et al., 2007, p. 218).

As indicated in the foregoing, relapse remains one of the major aspects of obesity (Latner & Wilson, 2007, p. 223) requiring a continuum of care above and beyond the approaches already considered above. Factors responsible for relapses may be a toxic environment and the costs of weight maintenance in such an environment (Milsom et al., 2007, pp. 224–226). There are obvious obstacles to the maintenance of continuing care, such as changes in training qualified personnel, prolonged financial support, and participants' motivation to remain in treatment "for the long haul." Various controlled randomized studies in Germany, Italy, and Sweden suggest somewhat positive results, especially when recipients of help become providers of help, supporting the evidence gathered by Post (2007) that "it helps to help."

Latner, Wilson, Stunkard, and Jackson (2002) examined the effectiveness of the Trevose Behavior Modification Program, a lay-directed, long-term, self-help weight-lost program. The high attrition rates associated with other extant weight-loss programs indicated a need for an economically feasible, long-term self-help treatment program for obesity. Latner et al. concluded that the Trevose model of weight control, a combination of self-help and continuing care, is an effective treatment for those who remain in treatment. Further, this program may be extended to a variety of settings with promising results.

The Trevose program has several unique characteristics that may explain its efficacy. For example: (1) lifelong treatment is offered at no cost, (2) the program is heavily behavioral in focus—a variety of rules are strictly enforced, (3) the initial 5 weeks of treatment demands a high degree of structure and involves a screening phase requiring participants to submit food records, attend all weekly meetings, and lose 15% of their total assigned weight loss goals. If individuals pass this phase, they are considered "members" and are allowed to continue in the program—those who fail to meet the foregoing requirements are permanently dismissed from the program. The remainder of the program is equally strict: (1) consistent attendance is required, (2) self-monitoring of food intake and specific weight goals each month, (3) if on vacation (requiring two week advanced written notice), members must weigh themselves and mail their weight record to their group leader on the day of their usual meeting. Members who fail to comply with these requirements are terminated and not permitted to rejoin. On the other hand, more experienced members who do not meet requirements are penalized by placement on "parole" and they are given an additional 2 months to meet goals. Reward for meeting goals includes graduation to higher levels of maintenance. Additionally, highly ranked members are encouraged to function as group leaders, assistant leaders, or office workers. When weight loss goals are maintained for at least 12 months, attendance at meetings is no longer mandatory but weight records must still be mailed monthly.

At 2 years, 43.8% of those initially enrolled in the Trevose program remained in treatment and lost approximately 19% of their body weight. After 5 years of treatment, 23.4% remained and lost approximately 18% of their body weight. Although attrition rates are high, for those who remained in treatment, gains were maintained for a period of 5 years. Given the difficulty involved in maintaining weight loss when traditional program are employed, it would appear that the demands of the Trevose program increases long-term success rates for a significant portion of people when compared to the more traditional short-term, less-directive approaches. Continuing care may be economically feasible when administered by laypersons through self-help treatment modalities. Additionally, self-help confers certain benefits such as self-reliance and an increased sense of self-efficacy (Latner, 2001).

Milsom et al. (2007) provided a detailed description of a self-help continuing care program that may be considered exemplary in this field (pp. 230–235). They also suggested that drop-out rates may not always indicate a negative outcome or treatment failure. Some individuals drop out because they have improved enough to consider themselves "cured" (p. 235). More practically, behavioral obesity treatment involves customizing a general overall CBT into a much more specific approach for obesity with an emphasis on self-monitoring of dietary practices, exercise behavior, and weight. Additionally, successful outcome is linked to the length of the program and the nature of contacts between helpers and participants, ranging from frequent face-to-face talk-based sessions to minimal contact (West et al., 2007). Programs of this type emphasize social support, problem solving, goal setting, dietary intervention with portion-controlled meals and meal patterns, increasing adherence to physical activity goals, motivation, and adapting behavioral weight control to minority populations.

The extent and impact of weight bias is so powerful that it is crucial to deal with the impact this stigma leaves on obese individuals (Puhl & Brownell, 2007). Coping with the stigma associated with weight problems should be an important component of any SH approach for obesity, including confirmation of self-acceptance, self-protection, strategies to compensate for negative consequences of being overweight, proper and even assertive confrontation and challenging of bias, social activism, and even avoidance and disengagement from bias. Methodological issues and detailed research recommendations are given to increase an understanding of coping strategies for weight stigma (pp. 356–359). It is important to recognize that the foregoing strategies dealing with the stigma related to obesity are not an endorsement of obesity as a healthy lifestyle. Indeed, obesity is a serious problem with definite physiological risks and highly probable negative psychosocial fallout—as such, an honesty-based component about obesity should be part of any treatment program, self-help or otherwise.

Prevention and Treatment of Overweight Children and Their Families

One of the major obstacles in successful prevention and treatment of overweight children involves a parent's denial of their child's excessive Body Mass Index (BMI). An excessive BMI in childhood may represent a risk factor for obesity in adulthood (Dolan & Faith, 2007, p. 265) necessitating preventive and sometimes therapeutic interventions. This conclusion makes one wonder whether "Obesity lies in the eyes of the beholder" (pp. 268–270) acknowledging that there are notable ethnic and socioeconomic differences in the perception and even acceptance of obesity (pp. 270–272). In an effort to deal with denial, a careful and detailed contextual and behavioral assessment is necessary, including assessment of BMI, and a simple "Self-assessment checklist for parents to examine their own readiness to implement individual lifestyle changes for their child" (p. 273). Parental modeling of healthy behavior (e.g., controlled eating, healthy meal choices, portion awareness, elimination of traditional junk/snack foods, exercise, etc.), as well as the monitoring of television watching (p. 274), with guidelines to help children learn to self-monitor behaviors (p. 274) should be included as well.

Consequently, parental feeding practices need to be assessed and when necessary corrected, such as breast feeding versus bottle feeding, chaotic, irregular, inconsistent and contradictory versus restrictive feeding practices, television viewing, including suggested parenting guidelines for pediatric obesity treatment (p. 278), ideas for alternative activities for television viewing (p. 278), and strategies to help reduce children's television viewing time (p. 279), beverage consumption (especially sodas), and fastfood consumption. The general behavioral change strategies recommended by Dolan and Faith (2007) include exposure to new and more helpful ideas and practices, role modeling suggestions for parents to eat healthier foods, and positive reinforcement for more appropriate and self-helpful behaviors. Additionally, Dolan and Faith provide a listing of helpful websites and popular books to guide parents on how to improve upon a child's eating skills (p. 282), as well as the American Academy of Pediatrics recommendations for the prevention of pediatric overweight and obesity (pp. 285–286).

Most treatment for overweight children needs to be mediated by their parents, including setting goals from the outset of treatment, creating a supportive environment, addressing weight bias, crafting healthy food menus, and promoting physical activity environments. In this context, physical activity is promoted over formal exercise and instruction on how to overcome obstacles in the promotion physical activity are provided. Physical activity would include sports, making activity a family goal, and strategies for increasing activity by decreasing sedentary behavior (Henderson & Schwartz, 2007). Presently, no outcome data are available to support the therapeutic efficacy of this program.

Night-Eating Syndrome

This is a relatively newly discovered disorder defined as an irregular pattern of eating behavior occurring when one is either unable to go to sleep without eating or they wake during the night to eat with the expectation that food will produce better sleep (Allison & Stunkard, 2007). Criteria for an operational definition of Night-Eating Syndrome (NES) on the basis of amount of food varies according to a ratio of how much food is eaten at night in comparison to how much food is eaten during the day (pp. 310–311). Operational problems inherent in this definition make it difficult to establish an exact notion of its prevalence, owing also to the fact that NES is a very private behavior that is not easily disclosed and may be co-morbid with other eating and non-eating disorders. In contrast to anorexia nervosa and bulimia nervosa, which occur mostly in women, NES occurs equally among men and women (Allison & Stunkard, 2007, p. 311). A recently published manual about overcoming NES has increased the public awareness and made it easier for many people suffering with this disorder to come forward and ask for professional help. Based on this model, treatment for NES consists of a variation of CBT primarily focused on detailed reports of thoughts and emotions experienced before eating, type and amounts of food/beverage consumed, number of calories involved in consumption, and thoughts and feelings experienced after eating (Allison & Stunkard, 2007, pp. 312–315).

Self-help strategies for NES include (1) regulating daytime eating patterns and preventing nighttime eating, (2) raising awareness of automatic thoughts and feelings, (3) considering alternatives to eating, (4) sleep hygiene and physical activity, and (5) inclusion of social support and pharmacotherapy (usually Sertraline). Unfortunately, night-eating syndrome is too new to provide longitudinal outcome data; however, as its scientific and professional popularity increases with an influx of new participants, there is no question that investigators will provide additional information about the nature and natural course of this syndrome over time.

Concluding Remarks

The eating disorders represent a complex group of diagnoses. Anorexia Nervosa is rare and the social/environmental explanations fall short of a convincing etiological explanation for the development of this disorder. Further, the relative failure of treatments aimed at anorexia nervosa would suggest that the problem has not been conceptualized properly. Additionally, the epidemic of obesity is inconsistent with a strong but widely held etiological social pressure among anorexics to be thin. Moreover, anorexia nervosa appears to have neurological correlates related to perceptual disturbances that have not been adequately explored or considered in most mainstream treatments. Relatedly, the known presence of anorexia nervosa for several centuries does not augur well for the proponents of sociological explanations for this disorder. Undoubtedly, this disorder is complicated—successful treatment on a wide scale has eluded some very brilliant clinicians. Perhaps it is time to strongly endorse a multi-disciplinary approach with the medical, neurological, psychiatric, and psychological communities contributing to a comprehensive, targeted treatment for AN.

Bulimia nervosa appears to respond better to psychosocial intervention. It represents a lesser form of psychopathology that lies closer to the healthy end of the continuum than does anorexia nervosa. Severity of a disorder, denial, and/or lack of insight (all hallmarks of AN) are poor prognostic indicators. If present in BN, they exist to a lesser degree. Bulimic patients have greater insight and the physical devastation that anorexia nervosa leaves in its wake is not characteristic of those who are exclusively battling bulimia nervosa. Additionally, individuals suffering from BN appear to have greater social support networks than those diagnosed with anorexia nervosa—social support is a positive prognostic indicator.

Unfortunately, individuals diagnosed with anorexia nervosa often isolate, perhaps due to the discomfort that individuals experience when in the presence of someone who appears emaciated. Moreover, anorexics may feel uncomfortable when individuals, sometimes strangers, attempt to convince them that they have a problem or offer well-intentioned but unsolicited and unwelcome solutions. The bottom line is that most with anorexia nervosa don't see their starvation and excessive exercise as a problem—they tend to experience it as reinforcing and necessary.

Obesity is by far the end result of the greatest eating disorder problem faced by Americans. It is striking that so many in the field of psychology focus on anorexia nervosa or bulimia nervosa and neglect obesity, a much greater psychological and physical problem. The high and increasing prevalence of obesity does not support the social-pressure-to-be-thin hypothesis. Diets do work, with varying degrees of success, if they are followed consistently and accompanied by exercise. Still, some may succumb to this politically correct "thinness pressure" hypothesis and find themselves on a road that is difficult to exit; however, it is not possible to convincingly argue that the thinness pressure is etiologically strong given the widely disparate prevalence rates for obesity when compared to AN and BN. Much like the problems with AN, and to a lesser extent, BN, obesity treatment should be multi-disciplinary and multi-modal. Parent training and consistent modeling is an important component in the establishment of healthy lifestyles for children.

Finally, there is absolutely no convincing evidence that eating disorders are due to "a patriarchy". Seemingly intelligent researchers extrapolate from a sex difference in the prevalence of a disorder and immediately invoke a "socialization effect" or patriarchy on these differential prevalence rates without any convincing supportive evidence. It is telling that disorders characteristically earned by men (e.g., substance use disorders, antisocial personality disorder, paraphilias, etc.) are frequently attributed to male pathology and the notions of "a matriarchy" or socialization pressures are often not considered by those in academia. What these seemingly intelligent researchers conveniently disregard is that any sex differences that may occur in socialization may simply be a function or reflection of true biological differences between the sexes. Some researchers indicate that boys and girls do not experience significant differences in socialization suggesting that sex differences are more biologically based than many would like to consider. Relatedly, the real-world effects of socialization cannot be determined by extant research methods and socialization occurs across sexes—how does one know if "male socialization" is more advantageous than "female socialization"? Attempts by feminists to socialize young males to be more feminine have failed. The same is true for young females socialized to be more masculine—success has not been forthcoming. Perhaps, if true and significant socialization differences really exist, they are a natural outcome of biological differences between the sexes.

Biological differences are generally ignored by social scientists and Women's Studies professors appear to be so deeply enamored or preoccupied with the victimization mentality that they neglect consideration of other possible explanatory variables; however, it is a mistake to suggest that a mind–body biological connection is not relevant in the genesis of psychopathology. It is a serious mistake to forget that men and women (especially at the group level) are different in a variety of ways (e.g., Mealey, 2000). For example, each cell in our bodies is different (males are XY and females are XX), on a macro-level, our brains are configured quite differently (e.g., Kimura, 1992; Pool, 1994; Rahman, Andersson, & Govier 2005); however, structural differences also exist on the micro level. Additionally, men and women respond to stress in different ways (e.g. Rohrmann, Hopp, & Quirin 2008; Tolin & Foa, 2006), hormonal change trajectories and the relative balances of hormones are different between the sexes—in other words, biological, cognitive, and behavioral differences are indisputable; Mother Nature is not a radical feminist—she is unbiased.

We briefly mention the following to support the argument that, when one examines the body of literature on the topic, society does not appear to be responsible for the sex difference in eating disorders (or other psychiatric disorders). When one is objective in their assessment, it is obvious that women are simply not oppressed in today's society; they are certainly not oppressed any more than males. Differential female oppression is a myth—sound empirical support to back up this claim is lacking. Women have not experienced disproportional oppression for decades and it is difficult to determine if significant oppression existed in centuries past based on what may have been a voluntary and necessary distribution of work responsibilities given the demands of survival and raising a family in pre-modern America and other societies. For example, for some time now, females have constituted the majority of college students, they continue to receive the lion's share of financial support both in college and when starting a business and they acquire both undergraduate and graduate degrees at a higher rate than males (and this trend is increasing). Females graduate from high school at a higher rate than males as well and there are more federal- and state-sponsored programs for females than for their male counterparts. Additionally, counter to conventional wisdom, women are represented in research at a greater rate than males. Relatedly, although prostate cancer kills many more people than breast cancer does, breast cancer research is funded at a much higher rate than research on prostate cancer.

The income gap is another popular myth—it hasn't existed since the passing of the equal pay for equal work act in the early 1960s and the pay difference was only about 10 cents on the dollar in decades prior—when controlling for explanatory variables, this pay gap probably never existed—see below. Presently, discrimination is in favor of women—women are now paid more than men for the same work (Farrell, 2005). Currently, the propaganda promoted by NOW is something like: Women only earn 75 cents on the dollar compared to men—this is dishonest and purposely misleading. When the overall group mean statistics are examined more carefully and controlled for explanatory variables such as seniority, hours worked, experience, part-time versus full-time, sick-leave, etc., the pay gap shrinks to 0.02 cents on the dollar and this difference is likely due to the hard manual labor and dangerous work that pays well because in a free market, not many people (and virtually no females) want this work (Nielsen, 2005; Keene, 2008). Speaking logically, if an employer could hire a female for 75 cents on the dollar and get her for the same work performed by a male, why would he or she ever consider hiring a male?

Additionally, males are more likely to be killed, victims of crime and violence (including domestic violence), and they are eight times more likely to die on the job than are females. Moreover, males continue to perform the work that is unacceptable to women (e.g., garbage collection, hard physical labor, and generally dangerous outdoor and unsanitary work), they utilize the health care system at a rate that is 50% lower than that of females and in the area of mental health, the system is utilized at a ratio of 3:1 female to male. Our military has accommodated women by reducing the physical requirements necessary to make it through basic training and females continue to be exempt from selective service draft registration. It is surprising to me that the myth of female oppression continues to be promulgated in academia and the popular media.

As the foregoing suggests, there is simply no convincing evidence for a "glass ceiling"—when females make the same career choices as men (e.g., become properly educated, actually use their degree, place priority on work instead of family, work long hours—sometimes 80 hrs a week, and don't take time off at rates higher than males), they become CEOs and CFOs at a slightly higher rate than males. The interested reader is directed to Christina Hoff-Summers (1995, 2000), Schlafly (2003), and Farrell (2005) for a research-based treatment of the foregoing topics and a host of other related issues. For a more entertaining, but immensely enlightening treatment of the foregoing issues, the reader is directed to Adams (2004, 2007). You will not find these volumes on the reading lists in the syllabi of social sciences or Women's Studies professors. This intentional omission is an embarrassment to the academic community and to the aforementioned disciplines and departments.

Social scientists, as a group, must become more open-minded and properly educated. Social scientists must consider all plausible explanatory variables in the development of a disorder and respond similarly in the development of a treatment or treatments for that disorder. They must disregard their personal or political agendas and focus on empirically supported findings and on the scientific process. The victimhood mentality is unhealthy and may be etiologically related to a variety of disorders. As a group, females should reject this mentality and recognize the myriad opportunities available to women. In a similar vein, men have not yet adopted this unhealthy mentality—may this mind-set continue unabated among males.

In closing, no single treatment is effective for all psychiatric disorders indicating that human complexity is greater than many realize—treatments need to be systematized, individualized, based on sound empirical support, and outcomes must be replicated. Additionally, all forms of treatment should remain on the table for consideration. In some cases a stepped-care model will suffice—in other cases, treatment will need to be more intense and multi-modal. Treatments with the most empirical support should be considered as first-line interventions and used in combination with other treatments that fit the unique characteristics of the individual and based on empirical findings. We are grateful to all the contributors in Latner and Wilson's volume (2007b) that covered the literature on SH with eating disorders in ways we could not have done ourselves. Their creative and helpful chapters represent a milestone in the SH and SC literature on obesity and eating disorders.

Chapter 10
Addictive Behaviors

> *By offering addicts treatment instead of jail, Drug Court was a conscious response by frustrated judges who were overwhelmed by the results of the '80s cocaine boom and felt that they were processing cases for the same drug-addicted criminals, again and again.*
>
> (Yeung, 2008, p. 62).

Addictive behaviors have the potential to disrupt the life of the individual who possesses the addiction; however, these behaviors also tend to produce a negative and cascading effect on everyone who may come into contact with the individual. More specifically, not only does an addiction produce misery for the addicted, it also creates misery for those who care for the individual, those who depend on the individual, and those who may be victims of the addicted individual's impaired judgment and behavior. As the foregoing suggests, addictive behaviors constitute a serious issue in mental health. For many addicts, their problems are chronic and complex; therefore, they have been long standing enough to produce a variety of related problems in a variety of contexts.

It is not uncommon for an addict to have problems in each of the following areas: (1) social and marital, (2) financial, (3) employment, (4) medical, (5) legal, and (6) psychiatric. Comorbidity is a common occurrence among the population of individuals struggling with addictions. Four million Americans suffer from comorbid serious mental illness and a substance use disorder (Magura, Cleland, Vogel, Knight, & Laudet 2007). Thus, treating individuals with addictive disorders typically requires intensive, multi-person, long-term treatment. Treatment often takes a multi-pronged approach and typically begins with a focus on the most problematic, high-risk, or dangerous behaviors in an attempt to provide some stability in the patient's life. Depending on the severity of presenting problems, connecting the patient with appropriate medical services, professionals who can help with legal issues, social workers who can direct the patient to necessary resources and programs, and attempting to establish a healthy system of social support may be simultaneous foci in a multi-pronged treatment plan. It is difficult to help an individual with an addiction, or keep them in treatment long enough to help, when their life is chaotic and social support is weak or non-existent.

T.M. Harwood, L. L'Abate, *Self-Help in Mental Health*,
DOI 10.1007/978-1-4419-1099-8_10, © Springer Science+Business Media, LLC 2010

Self-help treatments are particularly appropriate for individuals suffering from substance-related problems. Perhaps the most important element of self-help treatments for this patient group involves the concept of denial. "Addictions are characterized by massive denial of illness and rehabilitation must begin with a frank acknowledgement of the nature of the patient's addictive process" (Galanter, Hayden, Casteñeda & Franco 2005, p. 502). Many forms of self-help for addictions are delivered in a group format, an exceedingly effective method for receiving consensual validation and confrontation about denial.

As in many severe conditions and disorders reviewed in Section III, the topic of addictive behaviors is where the concept of self-change (SC), already discussed in Chapter 1 of this volume, comes into being, perhaps more prominently than in any other forms of dysfunctionality. While SH applies to both functional and dysfunctional populations, SC applies to most dysfunctionalities included in this Section. This conclusion means that while functional populations do not need to change themselves, they can add self-help activities to enhance themselves further. SH, in its specific as well as general meaning, is an addition to an already existing working or not working repertoire of adequate or inadequate skills. In dysfunctionalities, on the other hand, self-change means that a person's feelings and emotions, thinking, and behavior need to change, approaching and acquiring new skills and habits, and avoiding and giving up previously damaging habits as well as relationships with similarly disordered companions (L'Abate, Farrar, & Serritella, 1992). This conclusion assumes that SC can only occur with the help of professionals while there is substantive evidence that apparently a certain percentage of natural self-changes (e.g., "maturing out") occur for some who had struggled with addictive behaviors without any seemingly external professional, semi-professional, or non-professional helpers (Blomquist, 2007; Carballo et al., 2007; Klingemann & Sobell, 2007; Rumpf, Bishop, & John, 2007; Smart, 2007).

Addictive behaviors can be defined as "persistent and intense involvement with and stress upon a single behavior pattern, with a minimization or even exclusion of other behaviors, both personal and interpersonal" (L'Abate, 1992b, p. 2). Given this definition, addictive behaviors can be classified along a continuum of severity according to whether they are socially destructive and unacceptable, versus those that seem acceptable because they might not seem as destructive as others. This distinction grants that their social acceptability and destructiveness are relative criteria that may vary from culture to culture and even within a culture. This is the case in American society, according to socio-economic status (SES) and ethnicity lines (Barker & Hunt, 2007; Klingemann & Klingemann, 2007).

A major issue with addictive behaviors relates to whether they are viewed as being individual, intrapsychic and monadic, the traditional bad seed view, versus a relational view of addictive behaviors as having interpersonal causes and effects (L'Abate et al., 1992). For instance, recent contributions to the literature on self-change in addictive behaviors (Carballo et al., 2007; Klingemann & Sobell, 2007; Shaffer, 2007; Sobell, 2007) covered instances of natural remission supposedly without formal help. This remission has been called also spontaneous recovery, auto-remission, natural recovery, untreated recovery, and natural or spontaneous resolution to signify the disappearance of a disorder without any visible or documentable cause or source in a certain percentage of these disorders, as nuanced further down in this chapter (Sobell, 2007). However, evidence indicates that most addicts who successfully quit with little or no help, possess problems, histories, symptoms, and have experienced fewer negative consequences compared to addicts who were once in treatment and later recovered on their own (Smart, 2007, pp. 67–68; Sobell, 2007, p. 6).

Whether stuttering can be considered an addictive behavior, even if it diminishes with age, remains to be determined (Finn, 2007). The otherwise excellent contribution to the literature of Klingemann and Sobell (2007) on self-change in addictive behaviors include the passage of time or age as a major factor in this natural recovery; however, the role of the family (Lewis, 1992) and especially of co-dependent partners in such remission (L'Abate & Harrison, 1992) was not given due consideration. Consequently, even though the presence of such phenomenon as spontaneous remission in many addictive behaviors might be indisputable and amply documented, major contextual factors in the process of natural recovery have been over-looked, raising some important questions about the potentially interactive signal elements in spontaneous recovery (L'Abate, 1992c).

In general, only antecedent, intrapsychic "causes" are evoked to explain phenomena such as "health and cognitive appraisal" (Smart, 2007, p. 68); however, it seems overly simplistic to conceptualize self-change as a process purported to be entirely internal in nature—potentially relevant contextual factors, such as intimate relationships or even court-mandated treatment should be included in models of self-change (Klingemann & Klingemann, 2007). Given the complexity of addictive behaviors and the uniqueness of each individual and their contextual system, it would appear reasonable for one to formulate a process of self-change that is due to a variety of elements both internal and external operating in some form of interaction to the point that might make it difficult to attribute SC solely to any single factor or to one set of factors over another (L'Abate, 1992c; Smart, 2007, p. 68; Sobell, 2007). Nonetheless, Klingemann and Sobell's contribution (2007) includes valuable information as well as a "toolbox" containing materials and resources about evaluating and promoting self-change, also involving available web sites (Voluse, Korkel, & Sobell, 2007).

Destructive Addictive Behaviors

Addictive behavior that is destructive not only psychologically but also physically, potentially leading to mortality or serious morbidity are considered in the following sections.

Alcohol Abuse

Alcohol-use disorders (AUDs) constitute the most frequent psychiatric disorders encountered by mental health professionals (Schuckit, 2006, as cited in Doweiko,

2008). For a review of treatment approaches to alcoholism, the reader is referred to Lewis (1992) who included stages of recovery and how SC in alcohol means interrupting ongoing patterns, and facing the harsh reality of SC versus self-destruction, as well as the destruction of intimate relationships and the negative influence of this dependence on one's children. Lewis (1992) reviewed four different therapeutic methods that seem most successful with alcohol-dependent individuals: (1) structured family therapy, (2) the communication-system framework, (3) experiential/humanistic therapy, and (4) behavioral family therapy. For more recent coverage of the diagnosis and treatment of addictive disorders, the reader is directed to Schuckit (2006) and Frances, Miller, and Mack (2005).

It is important for any clinician to remember that alcohol-dependent individuals present some basic obstacles to treatment. For example, detoxification is necessary in a majority of cases and this should never be attempted without medical supervision. Preferably, detox should take place on an in-patient unit that specializes in alcohol withdrawal. Detoxification is a relatively brief component of the withdrawal process—some experts (e.g., Schuckit 2005) suggest that withdrawal symptoms and the physical/CNS readjustment period may last up to 6 months or more. Withdrawal from alcohol is more dangerous and claims more lives than withdrawal from any other substance of abuse. Fortunately, only about 20% of individuals with alcohol withdrawal syndrome (AWS) will require hospitalization; however, a physician needs to assess the patient to determine if hospitalization is indicated. The most frequently used and non-copyrighted measure for quantifying the severity of AWS is the Clinical Institute Withdrawal Assessment for Alcohol Scale-Revised (CIWA-Ar) (Doweiko, 2008). Vitamin therapy (e.g., immediate B-12, thiamine injections), controlled use of benzodiazepines (especially Diazepam or chlorodiazepoxide), and medical monitoring is typically required well beyond the 24-h detox period when treating individuals with AWS.

Because alcohol is a mild toxin, the complications of alcohol abuse are myriad and damage to one or more organ systems is common. Complications include avitaminosis, increased risk of cancer, alcoholic hepatitis, cirrhosis of the liver, pancreatitis, gastritis, glossitis, cardiopulmonary complications, cognitive deficits (e.g., transient global amnesia, Wernicke's encephalopathy, Korsakoff's psychosis), tardive dyskinesia, peripheral neuropathy, emotional instability, sleep cycle disturbance, fetal alcohol syndrome, and sexual dysfunction among males.

Spontaneous Recovery from Problem Drinking

Blomqvist (2007, pp. 41–43) includes in his review the characteristics of classic studies of SC in alcohol studies. Unfortunately, as the author admits, "...untreated alcohol abusers may differ from those who seek and receive treatment in important respects influencing diagnosis" (p. 44). One major factor cited by Blomqvist refers to "loss of control" (p. 47). He also raised the question on whether SC is "part of the natural history of alcoholism (pp. 50–53), admitting conclusively that" ..recovery rates are highly sensitive to measurement (p. 53); (Carballo et al., 2007; Smart, 2007; Rumpf et al., 2007). The relative emphasis on natural recovery or spontaneous remission might also trivialize the importance of self-change for a major portion of alcohol-dependent individuals, a component that is recognized in most mutual SH groups.

Mutual SH Groups for Problem Drinking

A general dissatisfaction with the efficacy and effectiveness of individual therapy for addictions spawned a variety of group therapy models for alcoholism and other addictions (Galanter et al., 2005). Differential assignment to specific group thera- pies is an important consideration—some patients simply do not respond well to certain groups and not all groups meet every patients needs. Group modalities for differential assignment include the following: (1) interactional, (2) modified inter- actional, (3) behavioral, (4) insight-oriented psychotherapy, and (5) supportive. A purely interactional group would involve a focus on interactional or interpersonal process, a promotion of self-disclosure, and emotional self-expression. The under- standing and resolution of interpersonal conflict is the primary treatment goal. The modified interactional group varies from the purely interactional group in that it places a strong emphasis on ancillary self-help groups devoted to abstinence such as AA and drug therapy such as Antabuse. Abstinence promotion and better interper- sonal functioning is the primary goal of treatment. Behavioral groups emphasize the reinforcement of any abstinence-promoting behaviors and punishment for engaging in undesirable behaviors. The treatment goal is modification of specific problematic behaviors. Insight-oriented groups target the exploration and understanding of group and individual processes. The primary treatment goal is to enhance the patient's abil- ity to tolerate distress without relying on alcohol. Supportive groups aim to bolster one's resources and encourage them to utilize their resources when necessary. The primary treatment goal in supportive groups is to promote adjustment to alcohol-free living (Galanter et al., 2005).

Galanter et al. (2005) point out that group therapy for alcoholism is typically more effective when all group members are problem drinkers and characteris- tic behaviors and the consequences of excessive alcohol consumption are specific foci. It is recommended that groups should be 5–12 members in size and meet at a frequency of 1–3 times per week (Galanter et al., 2005). Additionally, severe sociopathy, poor motivation for change, acute or treatment refractory psychosis, and cognitive deficits that interfere with information processing are useful crite- ria for exclusion from group treatment participation—after all, group process is powerful but easily disrupted when inappropriate members are involved in the treatment.

When comorbidity is part of the problem, patients should be directed to dual diagnosis groups and, in some cases, specialized settings (Galanter et al., 2005; Kelly, McKellar & Moos 2003). The foregoing should be tempered by the conclusion made by Bogenschutz (2007, p. 65S) that indicated the preponderance of evidence suggests that "...the benefits of 12-step attendance do not appear to be markedly different for those with psychiatric disorders." Poly-substance addicted individuals are best suited to multi-focused groups with members who are struggling with the same type of problem. Dependent and non-sociopathic patients are best suited to interactional group models while sociopathic individuals and others suffering from disorders of character are most appropriately placed in groups that focus on coping skills (Cooney, Kadden, Litt & Getter 1991; Poldrugo & Forti, 1988, as cited in Galanter et al., 2005). For patients suffering from major depression with comorbid substance abuse disorders, dual diagnosis self-help groups are recommended over traditional 12-step self-help groups, such as AA (Kelly et al., 2003).

As indicated in the foregoing, comorbidity is a common occurrence among individuals struggling with substance abuse. Some have promoted the notion that patients attempt to address their comorbidity by self-medicating. The most recent literature on this topic has not upheld the self-medication hypothesis in general; however, among women who abuse substances, there is some weak evidence suggesting that self-medication may be a motivating factor in their drug use.

An investigation by Magura et al. (2003) suggested that Double Trouble in Recovery (DTR), a 12-step dual-focus group addressing substance abuse and mental health issues, was effective at reducing alcohol use. More specifically, both drug and alcohol abstinence rates increased from 54% at baseline to 72% at follow-up. Helper therapy (assuming a helping role) and reciprocal learning activities (the learning of new attitudes, skills, and behaviors) were associated with improved abstinence rates. Bogenschutz (2005) found effects that were supportive of the foregoing general findings for a program developed for dually diagnosed individuals. Specifically, 12-step attendance significantly increased and substance use significantly decreased during the 12 weeks of treatment.

The 12-step programs are prototypical self-help groups for individuals suffering from substance abuse or addiction. The only requirement for membership is a desire to become abstinent from drugs or alcohol—total abstinence is the goal from the initiation of membership in a 12-step group. It is unclear why these groups tend to work so well for so many individuals—numerous elements of 12-step programs may have differential effects on patients. For example, praise for abstinence, self-monitoring and self-control strategies, adoption of new ways to cope and behave socially, support from group members/sponsor, the 12-step literature, and encouragement from group members to face painful feelings about themselves and others are all potentially effective strategies and interventions embedded in the 12-step model (Galanter et al., 2005). In any event, AA is considered to be the single most important element of a recovery program by many clinicians specializing in substance abuse treatment (Doweiko, 2008).

Moos and his collaborators (Humphreys, Finney, & Moos, 1994) developed a framework for studying SH groups. To elaborate on this framework, these researches followed up and examined the course of problem drinking among 439 adults involved in AA over a 3-year period; a life domains perspective was used that distinguishes chronic life stressors and social resources in different contexts. Participants completed measures of drinking status, chronic life stressors, social resources, and primary role incumbency. The severity of chronic financial stressors predicted, and was predicted by, more alcohol consumption and drinking-related problems. Among social resources, Alcoholics Anonymous (AA) was the most robust predictor of better functioning on multiple outcome criteria. Support from friends and extended family also predicted better outcome. This effect was stronger for individuals who were low on primary role incumbency, that is, they were unemployed and/or did not have a spouse or partner (Humphreys, Moos, & Finney, 1996). The frequency of avoidant behaviors was inversely related to work and partner resources. Alcohol is often involved in partner violence, especially when psychiatric comorbidity is present in one or both perpetrators or if the relationship itself is dysfunctional (Foran & O'Leary, 2008; James, 2003).

When Humphreys and Moos (2007, as cited in Doweiko, 2008) examined the effectiveness of 12-step, group-oriented treatment formats, they found that treatments including 12-step group involvement was 30% less expensive than CBT for substance abuse programs (the standard treatment). Additionally, among 12-step participants, 30% more patients were alcohol free at 2-year post-treatment compared to those who participated in CBT substance abuse treatment alone.

Additionally, differences in outcomes, alcoholic treatment utilization, and costs were examined between 135 alcoholics with no previous treatment history who chose to attend AA with 66 alcoholics who sought help from a professional outpatient alcoholism provider. At baseline, AA attendees had lower incomes and less education and experienced more adverse consequences of drinking compared to the other participants. Over the 3-year study, per-person treatment costs for the AA group were $1,826 (45%) lower than costs for the outpatient treatment group. Despite the lower costs, outcomes for the AA group at both 1 and 3 years were similar to those of the outpatient treatment group (Humphreys & Moos, 1996). Apparently, high-cost treatment is not necessary for all problem drinkers.

Kaskutas et al. (2005, as cited in Doweiko, 2008) examined the participation pattern of 349 individuals who sought formal treatment for AUDs. At 5-year post-treatment, AA involvement could be characterized by four subgroups: (1) low AA involvement characterized by individuals in their first year of post-treatment; (2) medium AA involvement characterized by individuals attending approximately 60 meetings in their first year of post-treatment with a gradual increase in attendance by year 5; (3) high initial AA involvement characterized by individuals attending 200 meetings in their first year post-treatment accompanied by a slight decrease in AA involvement by year 5 post-treatment; and (4) declining AA involvement characterized by approximately 200+ meetings a year initially but substantially reduced to about six meetings in their fifth year of post-treatment. At the end of their fifth year of AA involvement, 79% of those in the first subgroup were abstinent compared to 73% in the second subgroup, 61% in the third subgroup, and 43% in the fourth subgroup.

A medication aimed toward aversive conditioning is sometimes used as an adjunctive treatment for problem drinkers. Called disulfiram (Antabuse), this medication produces extreme discomfort if one ingests alcohol by blocking an enzyme (aldehyde dehydrogenase) that is an important step in the metabolic cycle of alcohol—the result is a build-up of acetaldehyde, a toxic substrate that creates symptoms of severe hangover. The clinical utility of this approach is questionable and some have died as a result of ingesting alcohol while on Antabuse. Additionally, the alcoholic must be compliant with disulfiram treatment—unfortunately, compliance rates are often problematic. To date, the clinical utility of Antabuse is questionable at best (Thaler & Sunstein, 2008). Naltrexone has been used to reduce cravings for alcohol and help prevent relapse—the results of this form of treatment suggest that it is best suited as an adjunct to more effective methods.

When the Internet and paper self-help materials are combined in the treatment of problem drinking, an additive effect appears to be present. Cunningham, Humphreys, Koski-Jännes, and Cordingley (2005) conducted an investigation that involved patients randomized to an Internet-based intervention or to an Internet-based intervention combined with an additional self-help book. Findings indicated that those who received the additional self-help book reported greater reductions in alcohol use and fewer consequences at follow-up compared to those only receiving the Internet-based intervention. This additive effect of an extra treatment component speaks to the importance of a multi-pronged approach to substance abuse treatment.

In another investigation of an Internet-based self-help treatment for problem drinkers (http://www.minderdrinken.nl), Riper et al. (2007) found that 17.2% of drinkers in the Internet intervention group had reduced their drinking to within guideline norms—only 5.4% the control group had achieved this level of success; the difference in change on drinking between the two groups is statistically significant. Further, intervention subjects reduced mean weekly alcohol consumption by a significantly greater amount compared to control group members. More specifically, the intervention group experienced a differential reduction of 12.0 standardized units. The authors concluded that the intervention was effective in reducing problem drinking in the community.

In an investigation involving alcoholics with comorbid anxiety disorder, a treatment involving cognitive-behavioral treatment (CBT) for panic disorder was integrated with content focused on the interaction of alcohol use and panic symptoms (Kushner et al., 2006). The authors concluded that this form of integrated treatment was well accepted by patients and offers significant clinical advantages over treatment for problem drinking alone. Additionally, this form of integrated treatment was suggested to be a practical and efficacious adjunctive form of treatment to the standard treatment for alcoholism. Some may conclude from the foregoing that the study supports the notion of self-medication; however, this conclusion is untenable for a number of reasons including small sample size, non-randomized treatment assignment, no report of sex demographics, the possibility that this type of comorbidity may lend itself more readily to reinforcement from self-medication, and the possibility that a multi-pronged treatment is necessary, or at least more effective, when comorbidity is an issue. Additionally, usefully framed, therapeutic insight into the real or imagined relationship between anxiety and alcohol use, coupled with effective CBT coping strategies, may be an important element for successful treatment in this patient group.

General Substance Abuse

Substance abuse represents a chronic and complex (pervasive) psychiatric diagnosis—comorbidity is the general rule and a complicating factor in any substance abuse treatment plan. As such, treatment plans for substance abuse need to be individualized and should include treatment strategies and interventions that are empirically supported, appropriate to the patient and their unique circumstances, and they should consider the use of online resources and self-help groups such as AA. In this section, substance abuse has been separated from alcohol abuse; however, this distinction is somewhat arbitrary—alcohol is a drug, it has psychoactive properties and addictive potential similar to those described below. The major distinction is that alcohol is a licit substance—most other drugs of abuse are not. In the following, we discuss stimulant abuse and drug abuse in general. We also cover tobacco use—a licit but highly addictive habit. Due to the scope of the problem, not all addictions or substances can be addressed or covered in-depth—the interested reader is directed to Abadinsky (2008), Schuckit (2006), and L'Abate et al. (1992) for a comprehensive coverage of treatment models and self-help resources.

In a large number of substance abuse cases, polysubstance abuse is present; however, individuals typically have a drug "of choice"—in other words, a particular substance or class of substances is preferred. Patients often seek their drug of choice with great vigor—other substances are typically abused in combination with their preferred drug, often resulting in a desired synergistic effect or to counteract unpleasant effects that may occur when their substance of choice is used at high doses. For example, alcohol, benzodiazepines, or other CNS depressants may be used to help a stimulant abuser get needed sleep or to take the "edge" off of some CNS stimulants. Further, non-preferred substances may be used as a substitute when preferences cannot be met.

Different personality types may experience higher rates of substance abuse, including alcohol abuse; however, to date, no specific personality type emerges as a strong predictor of substance abuse. On the other hand, individuals diagnosed with *DSM-IV-TR* Axis II Cluster B disorders appear to be more at-risk for substance abuse, perhaps due to the impulsivity that characterizes Cluster B diagnoses. Those diagnosed with antisocial personality disorders tend to experience relatively higher rates of substance abuse than other personality types—borderline personalities run a close second. This subset of substance abusers tends to mature in enmeshed families with inadequate or defective personal and generational boundaries (Ranew & Serritella, 1992). Individuals suffering from bipolar disorder and schizophrenia may experience relatively high rates of substance abuse as well. Substance abuse and mental disorder profiles of 310 long-term attendees of an MH SH agency indicates that the rates of these disorders bipolar and schizophrenia are equivalent to or exceed those found in clinical and community samples (Franskoviak & Segal, 2002).

Methamphetamine/Amphetamine Abuse

In the U.S., methamphetamine is the second most commonly abused illicit substance after marijuana (Doweiko, 2008). Methamphetamine, consumed by abusers, is typically produced in clandestine laboratories—quality assurance is not a top priority and drug potency is variable. Thus, overdose or other complications may result as a use of methamphetamine or other CNS stimulants produced in home laboratories. Tolerance to the euphoria produced by amphetamines develops rapidly requiring the addict to procure ever increasing amounts of the substance to achieve the desired effects.

The types of CNS stimulants that are popular today include amphetamine, methamphetamine, ephedrine, methylphenidate, Ice (a smokable form of methamphetamine), and Kat (aka, Cat, qat, Khat and Miraa). The most common forms of amphetamine are dextroamphetamine (d-amphetamine sulfate, twice as potent as the other common form of amphetamine) and methamphetamine (d-desoxyephedrine hydrochloride). Methamphetamine appears to be preferred over dextroamphetamine by abusers because it has a longer half-life and is better at crossing the blood–brain barrier. The variations within the category of stimulants cannot all be covered here—the interested reader is directed to Doweiko (2008) for CNS effects and consequences of abuse of various stimulants.

Cocaine

Cocaine is a topical local anaesthetic with psychoactive properties. When applied as a local anesthetic, cocaine begins to exert an effect in about 1 min with effects lasting as long as 2 hrs. In the past, cocaine was commonly used to aid surgical procedures involving the eye, ear, nose, throat, rectum, and vagina. The fast-acting anaesthetic effect coupled with strong vasoconstriction effects made cocaine the natural choice for delicate medical procedures. Today, we have other substances that provide surgeons with the same useful features cocaine possessed but without the abuse potential.

Cocaine, the active agent of the coca leaf, was isolated almost 160 years ago. Cocaine was once thought to be a miracle cure for many ailments including depression and later, narcotic withdrawal symptoms (Doweiko, 2008). Many lives were ruined before the medical community and U.S. government limited the availability of cocaine. Unfortunately, cocaine resurfaced in the 1980s as a major drug of abuse. Cocaine produces euphoria and makes the user feel full of energy; thus, the high addiction potential. Additionally, many users in the 1980s thought cocaine was a harmless drug even though historical evidence, forgotten by most, indicated otherwise.

Pharmacologically, cocaine quickly diffuses into the bloodstream and rapidly reaches the brain and other drug-rich organs (e.g., the heart). Cocaine creates a buildup of dopamine (DA) in the limbic system by blocking the re-uptake of this neurotransmitter. Cocaine has an affinity for at least five subtypes of dopamine receptors; however, the affinity appears stronger for some DA subtypes than for others. Cocaine also blocks the reuptake of the neurotransmitters norepinephrine (NE) and serotonin (SE); however, the significance of these effects is unknown at this time. Cocaine affects other receptors including the *mu* and *kappa* opioid receptors and this may explain the intense craving reported by cocaine-dependent individuals when they are unable to procure the drug.

Tolerance to cocaine's euphoric effect develops rapidly (Schuckit, 2006) and this may lead to a preoccupation with obtaining the drug—often to the detriment of social, marital, and employment obligations. Unfortunately, the problems with cocaine abuse do not end there—because cocaine is a vasoconstrictor and because it appears in high concentrations in heart tissue, the abuser may die from heart failure. More specifically, cocaine increases heart rate while reducing blood flow to the heart muscle—the end result is often death or heart damage.

Spontaneous Recovery from General Substance Abuse

Blomqvist (2007, pp. 35–36) reviewed all of the extant studies to date that examined the phenomenon of spontaneous recovery. He acknowledges, however, that the whole area of self-change in addictions is still marred in definitional and measurement problems of what constitutes "addiction" and "improvement" (p. 53). Smart (2007, p. 67) concluded that "those who recover with treatment may have fewer problems than those who do not seek treatment." On the basis of survey data, Rumpf et al. (2007, p. 76) concluded that "As a whole, . . . the evidence of untreated remission is supported by a substantial body of literature coming from cross-sectional, longitudinal and short- and long-term databases." However, some troubling questions remain: (1) What is the cost to the individual and society if they do not seek timely therapy from a professional and employ adjunctive self-help treatment? (2) what is the role of time, age, severity of addiction, substance of choice, polysubstance abuse, pervasiveness of the problem, chronicity of the abuse, level of social support and sex of the individual? and (3) what is the percentage of addicted individuals who achieve spontaneous long-term recovery on their own?

Self-Help Groups for Substance Abuse

Part of the literature on SH groups has been reviewed in Chapter 1 of this volume. In reference to substance abuse, a prospective, quasi-experimental comparison of five

12-step-based programs for substance abuse were compared with a five cognitive-behavioral (CB) treatment on the degree to which participants participated in SH groups, using also outpatient and inpatient mental health services. The experience of positive outcomes was evaluated at 1-year follow-up. Compared with participants treated with CB programs, participants in 12-step programs showed significantly greater involvement in self-help groups at follow-up. In contrast, participants treated in CB programs averaged almost as twice as many outpatient continuing care visits after discharge compared to those treated in 12-step programs, receiving significantly more days of inpatient care. Psychiatric and substance abuse outcomes were comparable across treatments. These results are relevant to cost-benefits analysis. If CB treatment is conducted by doctoral-level professionals while 12-step groups are conducted by non-professionals, given the same outcome, it looks like the latter may be less expensive than the former. Of course, the influence of self-selection must be assessed in order to accurately interpret outcome data in longitudinal evaluations of mutual SH organizations (Humphreys, Phibbs, & Moos, 1996).

Therapeutic Community (TC) models have been employed to treat substance abuse. The TC is a generic term for residential, self-help, drug-free treatment programs (Abadinsky, 2008). TCs share some common characteristics with 12-step programs; however, TCs incorporate a 24-h residential community with a structured behavioral approach of punishment and rewards. Therapeutic communities attempt to create a comprehensive change in lifestyle that promotes abstinence from illicit substances, the adoption of pro-social activities and values, and vocational training/employability enhancement (Abadinsky, 2008).

A variety of TCs exist including Synanon (founded in 1953) now found in several states, Phoenix House (located in the Bronx) that employs a strict daily schedule of activities beginning at 7:00 a.m. and ending at 9:00 p.m.—lights are out at 11:00 p.m. Odyssey House, located on New York's Ward's Island, is a TC that employs more professionals and medication-based withdrawal than most TCs. TCs have even been established in prisons located in New York and California. Unfortunately, the success rates of TCs are questionable—most research is poorly designed rendering findings of questionable meaning.

Chemical Dependency (CD) programs have increased in recent years. Some are for profit, others are non-profit. Outreach is central to these programs, marketing professionals are often employed, and individuals who possess insurance (such as employed cocaine or alcohol abusers) comprise the preferred patient population. Most often located in a health care facility, this tends to increase costs while reducing the number of vacant beds in the healthcare facility. Treatment is usually eclectic in nature and individual and group in format. Education, nutrition, relaxation training, recreation, counseling/psychotherapy, pharmacotherapy, and 12-step perspectives are often integrated into a comprehensive, intensive, and highly structured, 3- to 6-week in-patient treatment plan. Patients are encouraged to participate in 12-step programs after discharge. Outcome studies provide a mixed picture—in general, high-intensity/long-term residential treatment performs better than lower intensity, brief programs; however, for mild or moderate substance abuse of shorter durations, brief/low-intensity programs have proven effective and are more cost-effective (Abadinsky, 2008).

Tobacco Abuse

Smoking addiction has been reviewed by Serritella (1992a) who described "Nicotine is a fast-acting stimulant that triggers chemicals in the brain that stimulate pleasurable sensations that are inevitably reinforcing" (p. 97). Nicotine, the major psychoactive agent in cigarettes, was isolated in 1828 and it was known to have an effect on nervous tissue as early as 1889 (Doweiko, 2008). Almost a century later, scientists discovered the mechanism that nicotine employs to stimulate neurons and produce pleasurable affects. Each draw of cigarette smoke introduces a small dose of nicotine into the bloodstream that reaches the brain in less than 10 s. Nicotine reaches all blood-rich tissue; however, because it rapidly and easily crosses the blood–brain barrier, it is particularly well-suited to reaching the brain. This property of nicotine allows the substance to accumulate in the brain at a concentration that is about twice as high as the level found in the blood stream. The nicotine molecule is similar in shape to the ubiquitous neurotransmitter, acetylcholine—this similarity allows nicotine to create a rapid cascade of numerous neurochemical changes in the brain (Schmitz & Delaune, 2005). More specifically, a nicotine-induced rapid release of the neurotransmitter epinephrine produces a stimulatory/arousing affect. This is then followed by nicotine-induced release of the neurotransmitters dopamine and acetylcholine—the release of dopamine produces a sense of pleasure and relaxation through activation of the mesolimbic dopaminergic pathways that are part of the brain's reward system. Several other neurochemical changes occur as a result of nicotine's pharmacodynamics. Tobacco use is also covered in Chapter 12 (Severe Psychopathology)—the fact that tobacco use represents the single most preventable cause of death in the U.S. is the primary motivation for providing additional coverage on this topic.

Strong evidence exists indicating that cigarette manufacturers increased the nicotine content in cigarettes by as much as 10% between 1998 and 2004 (Brown, 2006). Cigarettes appear to have an addiction potential that is greater than cocaine's. Somewhere between 3 and 20% of first users of cocaine become addicted (Musto, 1991); however, between 33 and 50% of those who try cigarettes become addicted (Oncken & George, 2005). At present, approximately 4,700 chemical compounds have been identified in cigarette smoke—it is estimated that 1,00,000 additional compounds remain to be discovered (Schmitz & Delaune, 2005). Most tobacco smokers are not abusers of other chemicals; however, it is common for substance abusers to be heavy smokers (Doweiko, 2008). Methods to treat such an addiction vary from nicotine chewing gum, behavior modification, transdermal nicotine patch, hypnosis, and education. Most of these methods show similar success rates. Consequently, differential treatment selection depends on the proclivities of the patient, financial factors, and social acceptability. As with all addictive behaviors, cessation of smoking is subject to frequent relapses. Therefore, relapse rates are the most reliable indication of how successful any treatment method may be (Serritella, 1992).

Whether self-help interventions may change specific cognitions and the extent to which changes in such cognitions are related to behavioral changes was evaluated in a randomized field experiment following 2-week and 3-month follow-ups in 1,546 smokers. Smokers were assigned to one of four conditions offering smoking cessation self-help materials containing (1) outcome information alone, (2) self-efficacy enhancing information, (3) both sorts of information, and (4) no information. Results showed that (1) with regard to behavioral effects, only self-help interventions that included self-efficacy enhancing information were more effective than no information, (2) with regard to cognitive changes, outcome information led to increases in expected positive outcomes but also to increases in self-efficacy expectations, (3) self-efficacy-enhancing information led to increases in self-efficacy, (4) different cognitive changes between Time 1 and Time 2 were related to types of quitting activity at Time 3 in different types of smokers. Apparently, some types of information lead to specific cognitive changes, while other types seem to have more generalized cognitive effects. Furthermore, cognitive changes produced by self-help information may predict future quitting activity (Dijkstra & De Vries, 2001).

Lancaster and Stead (2005) evaluated the findings from over 60 studies on smoking cessation. These researchers concluded that standard self-help materials appear to increase quit rates only slightly when compared to quit rates of no treatment controls. Lancaster and Stead also failed to find any convincing evidence that standard self-help materials produce any significant incremental benefit when employed in combination with other interventions such as nicotine replacement therapy or information from healthcare professionals. When materials are tailored to the needs of individual smokers, their efficacy improves; however, the absolute size of effect remains unimpressive. In reality, only 30% of those who try to abstain from smoking remain smoke free for 48 hrs and only 5–10% achieve long-term abstinence (Hughes, 2005). Smokers typically attempt to quit five to ten times before finally achieving success and 50% of smokers are eventually able to stop (Hughes, 2005).

A novel self-help approach to smoking cessation, not included in the Lancaster and Stead (2005) review, is reported by Thaler and Sunstein (2008). The Green Bank of Caraga in Mindanao, Philippines has started a program called "Committed Action to Reduce and End Smoking." A would-be nonsmoker opens an account with a minimum balance of one dollar. For 6 months, participants deposit the amount of money they would otherwise spend on cigarettes into their account. After 6 months, participants must take a urine test to confirm that they have not smoked recently. If they pass the test, they get their money back. If they fail the test, the account is closed and the total amount is donated to charity. This program is supported by results obtained from MIT's Poverty Action Laboratory. More specifically, the MIT investigation found that opening up a bank account is associated with a 53% higher likelihood that smokers will achieve their goal of abstinence from tobacco. Apparently, no other anti-smoking approach, not even the nicotine patch, appears to be so successful.

Spontaneous Recovery from Tobacco Abuse

Floter and Kroger (2007) referred to this phenomenon in regard to smoking as "Self-Quitting" (p. 106) suggesting that "quitting without help is the best strategy to become a nonsmoker." These authors introduced the possibility of qualifying self-change in smoking as "self-healing," because the change does not require a total remaking of one's personality as required in self-change. This process is visible in individual self-quitters who demonstrate "...higher education, greater confidence in the ability to quit, i.e., 'self-efficacy,' lighter smoking, less alcohol consumption, fewer cigarettes smoked per day, and fewer slips in current quit attempts" (p. 109). The foregoing finding is counterbalanced by research indicating that the least successful method for smoking cessation is the one that is most common, "cold-turkey" (Patkar, Vergare, Batka, Weinstein & Leone 2003). Relapse rates are highest for those attempting a sudden discontinuation of smoking—cessation methods that utilize nicotine replacement therapy combined with psychosocial support produce higher success rates than the cold-turkey method (Patkar et al., 2003). It should be noted that among those who were successful "self-quitters" appear to have less severe, less chronic, are less likely to be polysubstance abusers, and less pervasive forms of the addiction. Additionally, higher levels of education and confidence would suggest that they may take a more proactive, informed role in their strategy to quit smoking.

Domestic Violence and Crime

Domestic violence and crime in general could be viewed as addictive behaviors because of their repetitive and reactive nature. Additionally, domestic violence and other criminal behavior often lack the presence of concrete, universal external circumstances that prompt them. It is extremely important to note that domestic violence occurs within a relationship; therefore, it is essentially a relationship problem with both parties sharing some responsibility for the initiation and maintenance of abuse. Interestingly enough and counter to conventional wisdom, the best research on the topic suggests a picture of domestic violence that is very different from the pictures presented in movies, the media, and by many feminists, and Women's Studies programs throughout the world of academia. More specifically, a meta-analysis by Archer (2000) found that women in heterosexual relationships were (1) more likely to use physical violence against their male partners and (2) were likely to use these acts more frequently than men. The one finding from Archer's meta-analysis consistent with conventional wisdom is that men were more likely than women to have injured their partner when they become involved in domestic violence. On the other hand, women are much more likely than men to use a weapon against their domestic partner (James, 2003).

The investigations included in the Archer (2000) meta-analysis were empirically sound and all published in peer-reviewed scientific journals. Unfortunately, much of the information widely disseminated at present is not based on sound empiricism. Inexperienced investigators often limit data collection to interviews involving women only or they interview women residing in women's shelters—this investigatory method does not allow for a representation of the population at hand for a number of reasons: (1) it fails to include men who historically under-report when they are victims of domestic violence, (2) the population in women's shelters represent the worst situations of domestic violence, and (3) there are very few "men's shelters" and males often leave the home to stay in a hotel or at a friends house when victimized by a violent spouse or girlfriend. To illustrate the phenomenon further, in the early 1990s, Seattle police instituted a "must arrest" policy when called to intervene in domestic violence situations. This policy was instituted because domestic violence was becoming increasingly prevalent and intervention in these types of situations is high-risk for officers. When arrest rates were computed, 51% of the arrests involved females as the perpetrators of the violence. This finding is striking due to the likelihood, strongly supported by research, that men under-report their domestic violence victim status.

Socialization may have a lot to do with this little-known phenomenon of domestic violence and this socialization appears to have a long history. For example, in France, when men were beaten by their wives, they were forced to don a dress and were paraded through the streets of France riding on horseback, backwards (James, 2003). Additionally, in our society, it is almost universally accepted that it is not alright for men to strike women; however, apparently, it is socially acceptable for women to strike men. For example, males may be struck if they say something a woman finds offensive—it is very rare for the opposite to occur. A cursory review of the popular media will reveal this behavioral double standard and it is relatively common place to see women/female adolescents strike men/male adolescents in public—especially in high school and on college campuses. According to Gregorash, *supra*, p. 89, "Patricia Overberg ranks fear of loss of relationship with children as one of the top three reasons that men choose not to leave abusive relationships. The remaining top two reasons for males to endure an abusive domestic relationship are (1) fear of ridicule and (2) sense of responsibility to provide and protect" (Cook, supra, p. 78) (Archer, 2000, p. 243). The fear of ridicule from society is still a powerful deterrent for males who are the victims of a violent domestic relationship.

Unfortunately, the empirically supported and peer-reviewed information on domestic violence is resisted and often rejected out of hand by those in academia—the worst offenders appear to be feminists and faculty in Women's Studies departments. At least one professor was actually prevented from teaching a particular course because he dared to present the findings from Archer's (2000) meta-analysis. The Women's Studies department at this professor's university threatened the chair of the "offending" professor's department with boycott should this professor ever be allowed to teach the course again. At this same university, this professor was dismissed from a thesis committee on domestic violence for stating that Archer's meta-analysis should be included in the literature review.

This is a disturbing development in academia where the free market-place of ideas should prevail. Additionally, society does not benefit from the failure of academics to present the best extant research on this topic. More specifically, the only logical and effective way to approach a problem and achieve effective results is to come at it from an informed perspective. Preventing the dissemination of scientific findings runs counter to the tenets of science (Beutler & Harwood, 2000). The reality is that violence against men is on the rise, violence against women is decreasing (James, 2003). As early as 1986, respected researchers published findings that domestic violence against men had been steadily increasing since 1975—unfortunately, this information has been suppressed (James, 2003). Mental health practitioners and others in the social sciences should not allow personal agendas or bias to prevent enlightened pursuit of change. Men, women, their children, and society all suffer when domestic violence occurs.

For the interested reader, Thomas James, J.D., wrote an exceptionally enlightening book on this topic titled *Domestic violence, the 12 things you aren't supposed to know*. The book is supported by primary sources obtained from peer-reviewed scientific journals and it is a must read for anyone with an open-mind and a willingness to do something effective about domestic violence in America. A model linking addictive behaviors in domestic relationships is presented below in this chapter and expanded further in a relational competence theory in Chapter 14 of this volume.

Treatments for domestic violence have traditionally not fared very well. Recidivism rates are high. One possible reason for this relative failure is that the problem has been conceptualized on faulty premise. In reality, both men and women engage in domestic violence. Although both sexes engage in domestic violence at rates that are approximately equal, females appear to exhibit slightly higher rates of physical aggression against their male partners. Finally, domestic violence manifests within the context of a dysfunctional relationship. A paradigm shift is necessary before effective treatments for domestic violence can be developed and employed.

Spontaneous Recovery

The issue with desistance in domestic violence lies in its definition as a crime, whether by official records, self-reports by victims who may dramatize the crime (and sometimes minimize the crime), and by perpetrators who tend to minimize it. Furthermore, once frequency, chronicity, and seriousness are taken into consideration, the definition becomes even more difficult to achieve through consensus among the various sources. The major measure of desistance is linked to the number of problems that probation officers reported about their probationers (Takala, 2007).

Nonetheless, desistance to domestic violence occurs as a function of age, maturation, growing aversion to the risk of being jailed again, changes in adult life, including more responsibilities and remarrying. The proportion of natural violence desisters may vary between 5 and 33% depending on the nature of the offense, a percentage largest among respondents who admitted burglary, vehicle-related thefts, shoplifting, and drug selling (Takala, 2007, p. 136). As a result, Takala concluded his review of the literature on crime desistance thus:

> Punishment and its threat, then, seem to have an effect on desistance from crime. However, they should be used wisely and moderately. They should express blame but not make it more difficult for the offender to go back to non-criminal way of life. Furthermore, they should not prevent the operation of the processes of spontaneous desistance (p. 136).

Sexual Abuses and Offenses

Children are the primary victims of sexual abuse and males commit sexual abuses more often than females. Perpetrators of sex-related crimes involving children typically earn the diagnosis of pedophilia. Clouding the issue of sexual abuse is the fact that many cases of claimed molestation or childhood sexual abuse, especially based on memories supposedly recovered during therapy, have received a necessary revision due to faulty memories created by overzealous therapists (Fine, 2006). Nonetheless, there are at least two different types of sexual molesters: (1) fixated ones, whose primary sexual orientation is toward children and beginning in adolescence, with males being the primary target, and (2) regressed ones, whose primary sexual orientation is toward age-mates in adulthood with precipitating stress usually evident, such as family abuse, educational failure, and occupational loss (Cooney, 1992).

Most treatment options focus on incarceration, treatment, a residential treatment facility, and community-based treatment programs. Additionally, aversive conditioning procedures and chemical castration are possible "treatment" options for pedophiles, rapists, and other sexual criminals; however, ethical concerns and effectiveness limit their use. For example, even the most radical treatments (e.g., chemical castration) are not 100% effective and recidivism rates are unacceptably high. The paraphilias may be conceptualized as disorders of intimacy—they appear to be deeply rooted, begin in childhood or adolescence, and tend to be long-standing. At present, no treatments for individuals diagnosed with any of the coercive paraphilias can be considered effective enough to reasonably ensure public safety.

An important issue with molesters and pedophiles lies in the perception of themselves as victims of external circumstances, rather than of persons in charge of their lives (Cooney, 1992, p. 138). This pattern is especially evident in incestuous families, where a triangle considered in Chapter 14 of this volume, might account conceptually for such a deviation and devastation. In spite of its importance and frequency, at least in the American culture, it is interesting that no data were given on the possible natural remission of these addictive behaviors in a contribution completely devoted to such a topic (Klingeman & Sobell, 2007). Additionally, the reinforcement potential associated with sexual behavior is powerful—countering this with psychosocial treatment or more invasive measures appears inadequate in the long term. In some cases, sex offenders simply mature-out of their problem. Unfortunately, it is impossible to know if and when an offender will mature-out and the long-term success rates of available treatments are so low, it is difficult to have any confidence in their effectiveness for any individual.

Sex Addiction

Some argue that sex addiction does not exist—it is not an official diagnostic category in the *DSM-IV-TR*; however, this does not mean that sex addiction is non-existent. Sex "addiction" may be more accurately characterized as a type of impulse control disorder. According to Schneider (2004), the prevalence of sexual addiction in America is about 6% and sexual addictions are often comorbid with other addictions, including drug and alcohol abuse and eating disorders.

A particular form of sexual addiction that is on the rise is cyber-sex. The typical cyber-sex addict is male, a heavy Internet user, married, frequently a college-educated professional, often a survivor of sexual abuse, and likely to be depressed (Schwartz & Southern, 2000). For some reason, males are more likely to seek and receive help for their cyber-sex addiction than females (Schwartz & Southern, 2000).

While individual psychotherapy and 12-step programs appear to constitute the best route to treating sexual addictions, the 12-step programs are effective as stand-alone treatments and they appear to have powerful effects on the addict's cognitions. In 12-step programs, self-esteem is often improved and spirituality often becomes an important component of the struggling sex addict's life (Fulton, 2004).

Programs developed for the treatment of sex addictions include: Sex and Love Addicts Anonymous (SLAA), Sex Addicts Anonymous (SAA), Sexaholics Anonymous (SA), and Sexual Compulsives Anonymous (SCA). SLAA was founded in 1976 and was the first of its kind to provide services for sexual addicts. This program is distinguished because it focuses on love addiction as well as sex addiction. Love addiction is defined as, ". . .extreme dependence on one or more love objects, being preoccupied with romantic fantasies, having serial relationships, or any combination of these" (Parker & Guest, 2002, p. 120). This focus on love addiction has attracted more females than any other sexually related 12-step program. SAA was founded by men who wanted more anonymity in the process of healing-this program appeals to a diversity of sexual orientations. SA began in California and advocates for a period of abstinence—they adhere to Judeo-Christian beliefs so divorced individuals or homosexuals are not recommended for this 12-step program. In 1982, SCA was founded specifically to support gay men.

Socially Based Addictive Behaviors

These addictive behaviors may not be as deadly as those reviewed in the foregoing; however, in many ways they may be just as deleterious or functionally impairing.

Codependency

Rather than focusing on individuals with evident addictive behaviors, L'Abate and Harrison (1992) focused on the partners of addicted individuals instead, considering co-dependency as another form of addictive behavior. They defined this position by offering three experimental checklists to evaluate objectively this process: one checklist for Primary Codependency (L'Abate, 1992d, p. 9), a second on Parenting Skills (p. 10), and a third on Workplace Codependency (p. 11). These authors defined codependency the way L'Abate defined addictive behaviors, as a process that controls an individual's behavior at the expense of more constructive spheres of activity (p. 286). They proposed to view co-dependency from a relational Selfhood Model 11 to be explained further in Chapter 14 of this volume. According to this model, addicted individuals, mostly men, could be characterized as being self-centered and "selfish" making themselves more important than others, by putting others down and "winning" at others' expense. These men tend to attract women who could be characterized by "selflessness," who make others more important then themselves, by putting themselves down. An experimental list of 13 discriminating signs was developed to identify the two personalities (L'Abate, 1992, p. 288) as well as behavior patterns that indicate the process of polarization that emanates from these personalities and produce reactive stances between the two parties (L'Abate, 1992, p. 289). In addition, L'Abate and Harrison suggested possible self-help strategies for codependents to avoid becoming involved, enmeshed, or "hooked" by provocation from the addicted partner (p. 294). Failing such strategies, these authors presented a Bill of Rights for Codependent Relationships (p. 296). All of these checklists, discriminating signs, and strategies could become part of a SH and SC program to help both partners (Jordan & L'Abate, 1995) that could be bolstered by specific practice exercises about co-dependency as homework assignments (L'Abate, 2010).

One important aspect about exercise from the viewpoint of self-help is that it is *Excessive Exercise:*

Exercise is an example of behavior that in its extreme form becomes an addiction when it interferes with social and occupational functioning. More specifically, compulsive exercise may occupy the focus of one's life at the exclusion of social or relational behaviors (Farrar, 1992a, b, c; Farrar et al. 1992). Excessive exercise is common among women suffering from anorexia nervosa. Further, Female Athlete Triad (FAT), which involves loss of menses, disordered eating, and osteoporosis, frequently accompanies excessive exercise by women, can be inexpensive and thus available to anyone who can walk, run, swim, or lie on a mattress to practice exercise routines. Another important aspect is that exercise has been shown to result in better mood and reductions in anxiety. On the other hand, physical injury and physical complications can result from *excessive* exercise—these can be costly both in monetary terms and in emotional and life-functioning terms. One web-based resource is Wellsphere, remedies, causes, and alternative treatments are provided with this web site. Another web site is Randy Schellenberg's—again, information and resources are available. A google search using "treatments for excessive exercise" yielded more than five million hits.

Calogero and Pedrotty (2007) made an important distinction between mindless and mindful exercise. The former becomes an addiction when taken to its extreme while the latter is one type of keeping in shape mentally and physically. Here is where the model of approach-avoidance presented in Chapter 1 of this volume suggests how one can approach an activity while avoiding other ones. Given the constant of time for all of us, we need to choose how to spend it. Whatever time we spend on an activity implies avoiding other ones. Excessive concern with compulsive doing needs to be balanced with concern for enjoying life while engaging in leisurely pleasant events. A behavior with similarities to excessive exercise is excessive spending.

Excessive Spending

Excessive spending is closely allied to material acquisition and hoarding, with strong gender differences in white collar crime seemingly more prevalent among women. For example, the criminal profile of an embezzler is a middle-aged white female. A major treatment strategy for reducing this addictive behavior is to teach money management by helping participants to work on a budget, lowering expectations, setting realistic priorities, and implementing workable strategies (L'Abate, 1992a). The other side of the coin of excessive spending and hoarding is accumulation of a great deal of money, as found in many business tycoons whose only priority is to make money. Excessive concern with both Doing, as in exercise, and with Having, such as money, goods, or possessions, as in excessive spending, will be covered in Model 7 in a relational competence theory related to SH and SC presented in Chapter 14 of this volume. A google search using "treatments for excessive spending" yielded more than 1,00,000 hits. One site that appears to provide useful information is "wrongdiagnosis.com"—see end of chapter for full web site address. This site provides symptoms/a diagnostic checklist of excessive spending and treatment options.

Gambling

There are two types of gambling addiction referred to across texts: pathological and problem. Pathological gamblers possess an intense impulse to bet in order to relieve anxiety and tension even in light of their losses and negative effects on daily functioning. Problem gamblers possess this proclivity to a lesser degree (Erickson, Molina, Ladd, Pietrzak, & Petry 2005). Elders are particularly vulnerable to gambling addiction—a number of studies indicate that the elderly go to casinos for the purposes of gambling with spending money on food as a secondary purpose

(Moufakkir, 2006). Casinos are fully aware of the characteristics and tendencies of elderly gamblers and they have developed strategies to market to and profit off the elderly. McNeilly and Burke revealed that two-thirds of senior-related facilities received packaged offers by local casinos—over half of the facilities accepted.

Wildman (1992, p. 226) summarized his review of available treatments for pathological gambling by concluding that "motivations are complex and vary from individual to individual. . . treatment procedures . . .should be selected and utilized only after the client/patient is assessed comprehensively." Individual therapy for gambling addiction does have its benefits, self-help organizations such as Gamblers Anonymous (GA) and the National Council on Problem Gambling (NCPG) help line have also proven helpful. NCPG educates callers about the dangers of gambling addiction and helps direct the caller to the most appropriate treatment (Potenza & Griffiths, 2004). GA is modeled after AA and is the first form of self-help treatment sought after by North Americans. The purpose of GA is to promote abstinence; however, GA is less spiritual-focused and more family-oriented compared to AA. Additionally, GA typically consists of smaller groups and teaches basic financial life skills (Petry, 2005). Behavioral self-help strategies identified as helpful in curbing the impulse to gamble include exercise, relaxation techniques, and breathing techniques.

Social gambling is widespread in the Chinese culture to the point of its being a preferred source of entertainment, involving circa 4% of the population. Chinese problem gamblers, ". . .consistently have difficulty admitting their [problem] issue and seeking professional help for fear of losing respect" (Loo, Raylu, & Oei, 2008, p. 1152).

Spontaneous Recovery

If one were to argue that a major characteristic of most self-destructive behaviors is inadequate awareness or denial of the destructive nature of the disorder and a failure to admit personal responsibility, then severe gambling is one of the most potentially destructive addictive disorders. Consequently, it is often difficult for individuals with this addictive behavior to initiate early intervention before the problem progresses. Instead, many rely on eventual spontaneous recovery or convince themselves that they will "hit-it-big". The less severely addicted do tend to seek treatment, but they are a relatively small proportion compared to those who compulsively gamble and eventually experience bankruptcy or inevitable criminal charges (Toneatto & Nett, 2007). This issue and the crucial importance of awareness in self-help and self-care will be discussed further in Chapter 14 of this volume.

Thaler and Sunstein (2008) report that several states, including Illinois, Indiana, and Missouri, have enacted laws enabling gambling addicts to put themselves on a list that bans them from entering or collecting gambling winnings. These laws have been created to deal with the fact that many addicts, including gambling addicts, are painfully aware of the problem but feel unable to control it without external help. With the help of state laws and exclusion of settings where they would be reinforced for their addiction, they are no longer able to gamble. However, if a gambler wants to gamble s/he can do it directly and immediately with a phone call. Consequently, this approach will need further evaluation of outcome before recommending it for enactment in other states.

An exhaustive review of research about SH treatments for problem gamblers (Raylu, Oei, & Loo, 2008) noted that: "Currently, very little is published about the application and efficacy of various forms of self-help treatments for problem gambling... [treatments] are still in their infancy" (p. 1372). According to these researchers, only two forms of SH treatments have been reported in the literature, that is: SH manuals (see Chapter 6 in this volume) and audiotapes. Relevant videos (The Hustler, The Color of Money, The Cincinnati Kid, The Champ, and a host of others) have been produced illustrating the destructive nature of pathological gambling—some may profit from the messages contained in these movies. Internet sites in the form of support groups are available and Gamblers Anonymous is an option for some. In general, an array of treatment approaches should be administered. For instance, written materials such as SH books (see Chapter 4 this volume), treatment manuals (see Chapter 6 this volume), computer-based SH treatments (see Chapter 5 this volume), including palmtop and desktop computers (see Chapters 3 and 5 this volume), telephone interactive voice response systems (see L'Abate & Bliwise, 2009), Internet (see Chapter 5 this volume), and virtual reality applications (North et al., 2008).

These approaches, according to these writers, might help "problem gamblers who are not accessing professional treatment due to shame, guilt, fear of stigma, privacy or financial concerns, as well as those living in rural areas or less severe gambling problems" (p. 1372). No evidence, however, was included about these possible reasons for the avoidance of seeking psychological or medical treatments. This review concludes with a statement about "...a need for a cohesive theory to guide research" (p. 1372) (see Chapter 14 this volume).

A google search using "treatments for excessive gambling" produced 72,000 hits. Examples of web sites include Harbour Pointe (www.lostbet.com), billed as the nation's premier gambling treatment center for 23 years (phone: 800-567-8238), and NonGambler.com (877-559-9355). Harbour Pointe provides an impressive array of support information.

Interpersonal and Love Relationships

Most addictive behaviors show their bottom line characteristic within this category. More specifically, over-dependence on a person or an object is signal and a pathological deep commitment or infatuation becomes an addiction when one partner is unreceptive to the termination of a relationship. Jealousy and fear of abandonment create psychic turmoil that is felt throughout all aspects of the relationship. In situations such as these, individuals are unable to set personal boundaries as well as accept boundaries set by a partner or ex-partner (Farrar, 1992). In situations such as these, group, couple, family therapies, and distance writing (Chapter 3 this volume) may be a welcome alternative or adjunct to traditional psychotherapeutic practices (Jordan & L'Abate, 1995).

One web site devoted to this topic is http://saferelationships.com/, involving The Institute for Relational Harm Reduction & Public Psychopathy Education for those in Pathological Love Relationships. A variety of educational resources and links to helpful information on topics such as free workshops, how to find an affordable therapist, and relationship quizzes are examples of what can be found here.

Spontaneous Recovery

M. B. Sobell (2007) makes an interesting analogy for most addictive behaviors as being "...understood as a love relationship" (p. 152). By taking this analogy one step further, he suggests that there are many ways to dissolve a relationship, i.e., "...many ways to leave one lover" (p. 152). He also suggests a list of factors most likely to influence decisions about what direction of change to purse (p. 156, Table 7.1) including the following: (1) Information about treatment programs, examples of how others have changed, SH groups in existence available for face-to-face talk-based psychotherapy or online interventions, trusting friends and family, and professionals, as outlined in Table 1.1; (2) environmental factors, such as availability of SH/SC sources, access to SH/SC services and agencies, distance, and community attitudes; (3) personal situation/pragmatic factors, such as costs and interference from other commitments and responsibilities; and (4) psychological factors, such as attitude toward independence, trust in others to give aid, beliefs on how one should recover, and past experiences.

The psychological factors outlined by M. B. Sobell are expanded in a relational competence theory outlined in Chapter 14 of this volume, where his analogy of a love relationship becomes an important model in terms of approach-avoidance, where dependency, denial of dependency, and interdependency are present (Fig 1.1).

Religious Fanaticism

Religious beliefs and practices may become addictive or problematic when there is an overuse of the deity and of religious practices that are obsessively and compulsively followed to the extreme. In this instance, the individual becomes consumed by these practices at the expense of other beliefs, practices, or behaviors (L'Abate, Hewitt, & Samples, 1992). Some academics at faith-based universities recognize this problem and refer to these types of behaviors as "spiritualizing". This phenomenon represents an unrealistic perspective not endorsed by faith-based institutions. L'Abate et al. (1992) argued that: "Religious addictions... have the function of filling up a weak, chaotic, inconsistent, and incomplete internal self-structure (i.e., self-definition and identification) with an externally given structure"

(p. 276). They suggested therapeutic guidelines to help those addicted with these beliefs and practices (pp. 277–283).

The line between appropriate religiousness and rigid fanaticism is not difficult to draw once religious fanaticism is viewed as an addiction to the point of becoming such a pervasive influence in one's life at the expense of other aspects. For instance: (1) demanding that employers conform to one's religious beliefs and practices, by refusing to work on certain holidays; (2) repetitive expressions of religious statements or quotes from a religious source; or (3) maintenance of dietary and physical regimes, even to the detriment of health in loved ones. However, one must distinguish among Western Christian versus Islamic religious practices. The latter are followed rigidly by the majority of its believers, such as kneeing and praying specific times of the day, to the point that they do not qualify as addictions. Hence, religious fanaticism must be considered within the cultural, social, and ethnic contexts in which they occur.

A recent investigation on compulsive prayer (Bonchek & Greenberg, 2009) represents a different perspective in religious fanaticism. More specifically, the foregoing investigators characterize religious fanaticism as a form of OCD. The primary treatment strategies for OCD (i.e., CBT/exposure and response prevention, and SSRIs) have demonstrated efficacy in the treatment of religious OCD. Within Judaism and Islam, the presentation of religious OCD poses unique challenges with respect to inaccessibility of personal prayer, sanctity of the symptom, fear of not having said prayers with sufficient devotion, and the religiosity of the therapist. Bonchek and Greenberg report on a therapeutically successful method of guided prayer repetition, a variant of ERP, in three cases of ultra-orthodox Jewish men. The method developed by Bonchek and Greenberg is promising and should be investigated further.

Spontaneous Remission

Anecdotally, the last few years have seen individuals who were able to escape abusive, fringe, religious communities where the name of the deity was used to control the behavior of blindly and uncritically conforming members. Usually, such "rebels" were rejected from the community and had to learn new ways of self-help and self-change to cope with a completely different reality. Often times, it is difficult to identify what internal or external factors might be responsible for such an avoidance of conformity and blind submission to an authority figure. However, various models of a relational competence theory in Chapter 14 may suggest different explanations for such a rebellion on one hand and conformity on the other hand.

Workaholism

The so-called Type A personality's over-involvement with work is the prototype for this addictive behavior, where individuals need to keep busy because they are unable to deal with free time and the discomfort of dealing with "unpleasant emotions", especially past hurts (Farrar, 1992). In addition to traditional individual, couple, group, and family therapies, the last generation has seen the growth of self-help groups in either face-to-face TB or online formats (see Chapter 5 of this volume).

Spontaneous Remission

Anecdotally, self-help and self-change occur in such individuals when they experience a heart attack, a failed relationship, or financial bankruptcy looms as a result of the destructiveness of such behavior.

Concluding Remarks

The treatment of addictive behaviors typically requires a multi-pronged, multi-person, individualized treatment plan delivered with high intensity. Medical management is often required when substance dependence is at issue, particularly when that substance is alcohol. A variety of self-help and self-change approaches are available for those dealing with addictions—failure to incorporate these into treatment represents a failure at the clinical level. Fortunately, as chapters in Part II attest, these types of self-help approaches have recently increased, opening up a new frontier of help for those who are suffering from complex, chronic, and destructive behaviors that may require more than traditional once-a-week sessions with a mental health professional.

Clinicians will be in a better position to serve the needs of their addicted patients if they are familiar with the array of self-help resources available. Online resources, bibliotherapy, 12-step programs, and other forms of group self-help treatment constitutes popular categories of self-help—manifold forms of self-help may be found in any of these categories and it should not be hard to find a variety of self-help materials that can be used in combination either as part of a patient-directed treatment approach, or more advisably, as part of a therapist-directed treatment plan for addiction.

Addictions have far reaching negative implications—lives are destroyed, health is ruined, finances are depleted, relationships are lost, employment is often unmanageable, and legal issues are often present in the addict's life. The complexity of most addictions suggest that the clinician should use whatever resources are at hand—for many, psychotherapy is cost-prohibitive and available resources are minimal. Self-help methods/materials are exceedingly important for those who are experiencing financial hardship—many of these resources are free. Moreover, even when one has adequate financial resources, self-help materials can function as adjunctive treatments that serve to help the addict between sessions.

Finally, much work needs to be completed on the clinical utility of some self-help resources. Findings as to the efficacy of some programs or resources are mixed in some cases while other cases have inadequate information to make any strong conclusions with respect to clinical utility. The self-help resource with the most empirical support appears to be those that fit within or approximate the 12-step model. Still, this should not be taken as a suggestion to ignore other forms of self-help treatment—individual preferences and other factors should be taken into account when considering the array of self-help options available today.

Additional Self-Help Resources for Addictions

Alcohol and Substance Abuse Resources

www.alcoholics-anonymous.org provides information on AA including policies, meeting locations nationwide, and how to contact local chapters.

www.na.org, the web site for Narcotics Anonymous, provides information similar to the AA web site.

www.al-anon.alateen.org for spouses of substance abusers and to meet the special needs of teenagers who abuse substances.

www.smartrecovery.org, Self-management and Recovery Training (SMART), an empirically supported self-help program for individuals struggling with a variety of substances, was founded in 1985, is abstinence oriented, intended for work with adults, and employs a CBT model. A 12-step involvement is also encouraged. SMART may be best suited to individuals with an internal locus of control.

www.cfiwest.org/sos/index.htm, Secular Organization for Sobriety (SOS) employs a CBT approach and stresses personal responsibility, critical thinking, and identification of one's unique cycle of addiction. It is for both chemical and alcohol problems.

www.womenforsobriety.org is an organization specifically for women. It was founded in 1976 by Jean Kirkpatrick based on the premise that men follow different recovery processes than do women. Self-esteem is an emphasis and research suggests that about 33% of members participate in AA. Focus is on alcohol.

www.moderation.org, Moderation management (MM) has the goal to "reduce" or "control" drinking—abstinence is not the goal of MM. Behavior modification is a primary component of the program. Unfortunately, the founder of the program, Shirley Kishline, was involved in a motor vehicle accident that killed a father and his 12-year old daughter. Kishline's BAL was 0.260, more than 3 times the legal limit for her state of residence. She was convicted of the crime of vehicular homicide.

www.unhooked.com is the web site for LifeRing, an alternative to 12-step programs, espouses sobriety, secularity, and self-help.

Smoking Cessation

www.guidetopsychology.com/stopsmok.htm is dedicated to helping individuals quit smoking. Self-help resources and information is available.

www.cochrane.org/reviews/en/ab001118.html, a site that reviews self-help methods for smoking cessation.

www.lungusa.org/site/c.dvLUK9O0E/b.33567/k.B594/Quitting_Smoking.htm, the American Lung Association site—a wealth of information on smoking and smoking cessation.

Excessive Exercise

www.wellsphere.com/wellpage/excessive-exercise provides a wealth of educational and self-help resources for excessive exercise and related disorders.

http://randyschellenberg.tripod.com/anorexiatruthinfo/id5.html is another site that provides information and links to important resources.

Excessive Spending

http://www.wrongdiagnosis.com/symptom/excessive-spending.htm, a site devoted to the dissemination of information, treatment options, and self-help resources.

Compulsive Gambling

www.lostbet.com provides a wealth of information and resources to help those struggling with gambling problems.

www.NonGambler.com is a web site devoted to treatment information and education.

Interpersonal and Love Relationships

http://saferelationships.com/ is devoted to providing education and resources to help individuals make good relationship choices.

www.loveaddicts.org/—Love Addicts Anonymous—for women and men.

www.allaboutlove.org/love-addiction.htm, an information site

Workaholics

www.workaholics-anonymous.org/knowing.html, a resource for self-diagnosis and self-help.

Sex Addiction

www.sexaa.org/—Sex Addicts Anonymous—self-help and support for both men and women.

www.psychcentral.com/lib/2006/what-is-sexual-addiction/ provides information on sex addiction and treatment.

Domestic Violence

www.endabuse.org devoted to early intervention before problems escalate to domestic violence.

www.nlm.nih.gov/medlineplus/domesticviolence.html, a comprehensive web site on domestic violence.

Chapter 11
Personality Disorders

Introduction

Professor Salvatore R. Maddi has provided one of the most comprehensive and concise conceptualizations of personality to date. According to Maddi (1980):

Personality is a stable set of characteristics and tendencies that determine those commonalities and differences in the psychological behavior (thoughts, feelings, and actions) of people that have continuity in time and that may not be easily understood as the sole result of the social and biological pressures of the moment (p. 10).

The implications of this definition are manifold; however, only a few of the more obvious are salient to our discussion of self-help for personality disorders. First, personality tends to be rather durable—as Maddi states, it has "continuity in time" (p. 10). Second, personality has a deterministic nature with respect to behavior. Finally, personality is the result of a stable constellation of characteristics and tendencies—this constellation is unique for each individual. The ramifications of the foregoing suggest that one's personality may be difficult to alter, it interacts with contextual/social elements, and if disordered, the reactive/interactive nature may pose unique obstacles or potential pitfalls in patient management and treatment compliance.

Among psychologists, the prevailing notions about personality disordered patients include the following: (1) They are difficult to treat; (2) they often lack insight and only come to treatment when co-morbidity, usually in the form of depression and/or anxiety motivate the patient to seek treatment; and (3) patients with antisocial personality disorder or borderline personality disorder (Linehan, 1993a) are the most difficult to treat—many therapists refuse to accept these individuals as patients. Some psychologists disagree with the foregoing notions about personality disorders and their treatment (e.g., Tyrer, 2005). An investigation by Perry (personal communication, 2001, as cited in Vinnars, Barbar, Noren, Gallop, & Weinryb, 2005) indicated that among personality disordered patients, recovery rates at 1-year follow up were 52 – 74% for cluster C patients, 30–46% for cluster B patients. Unfortunately, recovery rates for personality disorders were much lower in naturalistic studies (between 4 and 12%).

T.M. Harwood, L. L'Abate, *Self-Help in Mental Health*,
DOI 10.1007/978-1-4419-1099-8_11, © Springer Science+Business Media, LLC 2010

Some of the personality diagnoses pose particular problems with respect to the development and maintenance of a working relationship. For example, patients diagnosed with antisocial personality disorder may have a difficult time being truthful, establishing trust, or avoiding attempts to manipulate therapy/therapist. Borderline patients may experience dramatic shifts in feelings about the therapist ranging from idealization to loathing. Additionally, tendencies for self-harm, impulsivity, and instability in general all pose difficulties for the treating clinician. Due to the complex nature of most personality diagnoses (e.g., likelihood of co-morbidity, chronicity, pervasiveness of functional impairment, potential for self-destructive behavior, danger to others), we believe that stand-alone self-help treatments are contraindicated for the lion's share of personality disorders, especially those in which impulsivity is an issue. Further, we recommend that patients seek diagnosis and, if necessary, they should seek individualized treatment recommendations from a qualified mental health professional if a personality disorder is indicated.

Unfortunately, personality disorders do not have much self-help material associated with their treatment and we have been unable to find a stand-alone self-help treatment for personality disorders that has empirical support. In addition to the lack of empirical support, most competent clinicians would undoubtedly agree that extant self-help materials for personality disorders have a higher likelihood of producing negative effects if therapist involvement is inadequate. Still, treatment manuals for some personality disorders have received empirical support and some clinicians specialize in the treatment of personality disorders or some subset of this diagnostic category. In the vast majority of cases, responsible and high quality self-help for personality disorders carries a high degree of clinician involvement.

Self-Help Treatment for Personality Disorders

Treatment Utilization and Response

Bender et al. (2001) conducted an investigation into treatment utilization among patients with personality disorders. More specifically, they compared patients diagnosed with personality disorders to patients without personality disorder and carrying a diagnosis of major depressive disorder (MDD). The investigators found that individuals diagnosed with personality disorders were more likely than their depressed counterparts to have received every form of psychosocial treatment except for self-help groups. When broken down by personality disorder, patients diagnosed with obsessive-compulsive personality disorder (OCPD) utilized individual psychotherapy more than others in the study and they were almost three times more likely to utilize individual therapy than were patients diagnosed with MDD. Borderline personality disorder (BPD) patients were more likely to have utilized anxiolytics, antidepressants, and mood-stabilizing medications than any other group. Patients with BPD were also more likely to have utilized treatment at a higher rate with the exception of family/couple therapy and self-help treatment. Antipsychotic medications were more likely to be utilized by borderline and schizotypal patients.

Bender et al. concluded that patients should be assessed for the presence of a personality disorder to determine if they are receiving adequate treatment. Further, a personality disorder is an important factor to consider in treatment planning. Finally, patients diagnosed with BPD and schizotypal personality disorders utilized treatments at a rate that was higher than other diagnostic groups included in this investigation (diagnoses represented were major depressive disorder, BPD, OCPD, schizotypal, and avoidant personality disorder). When compared to patients with MDD, BPD patients utilized a wider variety of treatment modalities (individual, group, family/couple, day treatment, inpatient, and halfway house residence). The finding that BPD patients were more likely to utilize every modality of psychosocial treatment except for self-help groups, and they were more likely to have used psychotropic medications than were patients with MDD may be an indication that BPD patients may be resistant to or relatively uninterested in self-help treatments when compared to the other patient groups participating in this investigation. Additionally, the treatment of BPD patients is complicated by compliance and drop-out issues. The foregoing findings do not augur well for strong adherence to self-help treatment for BDP.

Of course, it is premature to make any strong statements about other forms of self-help for patients diagnosed with BPD such as therapist-guided, individualized self-help treatments. Linehan's original Dialectical Behavior Therapy (DBT, 1993a and 1993b) and subsequent variations may be the most effective extant treatment for patients suffering from BPD—this would suggest that an individualized, therapist-guided form of self-help treatment can be very effective for this group of patients. Therapist involvement is considerable in the application of DBT for BPD. For example, in all forms of DBT, patients have phone access to their therapist for skills coaching, crisis intervention, and general support between sessions—as such, DBT may be characterized as a maximum therapist involvement form of self-help treatment. On the other hand, the self-help component of DBT appears to be an extremely useful and effective element of treatment when therapist involvement is substantial (Scheel, 2000). Additionally, according to Westen (2000), DBT is especially efficacious at reducing para-suicidal behavior among patients diagnosed with BPD—an issue to be discussed in the following section on BPD.

In the Nottingham Study of Neurotic Disorder (Tyrer, Seivewright, Ferguson, Murphy, & Johnson, 1993), patients diagnosed with either generalized anxiety disorder (GAD), panic disorder (PD), dysthymic disorder (DYS), or personality disorder NOS were randomized to drug treatment, cognitive-behavioral therapy, or a self-help treatment program. Treatment methods, in particular self-help, were more efficacious among patients not diagnosed with a personality disorder. Patients diagnosed with personality disorder responded best to pharmacotherapy. The investigators in the Nottingham Study concluded that a diagnosis of personality disorder made prior to treatment may be useful information in treatment planning—that is, the decision to use pharmacotherapy, antidepressants in particular, may be the treatment of choice for these patients.

In a naturalistic longitudinal study on ethnicity and mental health treatment utilization by patients with personality disorders (Bender et al., 2007), investigators found that treatment utilization differed by ethnic group. More specifically, minorities, Hispanics in particular, were much less likely than their white counterparts to receive a variety of outpatient and inpatient psychosocial treatments—psychotropic medication use was also lower among Hispanic patients. Further, the more severe the personality disorder, the more pronounced the differential treatment by ethnic group. An attenuating factor in the foregoing findings was the quality of the therapeutic alliance. More specifically, the degree of positive support alliance predicted the amount of individual psychosocial treatment used by black and Hispanic, but not by white participants.

Borderline Inpatients

Borderline Personality Disorder (BPD) is a serious and durable mental disorder. Prevalence rates for BPD range from 0.2–1.8% within the general population. Among outpatients, the prevalence rates for BPD increase to 8–11%. Among inpatients, prevalence rates for BPD fall within the range of 14–20% (Modestin, Abrecht, Tschaggelar, & Hoffman, 1997; Widiger & Frances, 1989; Widiger & Weissman, 1991, as cited in Linehan, 2000). Suicide rates are high among patients diagnosed with BPD—according to Linehan, Rizvi, Welch, & Page, (2002) between 7 and 38% of all individuals who ultimately commit suicide meet BPD diagnostic criteria. Among those diagnosed with BPD, approximately 9% commit suicide (Frances, Fyer, & Clarkin, 1986, as cited in Linehan, 2000). When BPD is accompanied by Axis I co-morbidity, the likelihood of positive prognosis is attenuated (Kosten, Kosten, & Rounsaville, 1989; Phillips & Nierenberg, 1994, as cited in Linehan 2000).

Zanarini, Frankenburg, Khera, and Bleichmar (2001) compared the types and amounts of psychiatric treatment utilized by BPD inpatients to psychiatric treatments utilized by patients diagnosed with a variety of other personality disorders—53% of the sample earned a diagnosis of personality disorder NOS, 33% fell in the anxious cluster personality disorder, 18% met criteria for a non-borderline dramatic cluster personality disorder, and 4% met criteria for an odd cluster personality disorder as defined by the DSM-III-R. Consistent with an earlier study examining treatment utilization among patients suffering from personality disorders, Zanarini et al. found that BPD patients utilized enormous amounts of psychiatric treatment—more than 75% of BPD patients had received individual therapy, been hospitalized previously, and were on a long-term course of pharmacotherapy. In fact, BPD patient utilized individual therapy, group therapy, self-help groups, day treatment, residential treatment, inpatient treatment, and pharmacotherapy at a significantly higher rate than Axis II controls. Unlike the previous study by Tyrer et al. (1993), self-help group utilization was relatively high in comparison to Axis II controls, that is, more than 50% of BPD patients utilized this treatment format versus 32% of Axis II controls.

A number of tentative conclusions may be made based upon the foregoing. First, severity of BPD may increase the likelihood that self-help groups will become a component of treatment for these individuals. Additionally, and consistent with previous findings, BPD patients, especially those with more severe forms of the disorder, utilize treatments at a rate that is exceptionally high. The only treatment format not utilized frequently among both BPD and Axis II controls was ECT—less than 10% of personality disordered patients utilized this treatment modality.

Manualized Supportive-Expressive Psychotherapy

Vinnars et al. (2005) conducted a randomized controlled trial comparing manualized supportive expressive psychotherapy to a non-manualized community-delivered psychodynamic therapy for patients with DSM-IV personality disorders. At the end of treatment both forms of therapy produced improvement on indices such as Global Assessment of Functioning (GAF, DSM-IV, 1994), percentage of patients meeting a diagnosis of personality disorder, severity of personality disorder, and psychiatric symptoms in general. No significant differences were noted between therapies at the end of treatment; however, at follow-up, patients in the supportive-expressive condition made significantly fewer visits to the treatment clinic than those in the non-manualized community-delivered psychodynamic treatment condition.

An interesting finding from this investigation was that supportive-expressive psychotherapy and community-delivered psychodynamic therapy appeared to have differential effects on outcomes. More specifically, the former appeared to have a greater positive effect on personality disorder symptoms and functional impairment while the later had a greater positive effect on general psychiatric symptom severity and functional impairment. At 1-year follow-up, 33% of patients no longer met criteria for a personality diagnosis, a figure that compares well with the recovery rate observed for cluster B patients. Vinnars et al. (2005) concluded that, based on their investigation, "...there is no reason to recommend supportive-expressive psychotherapy over community-delivered psychodynamic therapy for personality disorder patients" (p. 1939). Unfortunately, neither of these treatments has been translated to a self-help format and therapist involvement is high for both forms of psychodynamic therapy. Of course, the treating clinician may integrate some self-help materials or exercises into an individualized treatment plan.

Dialectical Behavior Therapy

Developed for the treatment of BPD, DBT has received empirical support for its application in this complex patient population (Linehan, Armstrong, Suarez, Allmon, & Heard, 1991). Traditional DBT emphasizes the reduction of extreme emotional experience/expression and/or increases the patient's tolerance for extreme emotional experiences. Additionally, the reduction of impulsivity is part of DBT's primary emphasis (Lynch & Cheavens, 2008). DBT is a complex integration of a variety of treatment elements including components from behavior therapy, cognitive therapy, and client therapy (Nock, Teper, & Hollander, 2007). Linehan published her BPD treatment manual (1993a) and the companion skills training manual (1993b) and at least five different randomized clinical trials have demonstrated the efficacy of DBT for treating women suffering from BPD (see Linehan et al., 2006; Muehlenkamp, 2006 as cited in Nock et al., 2007). Still, DBT was relatively slow to receive a large body of research support, and some investigators (e.g., Levendusky, 2000; Scheel, 2000) indicated that research involving patients suffering from BPD was unusually challenging. Inpatient samples may attenuate some of the DBT treatment research challenges; however, issues of compliance including self-initiated discharge from inpatient units against medical advice, high drop out rates from research as well as therapy, and high treatment utilization in general are concerns that remain and need to be addressed in research investigating the efficacy of DBT.

Although DBT (Linehan, 1993a) requires a large degree of therapist involvement, the skills training manual contains handouts, forms, and worksheets that the therapist may copy and distribute to their BPD patients for use at home, between treatment sessions. As such, these materials comprise a self-help aspect of DBT that is probably best characterized as a therapist-guided self-help treatment component. A recent DBT manual has been published (Dimeff & Koerner, 2007) and a relatively new DBT self-help workbook is available (McKay, Wood, & Brantley, 2007). The Dimeff and Koerner manual, developed for application with a variety of diagnoses and treatment settings, appears to have an adequate amount of empirical support behind it and it has been endorsed by Linehan; however, the McKay, Wood, and Brantley workbook appears to be entirely without empirical support. Given the serious nature of many personality disorders, BPD in particular, using the self-help workbook to treat BPD sans competent therapist involvement should not be recommended.

Modified Forms of DBT

DBT for PPD and OCPD

Lynch and Cheavens (2008) conducted a case study on the efficacy of DBT for co-morbid personality disorders. Their version of DBT was modified to treat individuals who were suffering from personality disorders that represented the somewhat opposite dimension of emotional and behavioral regulation from BPD. More specifically, the targets of their efforts were emotional constriction, behavioral rigidity, restriction of experience, perfectionism, and highly risk aversive behavior and thinking. These investigators employed their modified form of DBT to treat an individual who was suffering from co-morbid paranoid personality disorder (PPD) and obsessive-compulsive personality disorder (OCPD).

The modified form of DBT consisted of strategies and interventions designed to increase the patient's flexibility and openness to new experiences, and reduce rigidity in cognition and behavior. The duration of individual treatment was at least 28 weeks with a frequency and intensity of weekly 50-min sessions. The group skills training module had a similar treatment duration (i.e., at least 28 weeks) and sessions met weekly for 2 hrs. Most of the traditional DBT skills as conceptualized by Linehan (1993b) were employed in the group skills training; however, tolerance of emotional distress was not emphasized due to the over-controlled nature of the personality disorders being treated—this component of treatment could be included if necessary. Skills modifications included a "Radical Openness Module" (Lynch & Cheavens, 2008, p. 155) that features a form of loving-kindness/forgiveness training, a mindfulness-fixed versus -fluid and fresh states of mind training (to help move the individual away from the rigid end of the behavior spectrum and closer to the openness end of the spectrum), and techniques that induce positive affect just prior to in-vivo exposure. A more complete description of these skills is provided elsewhere (see Lynch & Cheavens, in press).

Following 9 months of individual DBT and 6 months of group skills training, their patient "…reported significant reductions in judgmental thinking…, interpersonal sensitivity, interpersonal aggression, bitterness, and rumination/brooding" (Lynch and Cheavens, 2008, p. 165). In addition to the foregoing, the patient's baseline score on the Hamilton Rating Scale for Depression (HAM-D; Hamilton, 1960) dropped from 21 (moderate level of depressive spectrum symptoms) to 6 (asymptomatic) at 17-month follow-up. Further, the authors report that their patient no longer met diagnostic criteria for PPD or OCPD at the end of their case study.

DBT for Adolescents

DBT has been adapted for use with adolescents (Miller et al., 1997) and emerged as an empirically supported treatment for self-injurious behavior for this patient group. A variety of variations in treatment length and intensity exist and are assigned based on patient risk such as suicidal potential. Further, DBT has demonstrated efficacy for reducing the rates of suicidal and non-suicidal self-injury in both inpatient and outpatient settings (Katz, Cox, Gunasekara, & Miller, 2004; Rathus & Miller, 2002, as cited in Nock et al., 2007). Miller et al., (1997, 2007) developed a form of DBT adapted for suicidal adolescents—the first citation refers to a journal article and the latter refers to a book on the topic of DBT for suicidal adolescents. Although DBT has been a consistent performer in producing reductions in self-injury for both adolescents and adults, it has generally not outperformed standard treatments or treatments applied by experts in the community; instead, DBT has produced results that are similar to other credible treatments for self-injury (Nock et al., 2007).

Nock et al. (2007) examined the efficacy of DBT in the treatment of an adolescent who engaged in non-suicidal self-injury. Because DBT has been recognized as one of the most promising treatments for adolescent self-injury (Nock et al., 2007), these investigators conducted a case study on the use of DBT for the treatment of this increasingly pervasive problem among adolescents. After a 6-week course of DBT treatment, their patient's rate of self-injury was decreased to zero. Overall, 24 treatment sessions were delivered—approximately at session 20, substance abuse (other than alcohol) stopped and there was a reduction in alcohol use. Relationship satisfaction between the patient and her father improved and the patient also reported improved relationships with peers. Therapy terminated at the end of the contracted 6-month treatment period. Throughout treatment, the patient reported having thoughts of self-injury and she engaged in two incidents of self-injury between sessions 6 and 24.

The psychological correlates of self-injury include (1) a current mental disorder; (2) an Axis I disorder characterized as internalizing (52%), externalizing (63%), and substance use (60%) disorders; and (3) the following Axis II disorders: borderline (52%), avoidant (31%), and paranoid (21%) personality disorders (Nock, Joiner, Gordon, Lloyd-Richardson, & Prinstein, 2006, as cited in Nock et al., 2007). Although other factors (e.g., maladaptive cognitive styles, biological aberrations, and environmental elements) are undoubtedly involved in the genesis and maintenance of self-injurious behaviors, Nock and Prinstein (2004, 2005) found empirical support for a two-dimensional, four-function reinforcement model for self-injury. More specifically, one dichotomous dimension of reinforcement (positive v negative) and the other dichotomous dimension (intrapersonal/automatic or interpersonal/social) appear to capture some of the functions that self-injury serves. With respect to the dichotomous dimension of positive versus negative reinforcement, self-injury for the purpose of obtaining positive reinforcement appears to increase some desirable internal state; on the other hand, self-injury for the purpose of obtaining negative reinforcement appears to attenuate some aversive internal states. Examining the contrasting dichotomous dimension of intrapersonal/automatic versus interpersonal/social, research suggests that self-injury motivated by social negative reinforcement functions to decrease some activating external event; conversely, self-injury motivated by positive social reinforcement appears to amplify the likelihood of some desirable social outcome (Nock et al., 2007).

DBT for Opioid Dependency Among Women Diagnosed with BPD

Substance abuse or dependence is a frequent co-morbid diagnosis among individuals suffering from BPD. Linehan, Dimeff et al. (2002) conducted a head-to-head randomized clinical trial comparison of DBT versus comprehensive validation therapy plus a 12-step program for women diagnosed with BPD and opioid dependence. The treatments were geared toward substance abuse. Comprehensive validation therapy (CVT, Linehan et al., 1996) is a manualized form of treatment that employs a component of DBT. More specifically, CVT utilizes the primary acceptance-based strategies used in traditional DBT. In the study at hand, CVT was tailored for use with patients suffering from co-morbid BPD and substance abuse and was combined with participation in a variety of 12-step programs geared toward substance use issues. In a similar vein, DBT was adapted for treatment with substance abusers diagnosed with BPD (Linehan & Dimeff, 1997). Finally, both conditions utilized the opiate agonist ORLAAM (40 mg. of levomethadyl acetate hydrochloride oral solution) throughout treatment.

Although both treatments performed equally well with respect to urinalysis, a number of differential treatment outcomes were noted. For example, those assigned to CVT + 12-step had a significant increase in mean opiate use during the last 4 months of active treatment—those in DBT maintained their mean reductions in opiate use across the entire 12 months of active treatment. The foregoing needs to be tempered by the fact that patients randomized to DBT were more likely to drop-out from treatment (64% retention rate) than those assigned to CVT + 12-step; the CVT + 12-step condition had 100% retention throughout treatment.

The finding that those in the DBT condition had better maintenance of treatment gains throughout treatment must be evaluated in light of findings from an intent to treat analysis. That is, when drop-out and missing urinalyses were considered, CVT + 12-step performed as well or better than DBT. At 16-month follow-up, urinalyses indicated no significant differences between treatment conditions (percentage of positive urinalyses by condition: CVT + 12-step = 33%; DBT = 27%). The 100% retention rate and reduction in illicit drug use by those in CVT + 12-step is an important treatment consideration because CVT + 12-step is a less complex form of treatment than DBT; hence, CVT + 12-step would be easier to teach than DBT.

Guided Self-Help for Binge Eating Disorder and Co-morbid Personality Disorder

Masheb and Grilo (2008) conducted a randomized clinical trial of two guided self-help treatments for binge eating disorder (BED). Two treatment manuals, *Overcoming Binge Eating* (Fairburn, 1995) and *LEARN Program for Weight Management 2000* (Brownell, 2000; 2004), were used in the study. More specifically, these investigators compared the efficacy of a guided self-help CBT and a guided self-help behavioral weight-lost treatment with 75 patients who met DSM-IV-TR research criteria for BED. Fairburn's manual was employed in the CBT-guided self-help form of BED treatment and Brownell's manual was used in the behavioral weight-loss guided self-help form of BED treatment.

One of the more important findings in this investigation was that co-morbidity predicted poorer treatment outcomes. That is, the presence of personality disorder co-morbidity appeared to have an attenuating effect on treatment outcomes with respect to various dimensions of eating disorder psychopathology and negative affect. In other words, eating disorder psychopathology and negative affect was greater at end of treatment for participants with a personality disorder than it was for those without.

Negative affect was also a predictor of higher attrition—the foregoing coupled with the finding that a personality disorder was predictive of higher post-treatment levels of negative affect and eating disorder pathology does not augur well for successful treatment. The investigators suggested that clinicians should address negative cognitive styles and personality in pretreatment planning and throughout treatment in an effort to enhance outcomes for individuals who carry a personality disorder diagnosis and display a tendency for negative affect.

Social Problem-Solving Plus Psychoeducation

Social dysfunction is common among individuals with personality disorders (Skodol, Pagano, et al., 2005). The primary goal of Social Problem-Solving therapy (D'Zurilla & Nezu, 1999) is to increase social competence. The Social Problem-Solving approach employed in the investigation at hand (Huband, McMurran, Evans, & Duggan, 2007) was a modified version of "Stop & Think!" an empirically supported problem-solving program (McMurran, Egan, Richardson, & Ahmadi, 1999; McMurran, Fyffe, McCarthy, Duggan, & Latham 2001) when applied in a secure setting. In this relatively simple problem-solving approach, therapists endeavor to increase social competence through a psychoeducational process in which patients are taught how to craft solutions to the various social problems they encounter in life. Although not a self-help program per se, a psychoeducational approach may provide individuals with skills that allow them to engage in future self-help behaviors.

Huband et al. (2007) applied the foregoing problem-solving program, in a group format and a community setting, with adults suffering from personality disorders. The total duration of the intervention was approximately 20 weeks and a wait-list control served as the comparison condition. The group-based intervention had a frequency of one 2-hour session per week and a treatment duration of 16 weeks. Prior to the group-based intervention, brief individual psychoeducation was provided for each participant. More specifically, individuals were informed of their diagnosis, helped to prioritize problems that were highlighted through personality assessment, informed how their diagnosis was related to social dysfunction and difficulties in problem-solving, and to provide an understanding of the treatment's relevance to their particular problem(s) and instill hope for change. Psychoeducation was generally delivered in three 1-hour sessions.

Using an intent-to-treat analysis, investigators compared the intervention to the control group based on scores rendered by the Social Problem Solving Inventory-Revised (SPSI-R, D'Zurilla et al., 2002) and scores on the Social Functioning Questionnaire (SFQ, Tyrer et al., 2005). These researchers found that those in the intervention arm showed significant improvement in problem-solving skills, significantly higher overall social functioning, and a significantly lower amount of anger expression. Huband et al. concluded that their investigation was an advance in the understanding of problem-solving interventions for adults with personality disorders.

Are Personality Disorders Truly Resistant to Change?

Some researchers have questioned the notion that personality is relatively stable and resistant to change. As Tyrer (2005) points out, the prevailing wisdom on personality disorders was that they are persistent. Relatedly, the clinical perspective on personality disorders was that treatment, if it had any chance of success, would necessarily need to be intensive; i.e., long-term, frequent, and multi-person. Tyrer challenges the foregoing notions and indicates that, for some groups, personality change is not simply possible; personality change may also occur rapidly.

Tyrer (2005) attributes the initial development of the notion that personality is immutable to Koch (1981) who characterized personality disorders as a degenerative process of the nervous system. According to Tyrer, the notion of immutability finally coalesced with the work of Kretschmer (1922) and Schneider (1923). The next notable figure involved in the conceptualization of personality disorders was Henderson (1939) who suggested that emotional maturity explained personality dysfunction and, given time, this dysfunction might improve with age. Black, Monahan, Baumgard, & Bell (1997) later relegated all but antisocial personality disorder to the realm of temporal stability; however, Stone, Hurt, & Stone (1987) characterized borderline personality disorder as the exception to temporal stability—after all, instability is a hallmark feature of BPD.

Tyrer (2005) points to three articles published in the same issue of the *Journal of Personality Disorders* (2005, issue 19) as signal in the re-conceptualization of personality pathology and their treatment. He summarizes these as follows:

1. "Abnormal personality in childhood and adolescence is not stable but is a predictor of adult personality" (p. 547). Tyrer cites the Children in the Community Study (CIC, Bernstein, Cohen, Skodal, Bezirganian, & Brook, 1996; Cohen, Crawford, Johnson, & Kasen, 2005) and uses results of the foregoing to support his argument. More specifically, the CIC investigation found that a gradual decline in personality pathology is evident between the ages of 9 and 25. Further, the Axis I diagnosis of conduct disorder is conceptualized non-traditionally by the CIC team; i.e., "...it is increasingly our view that stable childhood conduct disorder is best viewed as a disorder of personality" (Cohen et al., 2005, p. 474). Additionally, among children or adolescents with personality pathology, regardless of whether or not the pathology diminished, the likelihood of manifesting adult personality pathology is much greater (Cohen et al., 2005). Finally, childhood personality should be assessed more frequently (Westen, Dutra, & Shedler, 2005, as cited in Tyrer, 2005).
2. "Personality disorder increases the odds of co-morbidity of other mental disorders" (p. 575). Tyrer (2005) points to findings from the Collaborative

Longitudinal Personality Disorders Study (CLPS, Gunderson et al., 2000) in support of the foregoing. More specifically, evidence, although preliminary, suggests that most personality disorders appear to delay remission of major depressive disorder (Skodol et al., 2005, as cited by Tyrer, 2005). Additionally, pre-morbid personality anomaly appears to have a long-term negative effect on social functioning despite marked changes in the status of personality within the same time period (Seivewright, Tyrer, & Johnson 2002; Seivewright, Tyrer, & Johnson 2004, as cited in Tyrer, 2005). Finally, some personality disorders appear to predispose an individual to behave in such a way that negative life events accrue resulting in higher rates of other mental disorders (Zanarini et al., 1998; Seivewright et al., 2000, as cited in Tyrer, 2005).

3. "Borderline personality disorder generally has a favorable non-relapsing course not found with other personality disorders" (p. 576). Differences between borderline personality disorder and other personality disorders are possible explanations in BPDs non-relapsing course. BPD shares features with other personality disorders; however, BPD appears to have higher rates of co-morbidity compared to other personality disorders (Tyrer, 2005). Additionally, BPD appears to present with greater heterogeneity than do other disorders, and patients with BPD utilize a wider variety of treatment resources and at a much higher rate than most other disorders (Bender et al., 2001). Further, BPD patients may present with marked affective and schizotypal symptomology as opposed to continuous behavior patterns, and marked, sometimes daily, fluctuations are more characteristic of those with BPD—a characteristic not typically observed in more stable disorders (Tyrer, 2005). Data from investigations, including the CLPS, indicate that BPD may be a variant of affective disorder (Coid, 1993; Gunderson et al., 2004). Zanarini, Frankenburg, Hennen, & Silk (2004) found that, once BPD patients have accrued significant treatment gains, the disorder tends to stay in remission (or run its course). In general, successful treatment of BPD requires extensive and varied mental health service involvement coupled with high rates of polypharmacy.

4. "Longitudinal changes in personality disorder are best assessed using a dimensional approach" (p. 577). Although there are problems associated with a dimensional approach to personality assessment, the existing classification system for personality disorders is not well-suited to longitudinal research. A useful guideline for adopting a dimensional approach to longitudinal research was suggested by Shea and Yen (2003): "Personality disorders, with remission rates higher than anxiety disorders, appear to be less stable than conceptualized" (p. 373, as quoted in Tyrer, 2005). When clinical investigations yield significant changes in personality following short-term treatment, these changes tend to be recorded via a dimensional scoring system (Black & Sheline, 1997; Ekselius & von Knorring, 1999, as cited in Tyrer, 2005)

Concluding Remarks

In this chapter, we were unable to do justice to the topic of self-help for personality disorders because this area is not yet well developed. Extant self-help materials with empirical support are few and significant clinician involvement remains a necessary component of treatment; however, the availability of self-help resources is increasing. With this in mind, one must be cautious about the self-help materials they select—the consumer takes a risk by adopting a self-help treatment without empirical support and lacking significant qualified clinician involvement, extant self-help materials are simply not well-suited as a stand-alone treatment for personality disorders. We hope that the future will bring us additional empirically supported self-help materials for at least a subset of personality disorders. Still, such a development does not take clinicians out of the treatment picture regardless of the self-help treatment's excellence—reliable and valid diagnosis remains necessary for pinpointing the elements of personality that produce and maintain dysfunction—important information for treatment planning. Additionally, personality characteristics such as coping style and reactance have implications for treatment planning.

Of course, many individuals with personality disorders are unaware that they are suffering from a dysfunctional personality and many do not seek treatment until co-morbidity and/or considerable functional impairment drives them to seek help from a mental health professional. The foregoing poses some problems with respect to gaining access to patients early in the developmental course of personality psychopathology. As Tyrer (2005) and others have suggested, early assessment is possible and important when indicators such as social functioning and behavioral cues point to the possibility of a pre-morbid personality abnormality. Early detection and intervention may make treatment for personality disorders easier, more successful, less costly, and co-morbidity may be less of an issue.

Finally, it is clear that many troubling questions remain about personality disorders and their treatment. It is encouraging that new information is surfacing with respect to personality disorders. The suggestion that personality disorders are markedly more malleable than previously thought is compelling and should encourage research into this important area of psychosocial treatments. Relatedly, the issue of early assessment, beginning in childhood, coupled with early intervention has implications for prevention and improved functioning in adulthood. Additionally, treatment costs may be reduced and valuable resources may be freed up if early intervention proves even minimally successful. Finally, self-help resources may become more available if the prevailing notion about the persistence of personality disorders is changed based on accumulating sound empirical evidence.

Chapter 12
Severe Psychopathology

Introduction

The more severe forms of psychopathology are perhaps the least amenable to pure, individually delivered, self-help forms of treatment. Patients suffering from severe psychopathology are characterized by chronic, complex problems that often result in a relatively large degree of functional impairment. Additionally, functional impairment, the degree to which planful behavior has been diminished by the patient's difficulties (Harwood & Beutler, 2008) is a prognostic indicator; social support is another prognostic indicator that is often insufficient for patients suffering from complex, chronic problems. Functional impairment, social support, and problem complexity and chronicity, all empirically supported indicators of patient prognosis (Harwood & Beutler, 2008), may impact upon how self-help treatments are applied and how efficacious they are. Essentially, when self-help materials are included in the treatment of individuals suffering with severe psychopathology, clinician involvement is expected and this involvement should be maximal in the majority of cases. In this respect, self-help treatments may be viewed as adjunctive to more intensive, multi-person, clinician-based psychosocial treatments and pharmacotherapy. Further, in some instance when the foregoing prognostic indicators are deficient, self-help treatments may be tailored predominantly for use with family members and significant others rather than to the patients themselves.

As indicated in the foregoing, patient problem complexity and chronicity (PCC) suggests the need for multi-person treatment (Beutler, Clarkin, & Bongar, 2000; Beutler & Harwood, 2000); as such, stand-alone, individually administered self-help is likely to be insufficient to achieve successful outcome or significant improvement due in large part to the pervasiveness of problems—broad band treatment is typically necessary to achieve a favorable treatment response. Problem complexity refers to treatment relevant elements such as co-morbidity and the pervasiveness of the problem. It is related to functional impairment in that co-morbidity and pervasive problems tend to result in higher levels of functional impairment. Patient problem chronicity refers to the rate of problem recurrence and the overall durability of these problems. Chronicity is also related to functional impairment in that long-standing, durable problems have a greater likelihood of generating functional impairment.

T.M. Harwood, L. L'Abate, *Self-Help in Mental Health*,
DOI 10.1007/978-1-4419-1099-8_12, © Springer Science+Business Media, LLC 2010

As with self-help for personality disorders, the empirically supported self-help resources available for patients suffering from severe psychopathology, the families of these patients and others who care about these individuals are relatively few. This is unfortunate for a number of reasons, primarily the following: (1) self-help skills and strategies, delivered particularly in the form of psychoeducation, can function as an important adjunct to treatment that has been shown to reduce the likelihood of re-hospitalizations; (2) related to the foregoing, adjunctive self-help treatment/psychoeduction increases treatment compliance and reduces stressful, negative interaction within the patient's social support network; and (3) family members or others charged with the care of patients suffering from severe psychopathology are able to better manage their own caregiver stress levels and recognize problematic symptoms (e.g., cognitive and behavioral changes indicative of relapse) early enough to prevent danger to self or others and reduce relapse or attenuate the degree of deterioration should relapse be unavoidable.

Self-Help Treatments

Bipolar Disorder

Bipolar disorder is a chronic condition with a high potential for co-morbidity. For example, substance abuse disorders are typical of patients suffering from bipolar disorder. Chung et al. (2007) reports substance abuse rates among bipolar patients at 60%. Additionally, bipolar disorder with co-morbid substance abuse is associated with fewer and slower remissions, higher rates of suicide and suicide attempts, and poorer outcomes. Patients with bipolar disorder and co-morbid substance abuse should be aggressively treated for both disorders (Chung et al., 2007). Additionally, co-morbidity within this patient group exists in the form of eating and personality disorders (Chung et al., 2007). As such, patients diagnosed with bipolar disorder are typically classified as suffering from a complex (pervasive) severe illness. Additionally, although pharmacotherapy is the standard treatment for bipolar disorder, treatment success rates are not very high for a significant number of patients (Lembke et al., 2004). Specifically, non-compliance with prescription, medical and psychiatric co-morbidity, problematic life events, and family stress may combine to attenuate the effectiveness of medications. The foregoing suggests that adjunctive psychosocial interventions may play a significant role in treatment efficacy for patients suffering from bipolar disorder and research support for this notion has been increasing (Lembke et al., 2004; Miklowitz et al., 2006, 2007).

Chung et al. (2007) stress the importance of psychoeducation for both the patient suffering from bipolar disorder and the patient's family or social support system. Two particularly important aspects of psychoeducation center on the characteristics of bipolar disorder and the nature to the most effective treatments available. Family involvement or the involvement of a strong network of social support is essential for the successful treatment of bipolar disorder. The recognition of early warning signs for relapse, helping the patient maintain treatment compliance, especially in the form of medication use, and helping to establish good sleep hygiene are important elements for the successful, long-term treatment of bipolar disorder. Rivas-Vasquez (2002) found similar results based on psychoeducation. More specifically, bipolar patients experienced significant improvements in levels of social adjustment and global functioning when their spouses received targeted psychoeducation.

Sajatovic (2002) points to the importance of multi-person treatment for bipolar disorder. More specifically, in addition to pharmacological interventions, psychosocial interventions enhance the positive effects of treatment with respect to outcome and duration of treatment gains. Psychosocial treatments found to be especially effective in combination with pharmacotherapy, include interpersonal psychotherapy (IPT, Weissman et al., 2000, 2007), cognitive-behavioral therapy (CBT, Basco & Rush, 2005), and family-focused therapy (FFT, Miklowitz et al., 2008). Additionally, group therapy can be an effective adjunctive treatment for patients suffering from bipolar disorder. Further, family members of patients diagnosed with bipolar disorder can benefit from group therapy and this benefit can extend to the patient. Participation in group therapy or support groups is an effective method for establishing a strong network of social support.

An example of a group therapy approach with demonstrated efficacy (de Andrés, 2006) is the Life Goals Program (Bauer & McBride, 2003), a structured, manual-based therapy program that consists of five weekly sessions of structured psychoeducation (Phase 1) and behavioral strategies developed to combat destructive effects of bipolar disorder in the social, occupational, or leisure realm (Phase 2). Another self-help approach to bipolar disorder was developed by Monica Ramirez Basco—she recently compiled a workbook titled *The Bipolar Workbook: Tools for Controlling Your Mood Swings* (2006). Basco's workbook provides easy-to-follow guidelines and worksheets to help patients manage their bipolar disorder, reduce recurrence rates of manic or depressive episodes, and attenuate the severity of symptoms. More specifically, patients are taught strategies and skills to moderate their pace of activity and practice good sleep hygiene when manic symptoms are presenting. On the other hand, patients are taught strategies and techniques to remain motivated and avoid procrastination when depressive spectrum symptoms are becoming evident. General intervention targets include methods to help fine-tune medical treatments in an effort to maximize benefits, strategies to better control emotional reactions, and skills developed to maintain focus and achieve treatment goals.

One primary aspect of Basco's workbook is that it allows for tailored treatments based on the predilections and contextual factors unique to each patient. For patients diagnosed with Cyclothymia, another workbook, *The Cyclothymia Workbook: Learn How to Manage your Mood Swings and Live a Balanced Life*, was authored by Price (2004). Price's workbook guides consumers through an educational program designed to increase insight about themselves and their disorder. Skills and strategies designed to self-manage symptoms and reduce the negative impact that mood swings have on relationships, careers, and daily life are central to this specific self-help treatment workbook. Empirical support for Price's workbook appears non-existent at this time.

In an investigation of psychosocial service utilization by patients suffering from bipolar disorder, Lembke et al. (2004) found that utilization rates, in decreasing frequency were (1) therapy with a psychologist, (2) self-help groups, (3) therapy with a social worker, and (4) therapy with some other mental health professional. Comorbidity was a statistically significant predictor of greater psychosocial service utilization. More specifically, bipolar patients suffering from co-morbid personality disorders received more psychosocial services than those without (80% versus 20%). Additionally, bipolar patients suffering from co-morbid alcohol/drug abuse disorders were statistically more likely to use psychosocial services at a higher rate than bipolar patients without co-morbidity (76% versus 24%). Finally, bipolar patients suffering from co-morbid anxiety disorders were statistically more likely to utilized psychosocial services than patients diagnosed with bipolar disorder alone (60% versus 40%). Marital status was a predicator of service utilization as well; however, being married *decreased* the likelihood of receiving multiple services. The authors concluded that psychosocial service utilization among patients diagnosed with bipolar disorder was correspondent with problem severity and complexity. The foregoing finding is consistent with what investigators have found to be most effective in the treatment of disorders characterized by high levels of PCC.

A study that taught bipolar patients to identify early symptoms of relapse and to develop a laminated, wallet-sized, personalized treatment-seeking plan obtained greater improvements in social functioning and employment and they maintained their gains significantly longer at 18-month follow-up when compared to bipolar patients receiving TAU (Rivas-Vasquez, 2002). Although pharmacotherapy is the standard treatment for bipolar disorder, there are many alternative avenues available for adjunctive treatment. Unfortunately, most of the extant self-help materials for the treatment of bipolar disorder lack empirical support. The following Internet-based self-help resources may prove to be useful as adjunctive treatment for bipolar patients and important supportive/informational resources for their family members. As already stated, bipolar disorder is a form of severe psychopathology that responds best to multi-person treatment. That is, psychiatry, psychotherapy, psychoeducation, group support, self-help resources, and a dependable social support network constitutes an example of a good multi-person treatment team. Stand-alone self-help treatment is not recommended for bipolar disorder or any of the severe forms of psychopathology.

Specific Internet-Based Resources for Bipolar Disorder

Depression and Bipolar Support Alliance, http://www.DBSAlliance.org, is based in Chicago and has a mission to educate patients, families, and professionals about bipolar disorder, provide self-help materials/resources for those suffering from bipolar and related disorders, reduce public stigma, and improve access to effective care.

More than 50,000 people attend DBSA patient-run support groups every year, and more than 5,000 calls are personally answered each month on the DBSA toll-free information and referral line. The BDSA has a good relationship with professionals and publishes brochures, books, and videotapes about the treatment of mood disorders.

The Depression and Related Affective Disorders Association (DRADA) (http://www.med.jhu.edu/drada) is an international organization that offers peer support and assists self-help groups by providing education, information, and supporting research.

McMan's Web (http://www.mcmanweb.com) and McMan's Depression and Bipolar Weekly (http://jmcnamanamy@snet.net) provide abstract information about bipolar and depressive disorders from a wide variety of professional journals and information about relevant public policy legislation in addition to a bookstore, reader's forum, and message boards.

National Alliance on Mental Illness (www.nami.org) provides education about the biological nature of the disorder and referral to national and community-based support and advocacy groups.

Mary Ellen Copeland's website (http://www.mentalhealthrecovery.com) contains a variety of self-help booklets and workbooks written by Copeland to help people cope with a variety of psychological disorders, and the booklets contain ideas and strategies that people from all over the world have used to help combat the effects of their illness. This website also has videos and audiotapes that may be useful to consumers suffering from severe mental illness.

The Walkers Web for Depression and Bipolar Disorder (http://www.walkers.org) includes many avenues for thousands of people suffering from severe mental disorders to communicate with each other—trained volunteers moderate discussions for about four hundred patient-contact hours a week.

The Bipolar Significant Others (BPSO) Bulletin Board (http://www.bpso.org) provides family and friends of patients suffering from bipolar disorder with an opportunity to receive support and communicate with others dealing with similar difficulties.

The Dually Diagnosed—Mental Health and Substance Abuse

Among patients suffering from chemical dependency disorders, co-morbidity is common. According to Kessler (1995), among patients suffering from life-time illicit drug dependence or abuse, 59% met criteria for an additional life-time mental disorder. As such, the dually diagnosed represent a patient population characterized by a high degree of problem complexity and chronicity. Three signal elements in self-help dual-focused groups have been hypothesized. More specifically, (1) helper therapy, (2) reciprocal learning, and (3) emotional-support processes have been associated with successful outcomes in Double Trouble in Recovery (DTR), a 12-step dual-focus self-help group format. Research literature supports the notion that self-help, particularly along the lines of 12-step programs, can improve abstinence rates for individuals suffering from alcohol and drug-use disorders (Magura et al., 2003). Moos, Finney, Ouimette, and Suchinsky (1999; as cited in Magura et al., 2003) found a number of predictors for successful outcome from participation in 12-step programs. Specifically, some predictors of success, operationalized as abstinence from alcohol and drugs, reductions in subjective distress, and better indices of employment at 1-year post–treatment, included (1) stronger 12-step affiliation in the form of better meeting attendance, (2) communication with sponsor, and (3) familiarity with the 12-step literature. According to Fiorentine (1999; Fiorentine & Hillhouse 2000a, 2000b) the benefits of 12-step affiliation pre-, during, and post-treatment have been documented. Relatedly, psychosocial treatment appears to have an additive effect on self-help treatments for drug-dependent individuals.

Following 1-year post-treatment follow-up, the DTR program was associated with abstinences increases (54% abstinence at baseline to 72% abstinence at follow-up). The self-help treatment elements associated with successful outcome were helper therapy and reciprocal learning—emotional support was not associated with outcome in the Magura et al. (2003) study that controlled for member attitudes and behaviors at baseline. Helper therapy, a component of the mutual help process, is defined as a helping role that reinforces a group member's emotional and behavioral commitment to change (Gartner & Reissman, 1979). Reciprocal learning is defined as the sharing of information about coping strategies, experiences, failures, successes, and hopes. Magura et al. (2003) conclude that dual-focus self-help participation and the elements of helper-therapy and reciprocal-learning activities are important to recovery and should be encouraged by clinicians and veteran DTR members for dually diagnosed patients and especially those suffering from co-morbid chemical dependency and other psychiatric diagnoses.

In a meta-analytic investigation on the effectiveness of bibliotherapy for alcohol problems, Apodaca and Miller (2003) analyzed the findings from 22 relevant studies. The weighted mean pre/post effect size for bibliotherapy was 0.80 among self-referred individuals and 0.65 among individuals identified through health screening. Between group comparisons of bibliotherapy with no-treatment controls rendered an effect size of 0.31 for self-referred drinkers. These authors found their findings based on meta-analysis supportive of the cost-effectiveness of bibliotherapy for problem drinkers.

Dually diagnosed individuals face more challenges than patients who have earned a single diagnosis because, as already stated, dual diagnosis is frequently associated with substance abuse and is characteristic of individuals with high levels of problem complexity and chronicity; i.e., severe and pervasive pathology. For example, patients suffering from substance abuse disorders often present with multiple problems including legal issues, employment problems, marital/relationship difficulties, mental and physical health-related needs, and financial concerns. The combination of psychotherapy/marital therapy/couple therapy, psychiatry, social work, medical treatment/physician supervised detox, legal help, and financial consultation may all be necessary components for successful treatment. Additionally, participation in self-help groups such as 12-step programs improves the likelihood of successful treatment. Many veteran 12-step members, typically functioning as sponsors, can provide helpful direction and motivation for patients attempting to pull their lives together. Magura et al. (2003) identified some mediators associated with the effectiveness of 12-step programs for the dually diagnosed as they relate to the domains of drug/alcohol abstinence and health-promoting behaviors. Magura et al. (2003) found that internal locus of control and sociability mediated the effects of 12-step programs for both domains in question. Mediators of health promoting behaviors were spirituality and hope. Twelve-step programs may not be compatible for all individuals with substance abuse issues; however, there is a great deal of variability within the 12-step community—with persistence, patients are often able to find a group they ultimately connect with. Additionally, non-12-step groups are easily accessible in most communities—these may prove acceptable for those unable to connect with the 12-step philosophy.

Attendance at 12-step and other self-help programs may help an individual cope with and reduce cravings by replacing potentially high-risk behaviors with healthy supportive ones. Additionally, self-help/support group participation exposes individuals to those who have been successful in maintaining abstinence, provides support and effective methods of coping, and can help motivate individuals to address the multiple problems that must be targeted as a part of the recovery process. Another possible mechanism for the success of 12-step programs involves self-efficacy. Twelve-step involvement appears to increase one's perception of self-efficacy, a construct found to be a mediator of the effects of self-help on abstinence, through an identification process with successful individuals who share characteristics similar to themselves (Magura et al., 2002; Morgenstern, Labouvie, McCray, Kahler, & Frey, 1997). The following is a brief listing of self-help resources for substance abuse found on the Internet—a google search revealed more than 7.5 million hits:

> www.PPBH.org provides substance abuse help for patients and their families.
>
> www.DrugAlcohol/help.com, an alternative to AA.
>
> www.helpguide.org/mental/drug_abuse_addiction_rehab_treatment.htm pro vides drug abuse, rehab, self-help, and treatment options for drug addiction including self-help for families.
>
> www.ncadi.samhsa.gov/referrals/ provides information on alcohol and drug abuse self-help programs.
>
> www.pubmedcentral.nih.gov/articlerender.fcgi provides substance abuse treat ment providers' referral to self-help.
>
> www.helpself.com/directory/abuse.htm provides substance abuse self-help and personal health directory.

Schizophrenia—Self-Help Internet Forums

Schizophrenia is a chronic psychiatric disorder with profound implications for social, academic, and professional functioning. Among adolescent and young adult males, the potential for suicide following a diagnosis of schizophrenia is high—this is apparently due to the fact that in the early stages of schizophrenia, reality testing and insight are relatively intact; therefore, the patient is able to fully understand the ramifications of the diagnosis and the likelihood that career and relationship dreams may go unrealized. It is rare for a patient to earn a diagnosis of schizophrenia and not have it interfere with social and occupational functioning—personality is affected, sometimes severely. Behavior is also changed by schizophrenia—these changes do not augur well for good social and occupational adjustment.

Great advances have been made in the pharmacological and psychological (primarily psychoeducational) treatment of schizophrenia. Second and third generation, atypical antipsychotics create fewer negative side effects and some, primarily anecdotal, evidence exists supporting the notion that negative symptoms improve with atypical antipsychotic drugs for some individuals. Early diagnosis and good pharmacotherapy are essential to the treatment of schizophrenia. Psychotherapy/psychoeducation/family therapy and self-help resources are important adjuncts to treatment by providing assistance with issues of treatment compliance, the establishment of a healthy home environment, education about the illness, reduction of stressors, and reintegration into society.

Schizophrenia, although subtyped, is heterogeneous within subtypes—that is, varying levels of symptom severity, differences in delusional framework, personality characteristics, receptivity to others, responsiveness to medications, and symptom clusters all create a unique presentation that requires an individualized treatment plan. Additionally, contextual differences are important considerations for treatment planning. Further, some patients present with differential deterioration of various brain structures while other patients diagnosed with schizophrenia show no signs of neurological deterioration. There is also evidence of variation in response to antipsychotic medication based upon race. For example, AfricanAmericans appear to require lower doses of antipsychotic medication to achieve the desired effect. Patients diagnosed with schizophrenia may be very different from one another while at the same time sharing common characteristics such as delusions, hallucinations, and changes in affect.

Males diagnosed with schizophrenia are rarely married and often homeless or institutionalized. On the other hand, females diagnosed with schizophrenia typically have a better outcome as measured by a variety of dimensions. More specifically, they are more likely to be married and to remain married—this is partially due to the fact that females manifest schizophrenia at a later age than males making marriage much more likely. Additionally, the social expectations surrounding family financial responsibilities are not as high for females as they are for males. Because social and family responsibilities may be less demanding and more forgiving, stressors tend to be fewer and less severe—this has implications for relapse and the likelihood that a patient will be re-institutionalized. Females suffering from schizophrenia tend to have fewer hospitalizations, are institutionalized less often, and the course of the disorder is not as severe as it is for males. This may be due to a variety of reasons including marital status, differential social expectations, and a relative difference in the severity and amount of stressors experienced between sexes.

With respect to self-help resources, Hacker, Lauber, & Rossler (2005) investigated 1,200 posting by 576 users in 12 international schizophrenia forums and analyzed the data with respect to communicative skills and self-help mechanisms (SHM). Forum participants were patients diagnosed with schizophrenia and to a lesser extent, relatives and friends. The self-help mechanisms employed most frequently were disclosure of experiences and information dissemination about daily problems characteristic of the illness such as symptoms, medication issues, and emotional involvement with their diagnosis. Emotional interaction/empathy and expressions of gratitude were relatively rare occurrences.

In general, Hacker et al. (2005) found that patients suffering from schizophrenia participate in online forums in a manner comparable to patients suffering from other psychiatric disorders. That is, they discuss similar topics and friends and relatives appear to interact in much the same way. The authors conclude that Internet forums appear to be a useful method for coping with alienation and isolation. Unfortunately, self-help forums for patients suffering with schizophrenia are rare relative to forums for depression and other psychiatric disorders. Additionally, many patients diagnosed with schizophrenia have experienced the "downward economic spiral" as a result of the functional impairment associated with psychosis—this is more common for males. The implications of the financial difficulties that many individuals with schizophrenia face has direct bearing on access to the Internet and may contribute to the social isolation that many patients face.

An impressive body of research suggests that family interaction has profound effects on the course that schizophrenia takes—prognosis is affected by family dynamics. Specifically, families of schizophrenics high in negative interpersonal exchanges have a higher rate of re-hospitalization. Negative interactions include criticisms toward the patient and a lack of understanding with respect to symptoms and behaviors characteristic of patients suffering from schizophrenia. Criticism often centers on the negative (diminutive) symptoms associated with schizophrenia—the very symptoms most resistant to pharmacological intervention. On the other hand, positive, supportive, and understanding family interaction greatly reduces the rates of re-hospitalization and improves compliance with pharmacological prescription. The progression of the disease may be halted or attenuated with a positive, supportive, and informed interactional family style.

In an investigation involving parents of 22 patients diagnosed with schizophrenia, family members and self-help groups were reported as being most helpful in the management of this chronic psychiatric illness (Ferriter & Huband, 2003). Police, friends, nurses, neighbors, and clergy were all rated higher than general practitioners, psychiatrists, social workers, and psychologists in terms of perceived helpfulness. Professional staff was reported as being the least helpful to parents in the management of their offspring's disorder. Of least importance among causation models were pathological parenting theories—these theories have also been discredited by the scientific community. The most important causal theory identified by the parents was the biological and life-event (diathesis-stress) model. In a related study (Knudson & Boyle, 2002), support from social networks and mental health services was generally perceived to have been wanting; however, informational sources and emotional support from self-help groups was available for both relatives and caregivers.

The importance of family member interaction and support groups is probably traceable to effective psychoeducation about the management of schizophrenia. This is particularly important based on the stressors that families bear when one or more of their offspring are diagnosed with schizophrenia. For example, worries about the present and future, financial concerns (especially among low income families), stresses involved in dealing with a potentially unpredictable and profoundly changed son or daughter, anxiety, grief, depression, and disruption to a family's social life, stigmatization, guilt, and self-blame all may contribute to a family's feeling of isolation and despair (Ferriter & Huband, 2003; Maurin & Boyd, 1990; Oldridge & Hughes, 1992; Winfield & Harvey, 1993).

A number of Internet-based support organizations are available to families with offspring diagnosed with schizophrenia and patients diagnosed with this chronic illness. The quality of the materials varies and the consumer should seek some verification of quality assurance either by searching databases for evidence of empirical support, accreditation, or consultation with experts who specialize in schizophrenia. The following constitutes a brief sample of some of the self-help sites and treatment information available on the Internet (a simple google search elicited over 600,000 results):

www.livingwithschizophrenia.com, a site that helps concerned individuals learn how counseling and training can help with schizophrenia.

www.Recover-Inc.org, a mental health recovery program.

www.HealthBoards.com provides free advice, opportunities to share experi ences and ask questions—over 500,000 members.

ManicDepression.us.com provides information on self-help for schizophrenia.

www.healthcentral.com/schizophrenia/c/120/9630/ provides self-help expert on schizophrenia, and Christina Bruni describes the top ten self-help books on schizophrenia.

www.mentalhelp.net/poc/view_doc.php?type=doc&id=8832&cn=7 provides housing assistance for patients suffering with schizophrenia.

www.psychcentral.com/disorders/sx31t.htm is a resource for family members or someone who lives with schizophrenia.

www.negativesschizophreniaselfhelp.com/ helps one cope with Type II (nega tive) schizophrenia and its medication regimes.

www.wellsphere.com/wellguide provides help for patients or families who think that the symptoms of schizophrenia are getting worse—ways to relive stress are provided.

Self-Help for Smoking Cessation/Tobacco Use

The topic of smoking addiction has been covered in Chapter 10; however, some additional information is provided here based on the potential severity of the consequences that smoking presents. Undoubtedly, most would not consider addiction to smoking/tobacco to be a serious form of psychopathology; however, this particular addiction has serious social implications. For example, smoking addiction has a strong psychological component and smoking is the single most preventable cause of premature morbidity and death in the United States (Curry, Ludman, and McClure, 2003). The manifestation of durable addictive psychopathology may take some time to develop—the manifestation of serious medical pathology may take decades. Virtually all body systems are negatively affected by cigarette smoking (Doweiko, 2006). Nearly half a million people die prematurely each year as a result of tobacco use; this number includes the 15,000–35,500 non-smokers who die each year due to passive smoke, environmental tobacco smoke, or secondhand smoke (Abadinsky, 2008; Doweiko, 2006). It is estimated that male smokers lose 13.2 years of their lives when compared to their non-smoking counterparts—for females, the loss in years of life is 14.5.

The cost that smoking confers on our society is staggering in terms of health care, quality of life, and productivity—estimates vary from a low of $138 billion (Schneider Institute for Health Policy, 2001) to $157 billion (Doweiko, 2006). Nicotine is a highly addictive drug—it has an addiction potential similar to cocaine or narcotics (Doweiko, 2006), and treatment success rates tend to be mediocre at best. A complicating factor in smoking cessation involves what appears to be a relationship between depression and cigarette smoking; however, although this relationship is poorly understood. Evidence suggests that individuals suffering from depression experience more reinforcement from cigarette smoking than non-depressed counterparts. Additionally, smokers appear to experience higher recurrence rates of depressive episodes following cessation of smoking. Finally, cigarette smoking appears to precede the manifestation of depression in teenagers (Doweiko, 2006).

The Centers for Disease Control found that only 19% of cigarette smokers have never attempted to quit—this means that more than 80% of cigarette smokers will attempt to quit at least once and each year, 15 million individuals quit smoking for a period of at least 24 hrs. Smoking prevention programs have not faired well; the prevalence rate among high school seniors is approximately 25%—a 15-year investigation of a school-based smoking-prevention program showed no effect. Adult smoking prevalence rates hover at about 24%. The least effective method of quitting smoking is "cold-turkey". Based on the foregoing, self-help for smoking cessation is an important area of attention. This short section will focus on self-administered behavioral and pharmacological treatments for smoking cessation.

As Curry et al. (2003) point out, self-administered treatments targeted on a reduction in, or abstinence from smoking, may increase access to treatment for a wider variety of smokers. Self-help materials for smoking cessation may take a variety of forms including brief motivational leaflets or brochures, comprehensive step-by-step manuals, audiotapes, videotapes, pharmacological agents, and computer programs. Manual-based behavioral treatments for smoking cessation have had mixed results and the use of behavioral manuals for smoking cessation have not been successful as a stand-alone treatment. On the other hand, when self-help manuals for smoking cessation are combined with personalized adjunctive forms of treatment (e.g., written feedback, telephone counseling), quit rates increase (Curry et al., 2003). Manuals have several advantages including the following: (1) state-of-the-art cognitive-behavioral treatment elements packaged for wide dissemination and relatively low cost, (2) manualized treatments can be tailored to fit the characteristics and predilections of the smoker, and (3) manuals remain a resource for future use should treatment ever prove unsuccessful (Curry et al., 2003).

Pharmacological treatments (e.g., nicotine patch or gum, bupropion) produce a doubling of smoking cessation rates when compared to placebo (Curry et al., 2003). Data gathered by the Centers for Disease Control indicate that the inhaler and nasal spray are among the least effective pharmacological agents; however, results of meta-analyses indicate that all pharmacological agents produce similar smoking cessation rates and double cessation in comparison to placebo. When pharmacological sales data collected in 1998 are used to estimate quit attempts, the figure exceeds eight million quit attempts using pharmacotherapy (Centers for Disease Control and Prevention, 2000, as cited in Curry et al., 2003). Curry et al. (2003) estimate that one-third of annual quit attempts are made with pharmacological agents—of these, almost 49% employ the nicotine patch, 28% employ the nicotine gum, 21% employ bupropion, and less than 3% involve an inhaler or nasal spray (Centers for Disease Control and Prevention, 2000). Demographic data indicate that females are more likely than males to utilize self-help smoking cessation methods.

Unfortunately, when self-administered treatments for smoking cessation are applied in the field, accuracy in documented success or failure rates are difficult to quantify—often compliance issues reduce their effectiveness. Among clinicians, the general consensus is that smoking rates decline when self-help treatments are administered, this is especially true if treatments are stacked such as when behavioral modification is combined with pharmacological intervention; however, many smokers do not combine treatments. Another problem with the literature on self-help treatment for smoking cessation is that many investigations were not thorough—utilization rates were collected sporadically. The 1996 California Tobacco Survey for adults found that among daily smoker adults 25 years or older, approximately 28% reported using some method for smoking cessation, approximately 9% used self-help materials, 2.5% use them alone, and 6.8% used them in combination with another form of treatment (Curry et al., 2003).

Published reviews of the efficacy or effectiveness of self-help materials for smoking cessation provides some indication of their utility. For example, group treatments appear to produce higher post-treatment cessation rates; however, relapse rates tend to hover around 80%. Abstinence rates among self-administered program participants appear to increase. The foregoing findings need to be interpreted with caution based on the findings from Curry et al. (1988)—that is, self-selection appears to play a role in successful treatment. Specifically, a RCT found that smokers assigned to either group or self-help formats achieved nearly identical abstinence rates. This finding is consistent with those reported in other RCTs.

Self-help treatments for smoking cessation seem to be most effective for those smokers who are less addicted, more highly motivated, confident, have experienced longer periods of abstinence, and have stronger social support networks.

Additionally, minimal support in the form of supportive telephone contact and computerized feedback appear to provide an incremental improvement in success rates. Unfortunately, the foregoing characteristic of success are relatively rare among the small (5%) number of individuals who employ self-help materials—in reality, prognostic indicators tend to lie at the opposite/negative end of the dimensions (Curry et al., 2003).

Based on the Cochrane Tobacco Addiction Review, a meta-analysis involving 39 randomized trials with at least 6-month follow-up assessment and at least one self-help intervention arm without repeated face-to-face therapist contact, self-help materials improved quit rates over no treatment controls. Further, self-help materials tailored to the unique needs of the individual are more effective than non-tailored, one-size-fits-all, forms of self-help treatment. Additionally, and consistent with the literature on problem complexity and chronicity, cessation rates improve by increasing the intensity of treatment via proactive telephone counseling or through a reactive quit-line. Randomized trials utilizing the new technologies (e.g., hand-held computers) to help in the administration of self-help treatments and improve surveillance with respect to compliance may prove useful in more accurately determining the effectiveness of self-help treatments for smoking cessation.

Concluding Remarks

In reality, most psychiatric disorders can meet the level of severe psychopathology depending on a variety of elements. For example, contextual conditions and related patient resources, social/family support, quality of coping mechanisms, level of psychiatric resilience/ability to adapt, the presence of co-morbidity, and the pervasiveness and chronicity of the problem all impact on the level of psychiatric severity. We have chosen to limit our discussion to a relatively few severe diagnostic categories in an effort to provide depth. It is important to note that when any diagnosis reaches the level of severe psychopathology, the treatment recommendations outlined in the foregoing will apply with consideration to fit.

The general rule is that multi-person, multi-modal, individualized treatment based on each patient's unique presentation is indicated when attempting to address severe psychopathology. As a general rule, an initial symptom-focused approach, developed in an effort to stabilize the patient/reduce self-destructive and high-risk behavior is indicated to help establish more planful behavior and effortful treatment participation. Once stabilization has been achieved to an adequate degree, in-depth, insight-focused treatment may be appropriate for some based on patient-matching dimensions such as coping style, (Beutler & Harwood, 2000; Beutler et al., 2000; Harwood & Beutler, 2008).

Self-help methods: 12-step programs, non-12-step support groups, Internet resources, treatment manuals/workbooks, psychoeduction, and the development of healthy social support networks are important adjunctive treatments whenever severe psychopathology presents. As the foregoing suggests, multi-person-tailored treatment should appropriately utilize psychiatry, social work, psychology, and other (e.g., legal, medical) professional involvement in an effort to provide success-ful treatment. It is recommended that patients seek professional guidance in the selection of specific self-help resources to employ—finding the resources that can be tailored to the patients' specific problem will increase treatment effectiveness. Additionally, patients should become as self-informed as possible with respect to the availability of empirical support and quality assurance for these self-help resources. Advances in treatments for severe psychopathology augur well for successful change—myriad empirically supported interventions exist today and individualized combined treatment formats and modalities will increase the likelihood of durable positive change.

Chapter 13
Medical Conditions

Introduction

Psychosocial interventions have application in a variety of areas where medical conditions are concerned. Charcot is credited as one of the founders of modern neurology and he played an important role in the identification of hysteria (Faber, 1997), the documentation of the mind–body connection through his work on hypnotized hysterics, and the suggestibility of some patients. In particular, one of his students, Babinski, demonstrated that the "grande attaque", thought by Charcot to be an expression of hystero-epilepsy, was actually an expression of epileptic symptoms observed by hysterical, highly persuasive, and suggestible patients. The diagnosis of hysteria was often a result of the practitioner's preferences and suggestions—a point that seems largely lost today, especially by clinicians who specialize in the treatment of suspected trauma patients. These therapists believe that their patients are destined to suffer until their repressed memories are brought to the surface— they appear to have no difficulty finding patients who respond to their various forms of trauma diagnoses (e.g., victims of sexual abuse). The persistence of these therapists has often resulted in the formation of false memories (Spanos, 1996) and the destruction that ensues can be devastating to families and relationships.

The evidence that physiological symptoms can be psychologically induced, or psychological factors are associated with the development and maintenance of physiological symptoms, has resulted in a phenomenon labeled psychosomatic "illness". Today this phenomenon is referred to in the DSM-IV-TR (2000) as conversion disorder. The label conversion suggests that the mind is able to transform traumatic experiences into bodily states (McWilliams and Weinberger, 2003). Well-documented phenomena such as hand-glove paralysis, a condition that occurs without any detectable trauma to the nerves that are responsible for hand movement and sensation, is physiologically impossible due to the localization of dermatomes and other relevant nerve physiology. This phenomenon and others like it are theorized as stemming from a repressive process that did not entirely succeed McWilliams and Weinberger (2003). In a similar vein, Griffin and Christie (2008) discuss how unexplained child physical illness may be due to the inability of children to adequately express emotional distress through verbal communication. These

T.M. Harwood, L. L'Abate, *Self-Help in Mental Health*,
DOI 10.1007/978-1-4419-1099-8_13, © Springer Science+Business Media, LLC 2010

authors call for a multi-disciplinary treatment approach that includes an integrated psychological treatment component.

Psychologists often play an important role in the medical care of patients. For example, psychologists are frequently involved in the preparation of patients for surgery—many hospitals routinely utilize mental health professionals to help improve upon the likelihood and magnitude of successful medical outcome. Relatedly, aftercare, treatment compliance, and a variety of adjustment issues often fall under the purview of mental health professionals, especially when problems with treatment compliance or adjustment present. Of course, psychiatrists and MDs appropriately licensed and with professional training in mental health notwithstanding, most mental health professionals do not have the appropriate level of medical training necessary for the prescription of medical interventions. Other possible exceptions include Licensed Clinical Psychiatric Nurses (LCPNs) or appropriately trained Licensed Clinical Social Workers; however, these individuals typically function under the close supervision of an MD. In a similar vein, family physicians (and physicians in general) often receive training through their medical schools in counseling and psychotherapy skills—the result is improved patient–physician relationships (Borins, Holzapfel, Tudiver, & Bader, 2007).

Therefore, except in rare cases, psychologists and other mental health professionals should not provide direct medical care and should only involve themselves in medical issues if they are being supervised by an MD. Relatedly, as the foregoing implies, psychologists often partner with physicians in the care and treatment of patients—psychology/psychiatry and medicine are complementary. It is good clinical practice for mental health workers to establish working relationships with psychiatrists and other MDs in the community. Further, a working relationship with local pharmacists is helpful as well. Relationships with medical professionals are all the more relevant to psychologists treating patients who are older adults and are likely to have medical overlay and polypharmacy, patients who are taking any types of medications (prescription, over-the-counter), and those struggling with substance abuse issues.

The development of a working relationship characterized in the foregoing is not uncommon; however, this development is hampered by differential health and behavior codes used for reimbursement of services. That is, medical personal use a reimbursement system that does not correspond with the system employed by psychologists. Efforts are underway to integrate behavioral health care coding systems with medical care systems to produce a more user-friendly, collaborative care model (Kessler, 2008a). When physicians and psychologists work collaboratively, patient care is significantly improved and health care costs are reduced (Kessler, 2008b)—this is accomplished primarily because relapse is less likely or severe and treatment benefits are enhanced. Carr (2008) has called for an emphasis on research focusing on the mechanisms of bio-behavioral interaction. According to Carr, interdisciplinary teaching, research, and health care have begun to revolutionize academic medicine—an increased emphasis is being placed on multi-disciplinary education and knowledge and collaboration between disciplines.

Generally speaking, psychologists see their patients on a more regular basis compared to physicians—they are more likely to observe changes in behavior, cognitive abilities, and often they are privy to information that has a direct bearing on their medical care or physical condition. It is good clinical practice to have patients sign informed consent agreements allowing the mental health practitioner to communicate with the medical professional(s) assigned to the patient. Multi-disciplinary treatment is key to patients who are suffering from comorbid medical and psychiatric diagnoses. Patients such as these are likely to fall into the category of complex/chronic problems—multi-person treatment is indicated in these instances.

Physicians and psychologists recognize that psychosomatic illness and conversion disorder represent the ability of the mind to produce, or influence the development of, significant physiological changes and conditions or disease states—in some instances, highly pathological in nature. With the foregoing in mind, psychological interventions, often delivered by health psychologists, are helpful in the treatment of a variety of medical conditions such as hypertension, some forms of gastric ulcers, immune system malfunction, pain management for conditions such as arthritis, fibromyalgia, and migraines. Additionally, skin conditions (e.g., inflammatory conditions such as rashes, hives, eczema,), pulmonary problems (asthma), endocrine problems (e.g., diabetes), and gastrointestinal disturbances (e.g., ulcerative colitis, irritable bowel syndrome) all respond favorably to interventions delivered by mental health professionals.

Patients may be supplied with self-help materials targeted on preparation for surgery, education about medical disorders and their psychological association, and aftercare/adjustment issues. Mental health professionals can review these materials upon arrival or after admittance to the hospital, preferably under an appropriate level of medical supervision and as part of a formal multi-disciplinary treatment team. Ongoing problems or new developments may be addressed through a clinician-delivered maintenance program supplemented with self-help resources and medical advice. Relapse rates, physical and psychological deterioration, and recovery rates are all positively impacted by interventions delivered by appropriately trained nurses, a variety of mental health professionals, and health psychologists.

A Brief Sample of Medical Conditions That Have Self-Help Resources Available

Arthroscopic TMJ	Fibromyalgia
Asthma	Gastrointestinal bleeding
Atrial fibrillation	Generalized anxiety disorder
Binge eating	Heart disease
BiPolar disorder	HIV and AIDS
Breast cancer	Insomnia
Bulimia nervosa	Irritable bowel syndrome

Cancers (in general)	Late Luteal phase dysphoric disorder
Celiac disease	Lupus erythematosus
Chronic fatigue syndrome	Mild head injury
Chronic obstructive pulmonary disease	Migraines
Chronic pain	Myocardial infarction
Clostridium difficile infection	Obesity
Cognitive impairment	Pulmonary conditions
Congestive heart failure	Panic disorder
Diabetes mellitus (Type I and II)	Sickle cell disease
Diabetic neuropathy	Social anxiety disorder
Disorders of consciousness	Temporomandibular disorder
Headache	Tinnitus

Traumatic Brain Injury

Schoenberg et al. (2008) conducted an investigation into the comparative efficacy of a computer-based cognitive rehabilitation teletherapy program and a face-to-face rehabilitation program for individuals with moderate to severe closed head traumatic brain injury. Participants were at least 1-year post-injury at the time of the investigation. Telemedicine, a guided, maximal contact, self-help treatment approach, provides health care services and information via telephone and computer—it is an effective method for providing services to remote or underserved areas (Schoenberg et al., 2008). According to Schoenberg, the computer-based teletherapy cognitive rehabilitation program and the comparative face-to-face speech-language therapy produced similar treatment outcomes. Additionally, cost for treatment delivery was similar across treatment programs; however, when the two treatments were analyzed using cost per hour of therapy as the unit of analysis, the computer-based teletherapy treatment method was less expensive to deliver than the face-to-face treatment method.

Cognitive Impairment

Homework, a primary treatment component in cognitive-behavioral (C-B) treatment, may be considered a therapist guided form of self-help. Coon, Thompson, and Gallagher-Thompson (2007) explained how C-B intervention strategies combined with tailored homework produced a successful outcome in the treatment of a depressed and cognitively impaired patient. Phase of treatment, patient variables, and specific strategies to improve homework compliance were discussed. More specifically, in the initial phase of therapy, sessions were prescribed at a higher frequency. This modification allowed the clinician to assign brief homework in an effort to increase the likelihood of successful homework completion while simultaneously increasing the reinforcement frequency of successful homework completion. Additionally, therapists were able to quickly identify any obstacles to homework compliance and develop strategies to improve compliance, if necessary.

A notebook and calendar, useful materials when working with older adults in general, were utilized to help organize materials, plan and schedule sessions, and to maintain a database of assignments and skills learned. These simple materials provided the patient with a centralized, user-friendly method for emphasizing crucial therapeutic concepts and made them readily available for ongoing review and reinforcement—it is likely that treatment gains were enhanced and maintained with the use of the notebook.

Additional methods used in this specific case included audiotapes of sessions for home review and skill/concept reinforcement (especially during the initial phase of treatment) and role-plays involving situations where memory failure might occur in public. The development of organizational skills and strategies and memory aids was a primary therapeutic focus. Finally, homework was used to gauge the point where patient overload/cognitive impairment became problematic—in this way, tasks and responsibilities could be tailored more accurately to the patient's ability level.

The final phase of therapy, the reinforcement and maintenance phase, involved review of previously learned material, the use of modified thought records to help attenuate the severity or frequency of unhelpful thoughts related primarily to memory. Booster sessions, three in this case, were spaced at monthly intervals and referrals to appropriate support groups and organizations (e.g., the local Alzheimer's Association) were entered into the patient's notebook to help the patient and family negotiate the next phase of the dementing process.

The treatment of post-concussion syndrome following mild head injury (Mittenberg Canyock, Condit, and Patton, 2001) often involves a variety of psychological interventions aimed toward recovery of cognitive functions and treatment of the psychological aftereffects associated with brain injury. Although medication is generally the treatment of choice for the symptoms of post-concussion syndrome (PCS) with non-steroidal analgesics and antidepressants toping the list of prescribed medications, depression, anxiety, and fear of permanent cognitive impairment are a few of the criteria for PCS—psychosocial interventions may be more effective than medications in the treatment of these post-concussive symptoms.

The distressing aftereffects of brain injury function to exacerbate or maintain the acute symptoms of PCS. Psychological treatment often involves "...education, reassurance, and reattribution of symptoms to benign causes" (Mittenberg et al., 2001, p. 829). According to some investigators (e.g., Goldstein, Levin, Goldman, Clark, and Altonen, 2001; Levin et al., 1987; as cited in Mittenberg et al., 2001), research suggests that cognitive impairments will resolve in 3–6 months—this supports the use of reassurance for patients suffering from fears of permanent cognitive impairment. Cognitive restructuring is a technique used to make acceptable/plausible reattributions of subjectively experience symptoms to normal causes. This is a common and effective technique for reducing patient distress and improving outlook; that is, patients often misattribute symptoms or are inaccurate about their premorbid level of symptoms such as headache, fatigue, inattention, faulty memory, and mood disturbances. Additionally, the distress caused by the misattribution of normal occurrences such as headache may serve to exacerbate what patients experience as distressing symptoms well beyond their premorbid level of severity (Mittenberg et al., 2001).

In an effort to reintegrate individuals back to a level of functioning consistent with their premorbid abilities, patients are often provided with a gradual, graded prescription for work, social, and general responsibilities (Mittenberg et al., 2001). For example, to combat fatigue, difficulty with concentration, and general cognitive inefficiency, patients may be provided with a variety of modifications including reduced work load, a shorter work day, fewer days of work per week, shorter social visits, greater spacing between social visits, and an assistant to help with duties should fatigue or difficulty become problematic in the middle of a project or other time-certain activity. With time, the patient would be expected to shoulder additional responsibility as appropriate to recovery status. Patients should be monitored for signs of overload, headache, irritability, and fatigue beyond what would be considered normal for the activity would suggest that the patient may be pushing herself too hard—some duties may need to be shifted to a support colleague or time limits for work or other activities may need to be considered.

An investigation conducted by Relander, Troupp, and Bjorkesten (1972, as cited in Mittenberg et al., 2001) compared the effects of education about concussion with treatment as usual (TAU). These investigators found that the group of patients randomly assigned to the education condition returned to work significantly sooner than those receiving TAU (18 versus 32 days). Similar result were obtained by Kelly (1975, as cited in Mittenberg et al., 2001)—that is, patients who were educated about diagnosis and prognosis experienced lower levels of post-concussive symptoms (PCS) while those receiving TAU accompanied with discharge/aftercare instructions experienced iatrogenesis by comparison. Minderhoud, Boelens, Huizenga, and Saan (1980, as cited in Mittenberg et al., 2001) conducted an investigation on recovery rates for patients who had experienced mild acute head injury. One group of patients was provided with written material and verbal information about the nature, causes, expected prognosis of various symptoms, and reassurance that symptoms could be expected to remit. This group also received instruction on gradual resumption of activity. The control group received TAU and reported significantly greater PCS symptoms than the experimental intervention group at 6-month follow-up. Additionally, those in the experimental condition returned to work or school earlier and they had lower rates of absenteeism than the control group. In a clinical trial involving patients with mild head injury, Gronwall (1986) reported findings similar to the foregoing. In the Gronwall investigation, interventions included a printed manual about concussion symptoms and coping strategies, a prescription for graded return to pre-injury levels of independent functioning, and stress management and relaxation training.

Cardiac Diseases

Psychocardiology, aka as behavioral cardiology, is the study of the biopsychosocial factors involved in the genesis, course or maintenance, and the rehabilitation of cardiac disease (Jordan Bardé & Zeiher 2006). A text predicated on the biopsy-chosocial model of cardiac disease, *Contributions toward evidence-based psychocardiology: A systematic review of the literature* (Jordan et al., 2006), provides comprehensive coverage of the sociological elements involved in the etiology of cardiac disease. Likewise, a variety of psychosocial interventions and lifestyle factors are covered. In a similar vein, the contribution of depression, anxiety, personality factors (e.g., Type A personality), and rehabilitation issues are covered.

Sickle Cell Disease

Sickle cell disease (SCD) is a common, chronic, blood disorder that affects 1 in 500 African Americans and 1 in 1000 Hispanic Americans. Although it's more common in these ethnic groups, sickle cell disease occurs in people of all races. Due to advances in treatment and disease management, life expectancies for individuals suffering from sickle cell disease ranges from 40 to 50 years of age. SCD is painful and potentially dangerous due to its tendency to impair circulation resulting in organ damage.

Medications for SCD that reduce symptomology are available; however, this is a chronic condition and medication response rates and severity of the disorder are variable. A structured and empirically supported cognitive-behavioral self-help manual for sickle cell disease was developed by Anie and Green (2002)—these authors report that their SCD self-help manual is available on the website: www.sickle-psychology.com (2002). Our inspection of the website revealed a rather commercialized and confusing information dissemination system—we were unable to find a resource specifically identified as a self-help manual for SCD; however, a wealth of information is available from the website. For example, one can access links for sickle cell disease facts, information about iron overload, chelation, Parkinson's Disease, pain relief, hormone replacement therapy, women's health, Lyme Disease, and Sickle Cell camp. Additionally, patients may access a link where they can ask questions specific to their condition. Despite the commercial aspect of the site, it appears that it offers a relatively comprehensive self-help resource for patients suffering from Sickle Cell disease and the complications that accompany this blood disorder.

Bulimia Nervosa and Binge Eating Disorder

Some may question the characterization of Bulimia Nervosa and binge eating disorder as medical conditions; however, medical complications are common among these disorders and progression to a serious medical/psychological condition, anorexia nervosa, is not uncommon. An empirically supported Internet-assisted cognitive-behavioral treatment for eating disorders was developed by Ljotsson

et al. (2007). The Internet-assisted treatment includes a guided self-help component involving minimal therapist contact via email. *Overcoming binge eating* by
Fairburn (1995) was the patient self-help resource. Homework tied to each chapter was assigned and tracked by graduate students who used the therapist manual,
Guided self-help for bulimia nervosa. Therapist's manual (Fairburn, 1999). Guided
self-help has tended to produce better outcomes when compared to pure self-help
treatments (Carter & Fairburn, 1998; Loeb, Wilson, Gilbert, and Labouvie. 2000; as
cited in Ljotsson et al. 2007). Additionally, patients who receive self-help treatments
are more likely to attribute their success outcomes to their own efforts (Fairburn,
1997, as cited in Ljotsson et al. 2007).

Pain, Headache, Breast Cancer, Tinnitus, Physical Disabilities, and Pediatric Brain Injury

Cuijpers, van Straten, and Andersson (2008) conducted a systematic review of
randomized controlled or comparative trials involving several Internet-delivered
cognitive-behavioral (C-B) treatments for health problems. Although the magnitude of effects varied across conditions, the general conclusion reached by these
investigators was that the Internet will become a prominent player in the delivery of
C-B interventions for patients suffering from a variety of medical problems. More
specifically, Internet-delivered C-B interventions for pain (mean effect $d = 0.58$)
and for headache (ranging from $d = 0.19$ to 0.56) produced effects comparable
to those achieved by face-to-face interventions. Additional findings indicated that
quality of life in breast cancer patients improved slightly ($d = 0.22$) with a similar
change indicated for patients suffering from tinnitus ($d = 0.26$). Further, a moderate effect was found for patients suffering from loneliness resultant of physical
disabilities ($d = 0.46$) to large for parental mental health in pediatric brain injury
($d = 0.70$). With respect to tinnitus, Weise, Heinecke, and Rief (2008) conducted
an investigation on the efficacy of a biofeedback-based behavioral intervention.
Their findings rendered medium to large effect sizes in support of the efficacy of
the psychological treatment of tinnitus. Clear improvements were found on ratings of tinnitus annoyance, diary ratings of loudness, feelings of controllability,
coping cognitions, and depression symptoms. Further, these improvements were
maintained at 6-month follow-up. These authors went on to state that, "Through
demonstration of psychophysiological interrelationships, the treatment enables
patients to change their somatic illness perceptions to a more psychosomatic point
of view."

Buenaver, McGuire, and Haythornthwaite (2006) conducted a study on
cognitive-behavioral self-help for chronic pain associated with scleroderma. Their
self-help treatment involved minimal support from a lay leader or professional facilitator and the authors recommended a stepped-care model approach unless otherwise
indicated. As these investigators note, self-help has been provided via group formats, books and companion workbooks, audiotapes or videotapes, telemedicine

systems, the Internet, and in minimal contact formats—self-help treatments have been successfully employed in the treatment of chronic pain, pain-related disability, depression, and anxiety associated with arthritis (Lorig & Holman, 1993; Lorig, Ritter, Laurent, & Fries, 2004), low back pain (Buhrman, Faltenhag, Strom, & Andersson, 2004; Moore, Von Korff, Cherkin, Saunders, & Lorig, 2000; Von Korff et al., 1998), headache (Andersson, Lundstrom, & Strom, 2003; Blanchard et al., 1985; Devineni & Blanchard, 2005; Haddock et al., 1997; Jurish et al., 1983; Strom, Petterson, & Andersson, 2000), and temporomandibular joint disorder (TMD) (Dworkin et al., 1994; Townsend, Nicholson, Buenaver, Bush, & Gramling, 2001). According to Buenaver et al. (2006) improvements in self-efficacy appear to be signal in achieving reductions in pain and disability; further, these reductions appear to be relatively durable over time.

In the case of self-help treatment for the chronic pain associated with scleroderma, a number of patient considerations must be taken into account: (1) The patient's level of motivation for treatment must be assessed. As Buenaver et al. (2006) point out, patients who have earned diagnoses of clinical depression, any Axis II diagnosis, are severely disabled or cognitively impaired, or socially isolated may pose a challenge to treatment compliance and the establishment of a working relationship. The TRT (Treatment Readiness) scale from the MMPI-2 (Butcher, 1990) is a useful indicator of one's status as a receptive psychotherapy patient; (2) a stepped-care approach should be considered—in this model, self-management of treatment is the primary focus and professional contact is minimal. The level of professional care is increased on an as needed basis based upon the results of ongoing assessment of patient change; (3) self-help supplemented with some level of therapist contact is preferred over self-help alone—the support for this may be strongest for self-help treatment for arthritis and headache; (4) workbooks and books are readily available and these resources have received empirical support; and (5) patients and clinicians should be vigilant to the clinical utility of any workbook or book—the therapist should be familiar with available resources or avenues to research the effectiveness or efficacy of these materials.

Buenaver et al. (2006) found that patients responded differentially to the type of treatment offered. For example, one patient needed a "hook" to become invested in therapy—it was up to the therapist to find this motivating element and put it to good use in the interest of the patient. In a separate case, the use of a workbook was especially well-suited to the patient. She was able to review and implement the C-B strategies laid out in her workbook on a regular basis. Finally, one patient had limited reading ability, in his case, a stepped-care approach may have been the most successful—a clinic-based individual or group treatment seemed indicated for this patient.

Buenaver et al. (2006) offer a list of available workbooks and books targeted on the treatment of chronic pain; however, the only workbook with significant empirical support at the time of publication is the Lorig et al. (2006) workbook that targets a variety of chronic conditions—the workbook is titled: *Living a healthy life with chronic conditions: Self-management of heart disease, arthritis, diabetes, asthma, bronchitis, emphysema, and others (2nd ed.).* A third edition was released in 2006 and is completely revised and updated—the authors and title have not changed and this is the edition we have referenced. Additionally, audio CD versions of the workbook are available from the publisher, Bull Publishing Company (800-676-2855).

Cuijpers et al. (2008) are positive about the future of Internet-delivered C-B interventions employed for medical problems. They note that investigations involving CBT interventions have steadily increased in recent years. This development will improve upon the effectiveness of this form of self-help and reduce the burden on our medical and mental health systems. Relatedly, they see how CBT may be effectively employed in a stepped-care model similar to that proposed by Scogin, Hanson, and Welsh (2003). In the foregoing application, patients would be referred for additional care if the Internet-delivered intervention was not sufficiently effective in providing long-term relief.

In an investigation focused exclusively on migraine and chronic daily headache, Peters, Abu-Saad, Vydelingum, Dowson, and Murphy (2004) found that participants engaged in five areas of problem management: (1) Access to medical care, (2) pharmacotherapy, (3) alternative (non-allopathic) therapies, (4) social support, and (5) lifestyle modifications and self-help. Included in lifestyle change and self-help were job changes, sleep hygiene, dietary changes, stress control strategies, involvement in self-education about medications and their use, and an analysis of the triggers that invoked their own headaches. These authors concluded that medical care, especially with respect to chronic diseases, is evolving toward a greater self-reliance on the part of the patient in their own care. Within another investigation into the efficacy of self-help treatment for headache, a meta-analysis involving minimal contact therapy (MCT) and controlled clinical trials, home-based behavioral treatment for headaches yielded treatment effects that were equivalent or superior to those produced through clinic-based treatments (Haddock et al., 1997).

Diabetes

Schachinger et al. (2005) examined the efficacy of blood glucose awareness training (BGAT; Lubeck) utilizing a psychoeducational approach specifically designed for patients with type I diabetes mellitus. The RCT investigation employed an approach focused on the recognition and management of glucose levels when they reach extremes on the dimension of blood glucose levels. In short, those in the BGAT condition experienced significant improvements in the recognition of high, low, and overall blood glucose levels. Additionally, those in the BGAT condition experienced reduced levels of severe hypoglycemia, a potentially deadly condition primarily due to seizure and general cognitive impairment. Another important result of BGAT training was the reduction in external locus of control and fear of hypoglycemia experience by this group. The authors concluded that BGAT was efficacious in both American and European participants.

Obesity

The relative contribution of genetics/physiology versus purely psychological factors in the development of obesity is difficult to gauge and some level of interplay between these causal factors probably explains the lion's share of obesity.

Aftercare Self-Help Interventions

Kreulen and Braden (2004) examined the relationship between self-help-promoting nursing interventions and self-care and health status outcomes. More specifically, nurse-delivered self-help promoting interventions were positively related to general and illness self-care practices and the changes in behavior relative to self-care practice were linked to positive changes in health status and negatively related to patient morbidity. Interestingly, but consistent with previous research (e.g., Andersen, 1992; Edgar, Tosberger, and Nowlis, 1992, as cited in Kreulen and Braden), intervention effects on behavioral indices remained non-significant until 3-month post-intervention.

Findings from the foregoing investigation suggested that advanced disease status should be an indicator for a more intensive and tailored intervention dose. Further, a variety of patient characteristics (e.g., age, social network size, uncertainty, and resourcefulness) explained additional variance (ranging from 9 to 25%) in illness self-care practice, 22–27% of additional variance explained in general self-care practice, and 31–45% of additional variance accounted for in client morbidity. Kreulen and Braden indicated that their investigation revealed a complex interplay between intervention, patient attributes, and contextual variables.

Most hospitals supply their patients with aftercare information of some form. One popular format for aftercare is "CareNotes", a trademarked web-based method of disseminating information relative to a specific disorder. General information, information on inpatient care, and discharge care are typically covered in the CareNotes system. CareNotes is one of the services provided by the Micromedex Healthcare Series, a comprehensive database of information for hospitals and physicians. Micromedex is part of a larger health care information provider, Thomson Healthcare Evidence. The Thomson website may be accessed via the following URL; however, the site is login and password protected:

https://www.thomsonhc.com/carenotes/librarian/ssl/true/ND_T/CNotes/CS/F1E411

According to the website, Micromedex provides unbiased information on referenced information about drugs, toxicology, diseases, acute care, and alternative medicine. In addition to other helpful links to useful information, the Thompson Healthcare Evidence website has an electronic PDR library allowing physicians easy access to information relative to medication use. Information appears to be available for virtually all medical and psychiatric conditions that may require hospitalization, at some point, as a component of their effective treatment.

Self-Help Groups

Self-help groups are popular and cover a wide range of problems. Unfortunately, these groups are often operated without the application of quality control measures. Therefore, the utility of these groups varies widely and some may be more harmful than good. Alcoholics Anonymous (AA) is one group that has allowed some investigation into the effectiveness of this organization—results have been mixed and serious methodological issues plague many of the investigations. Still, there is a growing body of research suggesting that AA is helpful to alcoholism treatment and the prevention of relapse for some patients. It is a free and easily accessible resource with multiple chapters available in virtually every community—each chapter has its own flavor, patients need to find the group(s) that appeal to their proclivities. In some instances, 12-step programs are one of the only treatment options available to those who have limited resources and lack social support. Other 12-step programs have not enjoyed the same level of scientific scrutiny so their effectiveness is questionable.

In general, 12-step programs were not designed as stand-alone treatments. They are best viewed as adjunctive to more active forms of treatment, and they may be part of the aftercare plan for patients completing inpatient treatment programs—in the later stages of formal treatment, they may be most useful to the maintenance of treatment gains and in the development of a strong social support network—this is especially true for AA.

In an investigation of self-help group participation for people with life-threatening diseases, Adamsen (2002) concluded that self-help groups exert their positive effects through a universalizing of personal problems, i.e., patients are not alone in their struggles. In the instance of self-help groups for those suffering from life-threatening diseases (cancer, HIV/AIDS), life expectancy does not appear to be improved; however, as Adamsen points out, this is not the central objective of these groups—instead, these groups appear to improve the patients' ability to cope with the psychological and social consequences of living with a serious life-threatening disease. Additionally, the formation of social networks, new friendships, increased self-confidence are life enhancing effects—perhaps these groups are best characterized as increasing the quality of life instead of the quantity of life.

Irritable Bowel Syndrome (IBS)

IBS is a functional gastrointestinal disorder that affects approximately 10 – 20% of the U.S. population—it is characterized by diarrhea and/or constipation with accompanying abdominal pain. The costs of IBS are significant—medical costs alone reach 80 billion dollars per year in the United States—loses to productivity and the impact on functional impairment in a variety of domains have not been factored into this figure. Medical treatment for IBS has some empirical support; psychological treatment is considered an important treatment component for this disorder (Lackner, Morley Dowzer, Mesmer, and Hamilton, 2004, as cited in Sanders, Blanchard, and Sykes, 2007). Unfortunately, IBS is often treated solely by a patient's primary care physician and referral for psychological treatment is often overlooked (Sanders et al. 2007).

Bogalo and Moss-Morris (2006) evaluated the efficacy of homework tasks in a brief, self-help Cognitive-Behavioral Treatment (CBT) for irritable bowel syndrome (IBS). Participants were provided with an initial consultation session with a CBT therapist, a detailed self-help manual that provided structured homework tasks on a weekly basis, and minimal telephone support consisting of two contacts, one at 3 weeks into treatment and one at 5 weeks into treatment. The key findings indicated that homework compliance, in either quality or quantity of homework completed, had no impact at end-of-treatment; however, at 3-month follow-up, quality and quantity of homework was significantly associated with positive changes in symptoms. The authors concluded that homework, in this case a minimal contact therapist-guided form of self-help, may have an enhancing effect on treatment outcomes correspondent with level of compliance. This finding is consistent with the results of a meta-analysis by Kazantzis and Lampropoulos (2002). More specifically, compliance with self-help tasks was associated with positive treatment outcome.

In a more recent study on IBS by Sanders et al. (2007), self-help treatments were seen as an important psychological approach that could increase treatment effectiveness while reducing health care costs and losses to productivity and other forms of functioning. The treatment used in the Sanders investigation involved a book titled *Breaking the Bonds of Irritable Bowel Syndrome* (Bradley-Bolen, 2000). According to Sanders, this book was written as a self-help, CBT-based guide for the symptom management of IBS. Another book that IBS sufferers may find useful is the guidebook authored by Kennedy, Robinson, and Rogers (2003). Although both books are deemed useful with information on the digestive system, diagnostic medical tests, diet, and available medical treatments, the Bradley-Bolen book expands upon the Kennedy text by including exercises developed to help readers identify foods, situations, emotions, and thoughts that influence IBS episodes. CBT techniques for IBS sufferers who must deal with difficult situations are provided. The Bradley-Bolen book has been subjected to a controlled randomized investigation involving a wait-list control—the results of the study support the efficacy of the Bradley-Bolen book as a self-help treatment for IBS. Treatment gains remained relatively durable at 3-month follow-up. Further, the principles and strategies embedded in the book have received empirical support from other independent researchers (Sanders et al., 2007).

Non-specific Self-Help (Complementary Therapy)

In a recent investigation on medical patient expectations and the expectations of parents with children being treated in the medical system, Shaw, Thompson, and

Sharp (2006) found that patients preferred that their health care providers know more about the array of available complementary therapy and services. Patients also indicated that they would like to see the health care system change in a way that enhances patient choices for health care and improves upon patient access to self-help resources.

An additional finding from Shaw et al. was that patients preferred their health care provider to have a more open attitude to complementary therapies than currently experienced. Put another way, conventional treatment was not generally viewed as negative by patients; however, complementary forms of treatment were seen as possible avenues for incremental improvement in their health status. Patients simply wanted their health care providers to be well-informed about, and give due consideration to, the range of non-allopathic and conventional forms of treatment available.

In a similar vein, some patients expressed concerns about negative attitudes that health care providers had toward non-conventional therapies. Others indicated that their concerns about conventional therapies and the side-effects they were observing as a result of this treatment (e.g., steroids used to treat asthma in children) had been disregarded by their physician. Chatwin and Tovey (2004) describe how complementary and alternative medicine for cancer has received resistance within the medical community. These authors rightly call for legitimate challenge to the efficacy and effectiveness of these non-traditional approaches to cancer treatment by employing the methodological tools utilized in the establishment of evidence-based medicine.

No doubt, non-conventional therapies or treatments are controversial. Some are ineffective, others are potentially dangerous, and some may interfere or negatively interact with otherwise effective and safe treatments. Still, a number of non-traditional therapies or treatments have received empirical support for a number of conditions (e.g., chiropractic, acupuncture). It is important for physicians and other health care professionals to be informed about the potential benefits or dangers associated with non-conventional treatments. Additionally, health care providers should be able to direct patients to resources that provide accurate information about non-traditional forms of treatment. It is not recommended that patients engage in self-treatment without qualified professional guidance. Finally, physicians and other health care workers should remain open to the array of treatments that are both effective and safe—being informed about the potential dangers, cost-benefit ratio, interaction effects, especially if polypharmacy or medical overlay is part of the picture, are necessary components of effective treatment and patient management. As one patient put it, "They can't know everything in fairness. . .but don't decry something if you know nothing about it. . ." (Shaw et al., 2006, p. 347).

We do not make the foregoing recommendations or assertions lightly—we recognize the difficulty involved in educating oneself about the myriad alternative therapies available—this is a daunting task. We also understand that the level of treatment complexity is significantly increased when additional treatments are involved in patient care. On the other hand, in some cases, benefit may outweigh these important considerations. Medical professionals have begun to embrace alternative treatments for a number of reasons—partly because of patient interest and partly because of empirical support for some non-traditional interventions. As a result, textbooks have been written to help keep the medical and mental health care provider up-to-date on the important issues at hand when complementary therapies are being considered or requested by their patients. For example, the Physician's Desk Reference (PDR) publishes a variety of resources on herbal therapies, non-prescription drugs, and dietary supplements (e.g., Gruenwald, Brendler, and Jaenicke, 2007; Murray, 2006). A similar PDR resource was published for mental health professionals (LaGow, 2007) and other publishers have produced resources that provide information on side-effects, adverse drug reactions, and contraindications for prescription medications.

There are literally dozens of resources for physicians working with patients considering or already self-administering alternative therapies—the physician and mental health professional (and lay person) must be a careful consumer of these resources by examining the credentials of the publisher, organization involved in the publication, editors, and contributors. One resource that may prove invaluable to physicians and other health care professionals struggling with this issue is *The desktop guide to complementary and alternative medicine: An evidence based approach* (Ernst, Pittler, and Wilder, 2006). When good resources have been obtained by professionals, they have important information with respect to the alternative treatment's efficacy at their fingertips. At the very least, these resources can help one determine if a non-conventional treatment is contraindicated given the patient's medical and prescription drug profile. As a further cautionary note, Hughes (2007) argues that complementary and alternative medicine practices should not be integrated into clinical psychology because for many of these treatments, the empirical efficacy has yet to be established.

Current Investigations

Diabetes

van Bastelaar, Pouwer, Cuijpers, Twisk, and Snoek (2008) are presently conducting a randomized clinical trial investigation on a web-based self-help course for adults suffering from diabetes with comorbid depression. Their self-help program consists of an individualized, 8-week, moderated self-help psychoeducational intervention tailored to the unique needs of patients suffering from diabetes.

Chronic Pain

Morley, Shapiro, and Biggs (2004) developed a series of pdf file versions of a treatment manual for attention management in chronic pain (http://www.leeds.ac.uk/medicine/divisions/psychiatry/attman.htm). To our knowledge, this manual has not yet been subjected to rigorous RCT investigation; however, investigation may be in process. The manual is based on expert review and empirically supported treatment components for chronic pain.

Part IV
Conclusions and Prospects

Chapter 14
Who Benefits by Self-Help and Why?

By now it should be clear to readers that the self-help movement in mental health is represented by an enormous range of resources available, along various continua of validity and reliability. One of the most important areas in need of investigation is the area of patient–treatment matching with respect to SH. More specifically, *who* is most likely to benefit by SH? *What* are the most reliable indicators of assignment to SH? *When* are SH interventions most indicated? To answer these questions, a theory of SH and SC based on what is known about patient–treatment matching might more likely prove beneficial in the assignment of the various SH resources available today (e.g., Harwood & Beutler, 2008; Beutler & Harwood, 2000; Beutler, Clarkin, & Bongar, 2000; Beutler & Clarkin, 1990). A verifiable theory of change, specific enough to include patient dimensions such as coping style, reactance, problem complexity and chronicity, subjective distress, social support, and functional impairment might be a promising direction in SH research. Theories of change are less common than theories of pathology—this statement begs the question: Which is more important to patients, a theory of change or a theory of pathology? We believe that theories of change are ultimately more clinically relevant than those focused on pathology. Unfortunately, even fewer theories of change exist for those considering SH. One notable exception involves the work by Webpsych Innerlife (2009). The foregoing investigators have developed a patient-driven computer-administered program for patient–treatment matching, patient change, and differential assignment to various levels of SH. No other theories of change or personality mention this topic nor do most personality theories include how one can change for the better with or without help.

The theories that have come out of the positive psychology movement notwithstanding, extant psychotherapeutic theories do not sufficiently cover health promotion, prevention, or SH. By the same token, prevention and promotion treatises tend not to include psychotherapy. The various disciplines and models operate separate from each other and lack an underlying theory to support change as a multi-factorial process requiring a host of interrelated factors to describe and explain SH and SC.

Models of self-change (Sobell, 2007, pp. 13–16) include (1) conflict theory that postulated change results from felt discrepancies between what one wants from what one is, (2) the trans-theoretical model of change postulated stages of change

T.M. Harwood, L. L'Abate, *Self-Help in Mental Health*,
DOI 10.1007/978-1-4419-1099-8_14, © Springer Science+Business Media, LLC 2010

that begins with pre-contemplation and potentially continues through stages of contemplation, preparation, action, and maintenance, (3) crystallization of discontent after continuous evaluation and reevaluation of where one is personally and contextually and where one wants to arrive, (4) role exit about changing the role one has adopted to move into a new more positive role, and (5) cognitive appraisal that seems the model of change most cited in the field of addiction (Klingemann & Sobell, 2007).

What might be relevant to SH and SC is relational competence theory (L'Abate, 2002, 2003a, 2005; L'Abate & Cusinato, 2007; L'Abate et al., 2010; L'Abate & De Giacomo, 2003). We shall endeavor to illustrate how this theory may be relevant to SH/SC by suggesting who might profit by SH and who might not. This theory has relevance to the topic at hand because it may specify under what conditions one may seek and implement SH and SC and explain who can be helped by SH or by SC and what possible avenues may be necessary to help people help themselves. In an effort to provide a cohesive and concise treatment of relational competence theory, a theory-derived structured interview and written practice exercises are available (L'Abate, 2010).

A Theory of Relational Competence for Self-Help in Mental Health

Definition of Terms

The terms of this subheading need to be explained one at a time.

What Is a Theory?

A theory is a conceptual framework of interrelated and verifiable models covering all the possible avenues to SH and SC. In this case, relational competence theory is composed of 16 models. Models are the irreducible parts of a theory consisting of dimensions.

Why Is the Theory Relational?

In contrast to traditional theories of personality, which are usually intrapsychic, pathology-based, and monadic, this theory assumes that competence is circularly the outcome and cause of intimate (close, committed, prolonged, and interdependent) relationships. SH and SC are produced by the continuous interaction of individuals with intimates and non-intimates.

What Is Competence and How Does It Relate to SH/MH?

Competence refers to how effective or ineffective an individual is in fulfilling practical and realistic task demands throughout the life cycle. Consequently, there are different levels of competence ranging from superior ability to function above the average in a variety of settings and situations, to an inability to function effectively in any setting except in a restricted, supervised environment. Extremely effective individuals may not require any form of SH or SC. If these individuals do become involved in some form of SH, the purpose tends to involve augmenting an already existing, varied and working repertoire of skills, as in enrichment and fun in play (L'Abate, 2009d).

As we descend the ladder of effectiveness into relative or severe ineffectiveness, as reviewed in Part III of this volume, there is a corresponding increasing need for SH; lower rungs of the ladder indicate a need for SC. An inverse relationship exists between effectiveness in a variety of settings and need for SH and SC. Therefore, the relational competence theory is specifically concerned with how effective we are in our interactions with others and with objects.

Requirements of Relational Competence Theory

This theory requires specific criteria that differentiate this theory from extant ones.

Comprehensiveness

This requirement implies that the theory should be able to cover a variety of functional and dysfunctional levels of competence in a variety of settings.

Functional and Dysfunctional Behaviors: These behaviors may range from superior to diagnosable disorders defined by symptoms and syndromes found in various versions and revisions of the DSM-IV-TR (2000), including Global Assessment of Functioning (GAF).

Settings: SH and self-change can occur in one setting at a time or in more than one setting. Usually, SH may occur in just one setting while SC implies change in more than one setting. Model 3 will deal with this topic in greater detail.

Clinical Settings: These may be a community clinic, a specialized mental health center, a hospital, or the private office of a medical or psychological practitioner. Such settings may also include jails and penitentiaries.

Verifiability

This requirement means that whatever is done to produce SH and self-change needs to be made available in a reproducible format. Without replicability there cannot be verifiability allowing independent researchers to check and evaluate whatever claims one makes about the validity and reliability of any idea, including this theory.

Paper-and-pencil self-report tests, including experimental questionnaires: The experimental questionnaire and method of evaluation presented in Table 1.1 and Fig. 1.2 are completely reproducible but are unrelated to the theory. However, a variety of theory-derived paper-and-pencil self-report tests are available to interested readers (Cusinato & L'Abate, in press; L'Abate, 2005, 2010). Many have been subjected to repeated verification over the years.

Tasks and Interactive Practice Exercises: Many interactive practice exercises introduced in Chapter 3 of this volume (L'Abate, 2010) are related to models of the theory, allowing one to match evaluation with interventions in a manner that could be difficult or expensive to implement in traditional psychosocial interventions.

Therapeutic Prescriptions: Examples of theory-derived promotional prescriptions are the 3HC described in Chapter 1 of this volume for Model 7, Drawing Lines for Co-dependent women for a Selfhood Model 11, a Sharing of Hurts in Model 15 for intimacy. All three models are described below.

Better to be specific and "wrong" than to be generally non-specific and supposedly "right": This is the motto of the theory that in order to be verifiable whatever needs evaluation and modification needs to be specific. Specific of hypotheses can be verified more easily than general ones. Grand but vague theories cannot be evaluated *in toto*. This is why relational competence theory is broken into 16 relatively smaller, different but overlapping models that need to be evaluated one model at a time. The validity of the whole theory can only be evaluated model by model. The total validity of the theory depends on the sum total of the validity of its models (positive, questionable, or negative). The face-validity of these models was related to similar topics in various treatises in communication, personality, and relationship science (L'Abate, in press).

Redundancy: This requirement means that whatever behavior needs to be understood or modified can be understood and modified according to different but overlapping models and different approaches. SH and self-change can be understood and implemented according to a variety of models representative of the theory, by evaluation instruments, and by practical interventions.

Fruitfulness: A theory should promulgate research by those who are not connected to it, as in the case of attachment theory (Mikulincer & Shaver, 2007).

Models of the Theory Relevant to SH

There are 16 models that compose relational competence theory relevant to SH and self-change.

Identifying Basic, Underlying Factors

This theory includes three factors or models that are necessary in any theory of human relationships because they encapsulate what is known and important from the patient's past.

Model 1, ERAAwC: These letters stand for five components of an information-processing model that are present in any relationship and that are the basis for a variety of schools of thought and of psychotherapy (L'Abate, 2005).

Emotionality: How one feels and experiences subjectively at the receptive, input side of an information processing continuum. As discussed in a model of intimacy, these feelings include joys as well as hurts that need to be approached and shared with intimate others in a functional manner but that are avoided, hidden, denied, repressed, or suppressed in dysfunctional relationships. Many individuals have difficulty being aware of these feelings and they need to learn through SH and self-change how to "get in touch" with these feelings, especially, as discussed in Model 15, even if these feelings constitute the "unconscious or preconscious."

Rationality: Refers to thinking as well as to how intelligent one is in planning and forecasting future behavior necessary for problem-solving in practical and relational tasks. This component is important in self-help and self-change to plan and to realistically anticipate and understand the consequences of one's behavior. Cognitive appraisal, for instance, a process considered crucial to SC, is based on this component.

Activity: Refers to observable behavior as defined more specifically by other models. Both SH and SC requires one to engage in a variety of behaviors including activity involving words; however, words should be accompanied by actions, and actions typically speak louder than words. Non-verbal-motor activity and writing are considered options in this model. Play is included in non-verbal activities and play may be one of the best sources of SH available at any sage of the life cycle (L'Abate, in press).

Awareness: Refers to a continuum of how insightful one is about reflecting on one's errors and mistakes and changing them to improve SH and SC on the basis of past experiences, that is, Aw of personal errors. This Aw, ideally a form of meta-cognition, may range from the unconscious to being somewhat available either pre-quasi or semi-conscious, to being completely conscious (a healthy meta-cognitive skill set). Aw is necessary to successful SH and self-change. Without this corrective feedback function, SH and self-change are likely to be minimal. The "dissonance" model used to loose weight (Chapter 9, this volume; Tavris & Aronson, 2007) can be included at this stage. Individuals with high levels of pathology may not be able to access this corrective mechanism, remaining unchanged, no matter what forms of SH or self-change are attempted.

Context: Involves whatever is being perceived subjectively and what is happening that is affecting the individual with respect to spatial and temporal surroundings. In many disorders, for instance, the Aw of personal errors and of the context immediately surrounding them may be limited, defective, or distorted.

Model 2, Levels of Interpretation: This model refers to the process of trying to understand and interpret behavior and relationships at different levels of occurrence.

Describing human relationships includes one's public façade: How we present ourselves publicly is called "Impression Formation" or "impression-management". Some individuals with addictive disorders can present themselves in an extremely charming manner—those with antisocial personality disorder may be motivated to present themselves favorably in an attempt to manipulate others. How we behave in the privacy of our home and with intimate others is called the phenotypical sublevel.

Explaining human relationships implies two sublevels: (1) how we feel and think about ourselves is called the genotypical sublevel, and (2) the derivation of this process from our transgenerational experiences is called the historical sublevel. Many individuals may present themselves superficially as "nice" to the public but behave abominably in the privacy of intimate relationships. Addicted individuals, for instance, may hide their behavior from public scrutiny but repeat it in the safety of their homes.

Model 3, Settings: In contrast to contexts that are subjectively perceived, settings can be photographed and measured objectively. There are five classes of settings: (1) wherever we reside the most, what we call our *home* or residence; (2) where we learn how to *work*, such as schools, and where we actually work for a good part of our lives; (3) *leisure*, or surplus time settings in our home, school, or work including; (4) transitory settings, such as bars, beauty parlors, churches, grocery stores, gyms, or shopping malls; and (5) transit settings include roads, hotels, airports, bus stations as well as means by which we go from one settings to another, such as bicycles, buses, cars, and airplanes.

Identifying Basic Processes and Contents

These processes are necessary to survive and to enjoy life. Without them it would be impossible to achieve both priorities: survival and enjoyment.

Model 4, Ability to love: We approach who and what we love and avoid who and what we dislike along a dimension of *distance*: We want to remain close to a loved partner by marriage and by doing so we forsake, i.e., avoid others. We approach work because we need to survive and avoid wasting time with people or activities that would detract from that priority. We approach healthy food and activities and avoid unhealthy activities and food. We approach friends and family members we love and we avoid individuals and events we do not love or like, as shown in Fig. 1.1. In some instances, we have to face approach–avoidance conflict such as approaching authority figures we do not like or events and activities we experience as contrasting or contradictory feelings. We might not like funerals but we know that our presence is required if not needed. By this token, we approach SH and SC and avoid remaining the same especially if remaining the same means being involved in self-defeating and destructive activities, such as those included in Part III of this volume. Approach in its extreme may become over-dependence on a person, an activity, an object, or a substance, as in addictive behaviors (Chapter 10 this volume). Model 4 applies directly to Cluster C in Axis II of the DSM-IV-TR classification system to the extent that dependent personality disorders are the prototype for extreme approach and dependency (as in childhood), while fears, phobias, and avoidant personality disorders are the prototype for avoidance along a continuum ranging from innocuous fears to extremes where more than one person or one object are avoided, as the avoidant personality disorder, where such a dependency is avoided, denied, or suppressed (as in adolescence). The normative aspect of this approach is acceptance as adults of our continuous interdependence on others.

Model 5, Ability to control self: This ability occurs along a dimension of *self-regulation* characterized by extremes of *discharge* or disinhibition at one end and *delay*, inhibition, or constraint, both emotionally and cognitively at the other end (Gorfain & MacLeaod, 2007). We may approach or avoid someone or something either too fast or too slow. The locus of control can be internal, leading to internalizations, or external, leading to externalizations. This is the dimension that is inadequate, defective, or even missing in many disorders included in Part III, where these extremes are present. Functionality is present when there is an appropriate balance of discharge–delay functions according to life-cycle demands. This ability is necessary to negotiate problem-solving for SH and SC with intimates and non-intimates, as discussed in Model 16 of this theory. Model 5 applies directly to Cluster B of Axis II in the DSM-IV-TR to the extent that personality disorders in this Cluster are prototypes for discharge, verbal or non-verbal, physical or otherwise. Cluster C personality disorders tend to congregate on the delay side of this dimension.

Model 6, Ability to use both Processes: Combining Models 4 and 5 allows us to classify competence according to an assessment of GAF in the DSM-IV-TR with functioning varying from 0 (inadequate information) to 100 (superior functioning). When abilities to love and to control are balanced appropriately, in the approximate middle of each dimension, levels of functioning generally vary between 70 and 100 points on the GAF. When one type of ability is compromised and the other ability is highly functional, levels of competence are attenuated, varying between 40 and 69 points on the GAF. When both abilities are dysfunctional, then levels of competence are severely impaired, below 39 on the GAF.

Model 6, Ability to Balance Processes through Contents: Thus far, Models 4 and 5 describe processes without contents. There are six classes of resources that represent the contents of competence: Importance, Intimacy, Information, Services, Money, and Possessions. Combining Importance (Model 11) with Intimacy (Model 15) produces a modality of *Presence*: Being available emotionally and instrumentally to loved ones without demands for perfection, performance, or production. Combining Information with Services produces a modality of Doing or *Performance*. Combining Money with Possessions produces a modality of Possession or *Production*. Combining Performance with Production produces a supermodality of *Power*. In functional relationships Presence and Power are balanced democratically. In dysfunctional relationships both Presence and Power are transacted inadequately or ineffectively. Combining the three modalities of Being, Doing, and Possession, produces the Triangle of Living.

Extremes of Being are related to dysfunctionalities to the point that when this modality is predominant it may decrease Doing and Having. When Being is small it may enlarge Doing and Possessing. Examples of positive extremes in Being are present in Indus who rests on a bed of nails; negative Being is present in alexithymia where there is an inability to deal with feelings and emotions to be close to intimate others. Extremes in Doing are found in A-type personalities as reviewed in Chapter 10 of this volume. One extreme is illustrated by excessive exercise, on one hand, and inadequate personalities who are unable to work, on the other hand. Extremes of Having or Possessing are found in excessive spending (Chapter 10 this volume), financial tycoons, and in hoarders on one hand, and in religious orders that forgo worldly goods to help others, on the other hand. However, we require additional models to specify who wants and can use SH and SC.

Models Derived from Basic Factors, Processes, and Contents

Model 8, Self-identity: This model is developmental, represented by a dialectical continuum of resemblance or likeness: "Who am I and how am I like or unlike those who nurture me?" In other words, how do we resemble intimates with whom we have had close, committed, prolonged, and interdependent relationships since birth. For instance, the AA requirement to admit publicly that one is an alcoholic goes directly to self-identity, just as it applies to how we define our identities according to gender, age, marital status, occupation, and leisure time activities. This continuum of likeness varies along a curvilinear distribution ranging from Symbiosis, Sameness, and Similarity on one side versus Differentness, Oppositeness, and Alienation on the other side (Cusinato & Colesso, 2008; L'Abate, 2005; L'Abate & Cusinato, 2007). When Symbiosis is combined with Alienation we obtain the lowest level of competence, below 39 on the DSM measure of Global Functioning. When Sameness is combined with Differentness we obtain scores between 40 and 69 on that measure. When we combine Similarity with Differentness we obtain scores above 70.

Model 9, Styles in Intimate Relationships: These styles are derived from combinations obtained in Model 8. Symbiosis and Alienation are characterized by an Abusive-Apathetic (AA) or neglectful style. Sameness and Oppositeness are characterized by a Reactive-Repetitive (RR) style, while Similarity and Differentness are characterized by a Creative-Conductive (CC) style. CC uses SH freely and spontaneously because is it flexible and open to external feedback without needing SC. RR uses SH and SC with occasional external support. AA needs SH and SC with continuous external support.

Model 10, Interactions: The classifications present in Models 8 and 9 are process oriented to the extent that we need to add and rely on Model 7 to produce five different levels of interactions described according to an arithmetical model (L'Abate et al., 2010): The positive relationships of CC produce positive outcomes, either *multiplicative* or *additive* interactions where growth and change are the norm. The questionable relationships of RR produce *static* outcomes, where there is no growth or no breakdown, with positive and negative interactions remaining the same. The adverse relationships of AA tend to produce either *subtractive* or *divisive* outcomes, where deterioration, personal, and relational breakdown are the norm.

Model 11, Selfhood, the Attribution of Importance: This is a very important model that has been verified repeatedly (L'Abate, 2005; L'Abate et al., 2010) because it deals with the most important resource that is continuously exchanged among people: The attribution of importance to self and others as shown by compassion, caring, consideration, and concern. When this attribution is bestowed positively toward self and intimate others, a relational propensity called *Selfulness* ensues, where Presence is balanced with Performance and Production, with CC styles being multiplicative and additive. This propensity is visible in volunteers and those who help others without any selfish motives (Post, 2007). When this attribution of importance is bestowed positively on self but negatively on others, a relational propensity for *Selfishness* ensues with emphasis on Performance and Production at the expense of Presence, the RR styles are static and variable but essentially remain the same. When this attribution is bestowed negatively toward self but positively toward others, a relational propensity called Selflessness ensues, where RR styles are prevalent to keep relationships static (Chang, 2008; Post, 2007). Both Selfishness and Selflessness were described and defined operationally by experimental a variety of paper-and-pencil self-report instruments about co-dependency cited in Chapter 10 of this volume (L'Abate & Harrison, 1992).When this attribution is bestowed negatively toward both self and others, a relational propensity called *No-Self* ensues, where neither Presence, Production, or Performance can be accomplished and AA styles are predominant with subtractive or divisive interactions most likely.

Selfulness includes non-diagnosable conditions and some selected use of self-enhancement rather than SH. Selfishness includes Cluster B personality disorders of Axis II based on discharge and externalizations, leading to acting-out, criminality, and murder, with the need for SC before one can use SH. However, these individuals are the most resistant to SH and SC, asking for help during periods of breakdown, possible or real jail sentence, emotional or financial bankruptcy. Selflessness includes Cluster C of Axis II based on delay and internalizations, leading to anxiety and depression with self-mutilation and eventually suicide, with the need for SC before using SH. As Schwartz (2007, p. 39) found: "Giving beyond one's resources is, however, associated with worse reported mental health." Most people in this cluster are amenable to SH and SC. No-self includes Cluster A of Axis II and the disorders of Axis I in the DSM, severe psycho-pathology, bipolar disorders, and schizophrenias. Here SH may consist of medication compliance, voluntary attendance in group and/or family therapy, and a variety of other SH approaches that may or may not lead toward SC.

Model 12, Priorities: This model includes a variety of motivational concepts such as desires, needs, wants, goals, or intentions. No matter what one calls these concepts, ultimately they need to be ranked according to their importance and urgency to the individual according to how important and urgent these activities or settings may be. SH, for instance, may be desired before SC can occur, or SC might need to occur before one can use SH. Within both SH and SC one needs to choose what is most important and urgent. While Model 11 deals with how importance is attributed to others, Model 12 deals with how people, activities, settings, or objects are ranked according to their importance and urgency.

Applications of Previous Models

Model 13, Distance Regulation: This model is an extension of Model 4, except that here a model is proposed in terms of three dysfunctional roles, *Pursuer*, *Distancer*, and *Regulator*. Pursuers may want personal pleasure and profit, experienced physically, sexually, or financially, as in many addictive behaviors described in Chapter 10 of this volume. Distancers are afraid of both pleasure or profit and keep away from

either one or both. Regulators control distance inconsistently and contradictorily
by moving close and moving away from either pleasure or profit or may approach
pleasure and avoid profit or avoid pleasure and approach profit. They may want help
but when help is offered it may not be "good enough." This approach–avoidance
conflict is seen in many relapses in addictive behaviors (Chapter 10 this volume).

Model 14, Drama Triangle: This is a pathogenic model meaning that it lies at the
bottom of most dysfunctionalities (L'Abate, in press). It is composed of three roles
(*Victim, Rescuer, and Persecutor*) played contemporaneously and simultaneously
by anyone involved in such a triangle. One may feel victimized by the Persecutor;
however, the apparent Persecutor may feel victimized by whoever plays the role of
Victim. Both need to be rescued, either by another person, the Rescuer, or by some
other activity, object, or substance. Many addictive behaviors could be interpreted
as being used to Rescue one from avoidance of hurt feelings (L'Abate, 2009b).
This Triangle is found especially in the lives of inmates and addicts, and abusive
and incestuous families (L'Abate, 2009c). This is why many helpers need to be
careful not to become implicated in such a triangle out of the naïve, uncritical, and
unreflective need to help others.

Model 15, Intimacy: This model is defined as the sharing of joys, hurts, and
of fears of being hurt (L'Abate, 2009b). SH and self-change occurs at this level
based on the ability and willingness of another with which to share those hurt feelings. In functional relationships there is an approach toward admission and sharing
of hurt feelings with and among loved ones, including crying together (Hendricks
et al., 2008; Nelson, 2008). A great deal of dysfunctionality may be present here,
as in the case of disorders reviewed in Part III, and especially eating disorders
(Chapter 9 this volume). In dysfunctional relationships, admission and sharing of
feelings is either difficult or feels impossible. Hurt feelings are avoided intraperson-
ally and interpersonally. Consequently, there is no sharing and disturbing feelings
fester inside the individual effecting relationships and health (Vingerhoets et al.,
2008). Therefore, in dysfunctional relationships, healthy emotional intimacy cannot
occur.

Forgiveness is needed to help provide individuals with the intimate sharing of
errors and transgressions (Root & McCullough, 2007; Witvliet & McCullough,
2007). Unfortunately, without the admission and sharing of hurt feelings there is
no possibility to obtain forgiveness. One needs to be aware of one's hurt feelings
present in oneself and intimate others and be capable to forgive oneself for erring
before one can forgive others' transgressions (L'Abate, 1986). One could say that
sharing of hurts and of fears of being hurt is the *conditio sine qua non* for forgiveness
(L'Abate, 2005).

Model 16, Negotiation: This model is composed of two aspects: the structure and
the process of negotiating problem-solving. Structure applies to whether decisions
are large orchestrational (Shall we move to another city?) or small instrumental ones
(What kind of toothpaste shall I use?) and by who makes those decisions (authority)
and who carries them out (responsibility). Process involves (1) level of functioning: the higher this level the easier the possibility of successful negotiation (III),

(2) existing abilities (contained in all previous models) necessary to negotiate effectively (Skill), and (3) motivation to want to negotiate (Will). Unless these factors are present it is difficult to attempt SH and to achieve self-change.

Does the theory of relational competence answer the question, "Who benefits from SH and why?" The relational competence theory is comprehensive, verifiable, and specific enough to allow qualitative and quantitative evaluation of its component models as they apply to SH and self-change. Nonetheless, a theory, no matter how comprehensive, verifiable, and specific it may be, is not a substitute for evidence (L'Abate et al., 2010) and reality.

Back to Reality

In Chapter 1 of this volume we suggested two self-report measures that may help determine what specific areas of functioning would benefit from SH and self-change interventions. In Chapter 10 of this volume, in referring to co-dependency, we have cited a variety of theory-derived or theory-free instruments available to evaluate levels of functioning in intimate relationships. Above and beyond such an identification, throughout the various chapters, we have directly or indirectly suggested that successive sieves, hurdles, or steps approaches may be necessary in SH and SC (L'Abate, 1990). These steps go above and beyond theory or any self-report and is based on actual performance and production by participants rather than by their words. By systematically activating SH or self-change interventions and observing who responds and how they respond is important and should supplement what they self-report. This is the model nuanced in Chapter 1 that is based completely on costs, going from the least to the most expensive SH/SC intervention.

Consequently, to spell this model out, the following sequence of intervention is suggested. Given the four criteria of (1) cost-effectiveness, (2) mass-orientation, (3) ease of administration, and (4) no significant identified side effects, then generally speaking, any mental health SH and self-change approach should preclude more expensive and intensive approaches based on a cost-benefits analysis. Of course, patient dimensions, such as subjective distress, problem complexity and chronicity, functional impairment, and social support—all prognostic indicators and indicators of treatment intensity should be considered before assigning a patient to SH alone. In other words, some patients present with problems that are inappropriate for SH interventions alone—various levels of therapist involvement, multi-person, multi-modal, and multi-format treatment may all be required for a safe and effective therapeutic outcome.

Step 1. This step acknowledges the importance of objective evaluation about the need for SH and for SC. If possible, administer questionnaires presented in Table 1.1, available in L'Abate (1992c), and from other sources, keeping in mind that the first one is experimental in nature. Additionally the

clinical interview (to gather information on problem complexity and chronicity), information gathered from the SCL-90-R, particularly the GSI (for
a measure of subjective distress), measures of social support (e.g., Social
Support Questionnaire, SSQ, Sarason, Levine, Basham, & Sarason, 1983),
and a measure of functional impairment (GAF, DSM-IV-TR, 2000) would
help guide the clinician in the appropriate level of intervention and, if indicated, the implementation of SH. If SH is contraindicated as the sole method
of intervention, the clinician may proceed to symptom prevention, psychotherapy, and rehabilitation according to the four previously mentioned
criteria. Generally, SH interventions should be assigned when working with
relatively healthy populations before promotion, prevention, and psychotherapy are assigned as needed based on presenting problem(s). Additionally,
rehabilitation for special populations should be considered.

Step 2. Promotion is proactive and pre-therapeutic overlapping with SH activities. If the application of promotion at step 2 fails, the clinician should consider implementing more expensive, intensive, multi-person, and preventive
interventions.

Step 3. Prevention is para-active and para-therapeutic, targeted for not yet diagnosed but at risk-populations (Farrar, L'Abate, & Serritella, 1992). Step 3
approaches include targeted written practice exercises for populations at risk
(L'Abate, 2010). If this approach fails, the clinician may move to Step 4.

Step 4. Psychotherapy is reactive and therapeutic for diagnosed clinical,
chronic, and critical populations. For some, group treatment may be most
effective; however, not all are ready to tolerate this experience and individual
psychotherapy may be the most appropriate method of intervention.

Step 5. To improve the likelihood of success in Step 4, some participants
should be evaluated for pharmacotherapeutic interventions. Medication monitoring should be on-going and should allow for communication between the
psychiatrist and the therapist.

Step 6. If previous steps fail, rehabilitation (primarily occupational and social)
may be implemented to facilitate learning and relearning of previously
existing skills.

Conclusion

SH and self-change are areas of dynamic innovation and great promise. The
following are examples of what effective self-help and self-change can produce:

1. Presently, therapists are our primary mental health resources. Often, therapists
   are in high demand and unable to meet the needs of all who seek their services.
   In many cases, patients may feel they need a therapist when in fact, a variety
   of SH resources are sufficient. The modal number of therapy sessions is one,
   indicating that many patients simply need to be reassured that help is available.
   Unfortunately, these single sessions may be prevented by appropriate assignment
   to SH resources. Some method of assessment is required to determine if a patient

is a candidate for SH or requires more structured or intensive forms of treatment. A computer-administered program (WebPsych & InnerLife, 2009) is available for this very purpose. This sophisticated program is patient-driven and provides treatment recommendations based on computer administered assessment that range from "no treatment indicated" to intensive, long-term, multi-person treatment. Of course, SH is one of the options between the two foregoing extremes. If SH is indicated, information on a variety of resources is forthcoming, empirical support status is provided, and patients may chose which form of SH suits them most. SH materials have the potential to free up mental health resources (therapists) for more appropriate use of their time.

2. SH resources provide the patient with lasting guidance—a resource they can access repeatedly. These resources may also provide a sense of security because they are at the patient's fingertips. Relatedly, SH resources may increase a patient's sense of self-efficacy—they may feel like they can help themselves with minimal support or guidance from a book, manual, video, film, audiocassette, Internet source, or brochure.

3. SH has the potential to reach into communities where therapists are in low concentration. Rural areas may benefit most from the array of SH resources available. Additionally, prisoners may find SH useful as therapists are often not available for therapy or not available at all in prisons.

4. SH may augment or serve as an adjunct to therapy. SH may also play an integral role in therapy by providing focus and direction. In either case, SH resources have the potential to accelerate the change process and promote deeper levels of self-reflection.

5. SH is relatively inexpensive, convenient, and user-friendly. The sheer variety of resources available increases the likelihood that a patient will find multiple forms of SH to their liking.

6. Some individuals are not well-suited to psychotherapy. For instance, the highly reactant individual may perceive therapists as controlling and threatening to their independence—SH may be perceived as non-threatening. Agoraphobics may not be ready to leave the safety of their homes to receive psychotherapy without a considerable amount of therapist-supported SH. Individuals with a sexual dysfunction may find the privacy afforded by SH materials attractive and safe. Patients suffering from dependent personality disorder may be better served through a SH format than through dependence inducing individual psychosocial treatment.

7. The SH movement may actually help de-stigmatize mental health treatment by bringing into the home examples of what psychotherapists do and what constitutes treatment. More individuals may come to understand that mental health treatment is common, not embarrassing or an indication of weakness, and it is generally safe and quite effective. Contrary to the fears of many professionals, SH treatment may actually increase certain types of patient flow, primarily the many who require psychotherapy but often suffer for fear of stigmatization.

8. The "stepped-care" model is improved by considering SH resources. Additionally, SH materials may reduce the need for more intensive treatments and they may reduce the frequency and severity of relapse.

9. For those who benefit from SH and avoid the therapist's office, we say "Well
   done"—our goals as psychotherapists are to maximize patient enjoyment while
   at the same time doing what we can to provide the skills that will allow the
   patient to function well independent of the therapist. If this can be achieved sans
   therapists or with minimal therapist involvement, we have treated our patients in
   the most ethical manner possible.

We can be confident in stating that the SH movement in mental health is here to stay.
Innovations, efficacy and effectiveness research, profit motive, benefits to patients,
and increasing popularity will undoubtedly propel this movement in many directions
and to greater heights.

At present, the consumer should be aware that sham treatments exist, some are
dangerous while other treatments simply remain unsupported. It is the responsibility
of the developers and publishers of these materials to respect truth in advertising.
Publishers or developers of products or programs should clearly indicate if empirical
support exists—if so, they should provide a balanced and comprehensive review of
the research findings in layman's terms. False or unsubstantiated claims should be
avoided.

Therapists and physicians should become familiar with the SH materials that
have received empirical support. They should be able to advise their patients in the
selection of materials or Internet/computer programs. Many therapists keep a library
of SH materials for lending to patients—this is good practice and should be encouraged. Psychotherapy is effective in many forms and patients respond differentially
to various forms of intervention—the greater the array of potentially therapeutic
interventions, the higher the likelihood of positive change and the greater the magnitude of change. Of course, the accuracy of the foregoing statement is dependent
on the skill of the therapist in matching intervention, strategy, or principle of change
to the patient.

If SH is assigned as homework (as is often the case), it is extremely important for the therapist to review the homework and provide feedback. Ideally, this
review would take place in the early stage of any session that homework is due.
If a patient presents for therapy in great distress, this obviously takes precedence
over the review of homework. In such instances, the therapist should do what she
can to reduce distress levels and only proceed to homework if appropriate. In some
instances, review of homework and feedback on the assignment may have to wait
for another session. In any event, if homework is assigned and the therapist is not
attentive and appropriately responsive to the patient's efforts, compliance will suffer.
Compliance with homework is an important positive prognostic indicator.

In closing, some form(s) of SH should be considered for every patient. The tim-
ing of SH implementation and the selection of SH resources depends upon the status
of the patient along a variety of dimensions (matching dimensions, stage of change,
treatment readiness, severity of disturbance, etc.); however, at some point in treatment (or as a substitute for treatment), SH can serve the goals of the patient and
therapist well.

Appendix

Medical and non-medical newsletters containing credible advice and useful information about health matters for laypersons and professionals have proliferated during the last decade. Even though, these newsletters originate from different sources, the publisher for some may be the same, judging from the same address for many of them.

Cleveland Clinic, *Men's Health Advisor,* P. O. Box 5656, Norwalk, CT, 06856-5656.

Duke University Medicine, *HealthNews,* P. O. Box 5656, Norwalk, CT, 06856-5656.

Environmental Nutrition. Belvoir Media Group, 800 Connecticut Ave. Norwalk, CT, 06854-1631.

Harvard Medical School

> *Exercise and age: A prescription for mature adults.* Pamphlet.
> *Men's Health Watch,* Dr. Harvey B. Simon, 10 Shuttuck St., Boston, MA. 02115.
> *Mental Health Letter,* Dr. Michael Miller, 10 Shuttuck St., Boston, MA. 02115.
> *Strength and power training at any age,* Harvard Health Publications, P. O. Box 9307, Big Sandy, TX, 75755.
> *Takind blood pressure to new lows.* Pamphlet.

Johns Hopkins Medicine, *Special Health Reports,* Baltimore, MD. Medletter

> Associates, LLC, 6 Trowbridge Drive, Bethel, CT 06801.
> *Antidepressants: If the first drug doesn't work, don't give up.*
> *Depression and Anxiety Bulletin*
> *Getting relief from light therapy*
> *Is it "normal" worrying or an anxiety disorder?*
> *Supplemental Mood Prescription*
> *The Memory Bulletin.* P. O. Box 420879, Palm Coast, FL 32142-9305.
> *Which type of talk-therapy is right for you?*

T.M. Harwood, L. L'Abate, *Self-Help in Mental Health,*
DOI 10.1007/978-1-4419-1099-8, © Springer Science+Business Media, LLC 2010

The Johns Hopkins White Papers 2008 are highly recommended for their summary of recent research findings in an easy-to-read format.

Heart Attack Prevention
Memory
Nutrition and Weight Control for Longevity
Vision

Massachusetts General Hospital, *Mind, Mood, & Memory.* P. O. Box 5656, Norwalk, CT, 06856-5656.

Mayo Clinic, *Healthletter,* P. O. Box 9302, Big Sandy, TX 75755-9302.

Minnesota Medical School, St. Paul, MN. Address to be found

Mount Sinai School of Medicine, *Focus on Health Aging,* P. O. Box 5656, Norwalk, CT, 06856-5656.

Nutrition Action Newsletter, *Center for Science in the Public Interest,* Suite 300, 1875 Connecticut Avenue, N.W., Washington, DC, 2009-5728.

University of California, Berkeley, CA. address to be found

University of California, Los Angeles. Division of Geriatrics, *Healthy/Years: Helping older adults lead happier, healthier lives,* P. O. Box 5656, Norwalk, CT, 06856-5656.

References

Abadinsky, H. (2008). *Drug use and abuse: A comprehensive introduction*. Belmont, CA: Thomson

Abadinsky, H. (2008). *Drug use and abuse: A comprehensive introduction* (6th ed.). Belmont, CA: Thomson.

Ackerson, J., Scogin, F., McKendree-Smith, N., & Lyman, R. D. (1998). Cognitive bibliotherapy for mild and moderate adolescent depressive symptomology. *Journal of Consulting and Clinical Psychology, 66*, 685–690.

Adams, M. S. (2007). *Feminists say the darndest things: A politically incorrect professor confronts "womyn" on campus*. New York: Sentinel.

Adams, M. S. (2004). *Welcome to the ivory tower of babel: Confessions of a conservative college professor*. Augusta, GA: Harbor House.

Adams, T. L., & Smith, S. A. (Eds.). (2007). *The virtual world of geeks, gamers, shamans, and scammers*. Austin: University of Texas Press.

Adamsen, L. (2002). From victim to agent: The clinical and social significance of self-help group participation for people with life threatening diseases. *Scandinavian Journal of Caring Science, 16*, 224–231.

Addis, M. E., & Cardemil, E. V. (2006). Psychotherapy manuals can improve outcomes. In J. C. Norcorss, L. E. Beutler, & R. F. Levant (Eds.), *Evidence-based practices in mental health: Debate and dialogue on the fundamental questions* (pp. 131–140). Washington, DC: American Psychological Association.

Akhondzadeh, S. (2007). Herbal medicines in the treatment of psychiatric and neurological disorders. In L. L'Abate (Ed.), *Low-cost approaches to promote physical and mental health: Theory, research, and practice* (pp. 119–138). New York: Springer.

Alaszewski, A. (2006). *Using diaries for social research*. London: Sage.

Allan, W. D., & Workman, J. O. (2006). PMT: Empirical evidence and clinical pragmatics. *Psyccritiques*, 51, 1037–1042.

Allison, K. C., & Stunkard, A. J. (2007). Self-help for night eating syndrome. In J. D. Latner & G. T. Wilson (Eds.), *Self-help approaches for obesity and eating disorders: Research and practice*
(pp. 310–324). New York: Guilford.

Allport, G. W. (1942). *The use of personal documents in psychological science*. New York: Social Science Research Council.

Andersen, B. L. (1992). Psychological interventions for cancer patients to enhance the quality of life. *Journal of Consulting and Clinical Psychology, 60*, 552–568.

Anderson, J. S. (2007). Pleasant, pleasurable, and positive activities. In L. L'Abate (Ed.), *Low-cost approaches to promote physical and mental health: Theory, research, and practice* (pp. 201–217). New York: Springer.

Anderson, T., & Strupp, H. H. (1996). The ecology of psychotherapy research. *Journal of Consulting and Clinical Psychology, 64*, 776–782.

Anderson, P., Rothbaum, B. O., & Hodges, L. F. (2003). Virtual reality exposure in the treatment of social anxiety. *Cognitive and Behavioral Practice*, 10, 240–247.

Andersson, G., Bergström, J., Holländare, F., Carlbring, P., Kaldo, V, & Ekselius, L. (2005). Internet-based self-help for depression: Randomized controlled trial. *British Journal of Psychiatry, 187*, 456–461.

Andersson, G., Carlbring, P., Holmström, A., Sparthan, E., Furmark, T., Nilsson-Ihrfelt, E., et al. (2006). Internet-based self-help with therapist feedback and in-vivo group exposure for social phobia: A randomized controlled trial. *Journal of Consulting and Clinical Psychology, 74*, 677–686.

Andersson, G., Lundstrom, P., & Strom, L. (2003). Internet-based treatment of headache: Does telephone contact and anything? *Headache, 43*, 353–361.

Andrews, G., & Slade, T. (2001). Interpreting scores on the Kessler population. *Australian and New Zealand Journal of Public Health, 25*, 494–497.

Anie, K. A., & Green, J. (2002). Self-help manual-assisted cognitive behavioural therapy for sickle cell disease. *Behavioural and cognitive psychotherapy, 30*, 451–458.

Antony, M. M., & Swinson, R. P. (2000). *The shyness and social anxiety workbook: Proven techniques of overcoming your fears* . Oakland, CA: New Harbinger.

Antshel, K. M., & Barkley, R. (2008). Psychosocial interventions in attention deficit hyperactivity disorder. *Child and Adolescent Psychiatric Clinics of North America, 17*, 421–437.

Apodaca, T. R., & Miller, W. R. (2003). A meta-analysis of the effectiveness of bibliotherapy for alcohol problems. *Journal of Clinical Psychology, 59*, 289–304.

Archer, J. (2000). Sex differences in aggression between heterosexual partners: A meta-analytic review. *Psychological Bulletin, 126*, 651–680.

Areán, P. A., McQuaid, J., & Muñoz, R. F. (1997). Mood disorders: Depressive disorders. In S. M. Turner and M. Hersen (Eds.), *Adult psychopathology and diagnosis*, (pp. 230–255). New York: John Wiley and Sons.

Arntz, A., & Lavy, E. (1993). Does stimulus elaboration potentiate exposure in vivotreatment? Two forms of one-session treatment of spider phobia. *Behavioural Psychotherapy, 21*, 1–12.

Ash, E. L. (1920). *Mental self-help*. New York: The Macmillan Company.

Bachofen, M., Nakagawa, A., Marks, I. M., Park, J., Greist, J. H., Baer, L., et al. (1999). Home self-assessment and self-treatment of obsessive-compulsive disorder using a manual and a computer-conducted telephone interview: Replication of a U.K.-U.S. study. *Journal of Clinical Psychiatry, 60*, 545–549.

Baer, R. A. (2003). Mindfulness training as a clinical intervention: A conceptual and empirical review. *Clinical Psychology: Science and Practice, 10*, 125–143.

Bailer, U., de Zwaan, M., Leisch, F., Strnad, A., Lennkh-Wolfsberg, C., El-Giamal, N., et al. (2004). Guided self-help versus cognitive-behavioral group therapy in the treatment of bulimia nervosa. *International Journal of Eating Disorders, 35*, 522–537.

Baillie, A., & Rapee, R. M. (2004). Predicting who benefits from psychoeducation and self help for panic attacks. *Behaviour Research and Therapy, 42*, 513–527

Baker, B. L., Cohen, D. C., & Saunders, J. T. (1973). Self-directed desensitization for acrophobia. *Behaviour Research and Therapy, 11*, 79–89.

Banasiak, S. J., Paxton, S. J., Hay, P. J. (2007). Perceptions of cognitive behavioral guided self-help treatment for bulimia nervosa in primary care. *Eating Disorders: The Journal of Treatment & Prevention, 15*, 23–40.

Bara-Carril, N., Williams, C. J., Pombo-Carril, M. G., Reid, Y., Murray, K., Aubin, S., et al. (2004). A preliminary investigation into the feasibility and efficacy of a CD-ROM-based cognitive-behavioral self-help interventions for bulimia-nervosa. *International Journal of Eating Disorders, 35*, 538–548.

Bargh, J. A., & Williams, L. E. (2007). The noncoscious regulation of emotions. In J. J. Gross (Ed.), *Handbook of emotion regulation* (pp. 429–444). New York: Guilford Press.

Barker, J. C., & Hunt, G. (2007). Natural recovery: A cross-cultural perspective. In H. Klingemann & L. C. Sobell (Eds.), *Promoting self-change from addictive behaviors: Practical implications for policy, prevention, and treatment* (pp. 213–237). New York: Springer.

Barkley, R. A. (1997). *Defiant children: A Clinician's Manual for Assessment and Parent Training* (2nd ed.). New York: Guilford Press.

Barkley, R. A. (2005) *Attention-deficit hyperactivity disorder, a handbook for diagnosis and treatment* (3rd ed.). New York: Guilford.

Barkley, R. A., & Benton, C. M. (1998). *Your defiant child: 8 steps for better behavior*. New York: Guilford Press.

Barlow, D. H., & Craske, M. G. (2007). *Mastery of your anxiety and panic: Workbook*. New York: Oxford University Press.

Barrera, M., & Rosen, G. M. (1977). Detrimental effects of a self-reward contracting program of subjects' involvement in self–administered desensitization. *Journal of Consulting and Clinical Psychology, 45,* 1180–1181.

Barrett, P. M. (2004). *Friends for life! For children. Participant workbook and leader's manual*. Brisbane, Australia: Australian Academic Press.

Barrett, P. M. (2005). *Friends for life! For youth. Participant workbook and leader' manual*. Brisbane, Australia: Australian Academic Press.

Basco, M. R. (2006). *The bipolar workbook: Tools for controlling your mood swings*. New York: The Guilford Press.

Basco, M. R., & Rush, A. J. (2005). *Cognitive-behavioral therapy for bipolar disorder* (2nd ed.). New York: Guilford Press.

Bauer, M. S., McBride, L., (2003). *Structured group therapy for bipolar disorder: The Life Goals Program* (2nd ed.). New York: Springer

Baum, A., & Singer, J. (Eds.). (2001). *Handbook of health psychology*. Mahwah, NJ: Lawrence Erlbaum Associates.

Beck, A. T., & Steer, R. A. (1993). *Manual for the beck depression inventory*. San Antonio: The Psychological Corporation.

Beck, A. T., Epstein, N., Brown, G., & Steer, R. A. (1998). An inventory for measuring clinical anxiety: Psychometric properties. *Journal of Consulting and Clinical Psychology, 56,* 893–897.

Beck, A. T., Rush, A. J., Shaw, B. F., & Emery, G. (1979). *Cognitive therapy of depression: A treatment manual*. New York: Guilford Press.

Beck, A. T., Steer, R. A., & Brown, G. K. (1996). *Beck depression inventory manual* (2nd ed.). San Antonio, TX: Psychological Corporation.

Beck, A. T., Steer, R. A., & Brown, G. K. (1996). *Manual for beck depression inventory-II*. San Antonio, TX: Psychological Corporation.

Beck, A. T., Wright, F. D., Newman, C. F., & Liese, B. S. (1993). *Cognitive therapy of substance abuse*. New York: Guilford.

Bein, E., Anderson, T., Strupp, H. H., Henry, W. P., Schacht, T. E., Binder, J. L. et al. (2000). The effects of training in time-limited dynamic psychotherapy: Changes in therapeutic outcome. *Psychotherapy Research, 10,* 119–132.

Bekker, M. H. J., & Spoor, S. T. P. (2008). Emotional inhibition, health, gender, and eating disorders: The role of (over) sensitivity to others. In A. Vingerhoets, I. Nyklicek, & J. Denollet (Eds.), *Emotional regulation: Conceptual and clinical issues* (pp. 170–183). New York: Springer.

Belack, A. S., Bennett, M., & Gearon, J. (2007). *Behavioral treatment for substance abuse in people with serious and persistent mental illness: A handbook for mental health professionals*. New York: Brunner-Routledge.

Bender, D. S., Dolan, R. T., Skodol, A. E., Sanislow, C. A., Dyck, I. R., McGlashan, T. H., et al. (2001). Treatment utilization by patients with personality disorders. *American Journal of Psychiatry, 158,* 295–302.

Bender, D. S., Skodol, A. E., Dyck, I. R., Markowitz, J. C., Shea, M. T., Yen, S., et al. (2007). *Journal of Consulting and Clinical Psychology, 75,* 992–999.

Benson, H. (1982). The relaxation response: History, physiological basis and clinical usefulness. *Acta Medica Scandinavia-Supplementum, 660,* 231–237.

Benson, H., Kornhaber, A., Kornhaber, C., LeChanu, M. N. (1994). Increases in positive psychological characteristics with a new relaxation-response curriculum in high school students. *Journal of Research & Development in Education, 27,* 226–231.

Benson, H., Wilcher, M., Greenberg, B., Huggins, E., Ennis, M., Zuttermeister, P. C., et al. (2000). Academic performance among middle-school students after exposure to a relaxation response curriculum. *Journal of Research & Development in Education, 33,* 156–165.

Bentley, K., Walsh, J., Boyd, A., & Taylor, M. (2007). Schizophrenia. In B. A. Thyer & J. S. Wodarski (Eds.), *Social work in mental health: An evidence-based approach* (pp. 251–285). Hoboken, NJ: John Wiley & Sons Inc.

Bergin, A. E., & Garfield, S. L. (Eds.). (1994). *Handbook of psychotherapy and behavior change.* New York: Wiley.

Bernstein, D. P., Cohen, P., Skodol, A., Bezirganian, S., & Brooks (1996). Childhood antecedents of adolescent personality disorders. *American Journal of Psychiatry, 153,* 907–913.

Beutler, L. E. (1991). Have all won and must all have prizes: Revisiting Luborsky et al.'s verdict. *Journal of Consulting and Clinical Psychology, 59,* 226–232.

Beutler, L. E. (2000). David and Goliath: When psychotherapy research meets health care delivery systems. *American Psychologist, 55,* 997–1007.

Beutler, L. E. (2009). Making science matter in clinical practice: Redefining psychotherapy. *Clinical Psychology: Science and Practice, 16,* 301–317.

Beutler, L. E., Brookman, L., Harwood, T. M., Alimohamed, S., & Malik, M. M. (2002). Functional impairment and coping style. *Psychotherapy, 38,* 437–442.

Beutler, L. E., Castonguay, L. G., & Follette, W. C. (2006). Integration of therapeuticfactors in dysphoric disorders. In L. G. Castonguay & L. E. Beutler (Eds.), *Principles of therapeutic change that work* (pp. 111–120). New York: Oxford University Press.

Beutler, L. E., & Clarkin, J. E. (1990). *Systematic treatment selection: Toward targeted therapeutic interventions.* New York: Bruner/Mazel Publishers.

Beutler, L. E., Clarkin, J, F., & Bongar, B. (2000). *Guidelines for the systematic treatment of the depressed patient.* New York: Oxford University Press.

Beutler, L. E., & Harwood, T. M. (2000). *Prescriptive psychotherapy: A practical guide to systematic treatment selection.* New York: Oxford University Press. Translated to Italian: (2002) *Psicoterapia Prescrittiva Elettiva.* Roma: Sovera.

Beutler, L. E., & Harwood, T. M. (2000). *Prescriptive psychotherapy: A practical guide to systematic treatment selection.* New York: Oxford University Press.

Beutler, L. E., & Harwood, T. M. (2004). Virtual reality in psychotherapy training. *Journal of Clinical Psychology (special issue),* on "Technological Developments and Applications", *60,* 317–330.

Beutler, L. E., Kim, E. G., Davison, E., Karno, M., & Fisher, D. (1996). Research contributions to improving managed health care outcomes. *Psychotherapy, 33,*197–206.

Beutler, L. E., Malik, M. M., Alimohamed, S., Harwood, T. M., Talebi, H., Noble, S. et al. (2004). Therapist variables. In M. J. Lambert (Ed.), *Bergin and Garfield's handbook of psychotherapy and behavior change* (5th ed., pp. 227–306). New York: John Wiley & Sons, Inc.

Beutler, L. E., Moleiro, C., Malik, M. & Harwood, T. M. (2003). A new twist on empirically supported treatments. *International Journal of Clinical and Health Psychology, 3,* 423–437.

Beutler, L. E., Moleiro, C., Malik, M., Harwood, T. M., Romanelli, R., Gallagher, et al. (2003). A comparison of the Dodo, EST, and ATI factors among co-morbid stimulant dependent, depressed patients. *Clinical Psychology and Psychotherapy, 10,* 69–85.

Beutler, L. E., Williams, O. B., & Norcross, J. C. (2009). *Systematic treatment.* A proprietary software program.

Bilich, L. L., Deane, F. P., Phipps, A. B., Barisic, M., & Gould, G. (2008). Effectiveness of bibliotherapy self-help for depression with varying levels of telephone helpline support. *Clinical Psychology and Psychotherapy, 15,* 61–74.

Black, D. W., & Sheline, Y. I. (1997). Predictors of long-term outcome in 45 men with antisocial personality disorder. *Annals of Clinical Psychiatry, 9,* 211–217.

Black, D. W., Monahan, P., Baumgard, C. H., & Bell, S. E. (1997). Predictors of long-term outcome in 45 men with antisocial personality disorder. *Annals of Clinical Psychiatry, 9,* 211–217.

Blanchard, E. B., Andrasik, F., Appelbaum, K. A., Evans, D. D., Jurish, S. E., Teders, S. J., et al. (1985). The efficacy of cost-effectiveness of minimal-therapist-contact, non-prescription drug treatments of chronic migraine and tension headache. *Headache, 25,* 214–220.

Blomquist, J. (2007). Self-change from alcohol and drug abuse: Often-cited classics. In H. Klingemann & L. C. Sobell (Eds.), *Promoting self-change from addictive behaviors: Practical implications for policy, prevention, and treatment* (pp. 31–57). New York: Springer.

Bloom, B. L. (1992). Computer-assisted psychological interventions: A review and commentary. *Clinical Psychology Review, 12,* 169–197.

Bogalo, L., & Moss-Morris, R. (2006). The effectiveness of homework tasks in an irritable bowel syndrome self-management programme. *New Zealand Journal of Psychology, 35,* 120–125.

Bogenschutz, M. P. (2005). Specialized 12-step programs and 12-step facilitation for the dually diagnosed. *Community Mental Health Journal, 41,* 7–20.

Bogenschutz, M. P. (2007). 12-step approaches for the dually diagnosed: Mechanisms of change. *Alcoholism: Clinical and Experimental Research, 31,* 64S–66S.

Bohart, A. C., & Tallman, K. (1999). *How clients make therapy work: The process of active self-healing.* Washington, DC: American Psychological Association.

Borins, M., Holzapfel, S., Tudiver, F., & Bader, E. (2007). Counseling and psychotherapy skills training for family physicians. *Family Systems and Health, 25,* 382–391.

Bowman, D., Scogin, F., & Lyrene, B. (1995). The efficacy of self-examination therapy and cognitive bibliotherapy in the treatment of mild to moderate depression. *Psychotherapy Research, 5,* 131–141.

Bradley-Bolen, B. (2000). *Breaking the bonds of irritable bowel syndrome: A psychological approach to regaining control of your life.* Oakland, CA: New Harbinger Publications, Inc.

Breitholtz, E., & Öst, L. (1997). Therapist behaviour during one-session exposure treatment of spider phobia: Individual versus group setting. *Scandinavian Journal of Behaviour Therapy. 26,* 171–180.

Breslau, N., & Anthony, J. C. (2007). Gender differences in the sensitivity to posttraumatic stress disorder: An epidemiological study of urban young adults. *Journal of Abnormal Psychology, 116,* 607–611.

Brown, R. (2006). Speaking of "poppycock". . . a reply to the wall street journal. *ASAM News: Newsletter of the American Society of Addiction Medicine, 21,* 5–6.

Brown, V. (2008). No weighting. *Miller-McCune: Turning Research into Solutions, August,* 18–21.

Bryant, R. A., & Harvey, A. G. (2003). Gender differences in the relationship between acute stress disorder and posttraumatic stress disorder following motor vehicle accidents. *Australian and New Zealand Journal of Psychiatry, 37,* 226–229.

Buchanan, L. P., & Buchanan, W. L. (1992). Eating disorders: Bulimia and anorexia. In L. L'Abate, J. A. Farrar, & D. A. Serritella (Eds.), *Handbook of differential treatments for addictions* (pp. 165–188). Boston: Allyn & Bacon.

Buenaver, L. F., McGuire, L., & Haythronthwaite, J. A. (2006). Cognitive-behavioral self-help for chronic pain. *Journal of Clinical Psychology: In Session, 62,* 1389–1396.

Buhrman, M., Faltenhag, S., Strom, L., & Andersson, G. (2004). Controlled trial of internet-based treatment with telephone support for chronic back pain. *Pain, 111,* 368–377.

Burgoon, J. K., & Bacue, A. E. (2003). Nonverbal communication skills. In J. O. Greene & B. R. Burleson (Eds.), *Handbook of communication and social interaction skills* (pp. 179–219). Mahwah, NJ: Lawrence Erlbaum Associates.

Burns, D. D. (1980). *Feeling good: The new mood therapy.* New York: Signet.

Burns, D. D., & Noel-Hoeksema, S. (1992). Therapeutic empathy and recovery from depression in cognitive-behavioral therapy: A structural equation model. *Journal of Consulting and Clinical Psychology, 60,* 441–449.

Burti, L., Amaddeo, F., Ambrosi, M., Bonetto, C., Cristofalo, D., Ruggeri, M., & Tansella, M. (2005). Does additional care provided by a consumer self-help group improve psychiatric outcome? A study in an Italian community-based psychiatric services. *Community Mental Health Journal, 41,* 705–720.

Busuttil, W. (2004). Presentations and management of Post Traumatic Stress Disorderand the elderly: A need for investigation. *International Journal of Geriatric Psychiatry, 19*, 429–439.

Butcher, J. N. (1990). *The MMPI-2 in psychological treatment.* New York: Oxford University Press.

Butcher, J. N. (Ed). (2000). *Basic sources for the MMPI-2.* Minneapolis: University of Minnesota Press.

Butryn, M. L., Phelan, S., & Wing, R. R. (2007). Self-guided approaches to weight loss. In J. D. Latner & G. T. Wilson (Eds.), *Self-help approaches for obesity and eating disorders: Research and practice* (pp. 1–20). New York: Guilford.

Calogero, R., & Pedrotty, K. (2007). Daily practices for mindful exercise. In L. L'Abate (Ed.), *Low-cost approaches to promote physical and mental health: Theory, research, and practice* (pp. 141–160). New York: Springer.

Campbell, L. F., & Smith, T. P. (2003). Integrating self-help books into psychotherapy. *Journal of Clinical Psychology, 59*, 177–186.

Carbolla, J. L., Fernandez-Hermida, J. R., Secades-Villa, R., Sobell, L. C., Dum, M., & Garcia-Rodriquez, O. (2007). Natural recovery from alcohol and drug problems: A methodological review of the literature from 1999 through 2005. In H. Klingemann & L. C. Sobell (Eds.), *Promoting self-change from addictive behaviors: Practical implications for policy, prevention, and treatment* (pp. 87–102). New York: Springer.

Carducci, B. J. (1999). Shyness: A bold new approach. New York: Harper Collins.

Carducci, B. J. (2005). *The shyness workbook: 30days to dealing effectively with shyness.* Champaign, IL: Research Press.

Carducci, B. J., & Fields, T. H. (2007). *The shyness workbook for teens.* Champaign, IL: Research Press.

Carlbring, P., & Andersson, G. (2006). Internet and psychological treatment: How well can they be combined? *Computers in Human Behavior, 22*, 545–553.

Carlbring, P., Bohman, S., Brunt, S., Buhrman, M., Westling, B. E., Ekselius, L., et al. (2006). Remote treatment of panic disorder: A randomized trial of Internet-based cognitive behavior therapy supplemented with telephone calls. *American Journal of Psychiatry, 163*, 2119–2125.

Carlbring, P., Furmark, T., Steczkó, J., Ekselius, L., & Andersson, G. (2006). An open study of Internet-based bibliotherapy with minimal therapist contact via email for social phobia. *Clinical Psychology, 10*, 30–38.

Carlbring, P., Gunnarsdottir, M., Hedensjö, L., Andersson, G., Ekselius, L., & Furmark, T. (2007). Treatment of social phobia: Randomized trial of internet-delivered cognitive-behavioral therapy with telephone support. *British Journal of Psychiatry, 190*, 123–128.

Carlbring, P., Nilsson-Ihrfelt, E., Waara, J., Kollenstam, C., Buhrman, M., Kaldo, V., et al. (2005). Treatment of panicdisorder: Live therapy vs. self-help via the internet. *Behaviour Research and Therapy, 43*, 1321–1333.

Carr, J. E. (2008). Advancing psychology as a bio-behavioral science. *Journal of Clinical Psychology in Medical Settings, 15*, 40–44.

Carrard, I., Rouget, P., Fernandez-Aranda, F., Volkart A. C., Damoiseau M., & Lam T. (2006). Evaluation and deployment of evidence based patient self-management support program for bulimia nervosa. *International Journal of Medical Informatics, 75*, 101–109.

Carrington, P., Collings, G., Benson, H., Robinson, H., Wood, L. W., & Lehrer, P. M. (1980). The use of meditation-relaxation techniques for the management of stress in a working population. *Journal of Occupational Medicine, 22*, 221–231.

Carter, J. C., & Fairburn, C. G. (1998). Cognitive-behavioral self-help for binge eating disorder: A controlled effectiveness study. *Journal of Consulting and Clinical Psychology, 66*, 616–623.

Castonguay, L. G., & Beutler, L. E. (2006a). Common and unique principles of therapeutic change: What do we know and what do we need to know? In L. G. Castonguay & L. E. Beutler (Eds.), *Principles of therapeutic change that work* (pp. 353–369). New York: Oxford University Press.

Castonguay, L. G., & Beutler, L. E. (2006b). Principles of therapeutic change: A TaskForce on participants, relationships, and technique factors. *Journal of Clinical Psychology, 62*, 631–638.

Castonguay, L. G., & Beutler, L. E. (2006c). Therapeutic factors in dysphoric disorders. *Journal of Clinical Psychology, 62,* 639–647.

Castonguay, L. G., Goldfried. M. R., Wiser, S., & Raue, P. J. (1996). Predicting the effect of cognitive therapy for depression: A study of unique and common factors. *Journal of Consulting and Clinical Psychology, 64,* 497–504.

Centers for Disease Control and Prevention (2000). Use of FDA-approved pharmacological treatments for tobacco dependence—United States, 1984–1998. *Morbidity and Mortality Weekly Report, 49,* 665–668.

Chambless, D. L. (1990). Spacing of exposure sessions in treatment of agoraphobia and simple phobia. *Behavior Therapy, 21,* 217–219.

Chambless, D. L., & Ollendick, T. H. (2001). Empirically supported psychological interventions: Controversies and evidence. *Annual Review of Psychology, 52,* 685–716.

Chambless, D. L., Baker, M. J., Baucom, D. H., Beutler, L. E., Calhoun, K. S., Crits-Christoph, P., et al. (1998). Update on empirically validated therapies, II. *The Clinical Psychologist, 51,* 3–16.

Chambless, D. L., Sanderson, W. C., Shoham, V., Johnson, S. B., Pope, K. S., Crits-Christoph, P., et al. (1996). An update on empirically validated therapies. *Clinical Psychologist, 49,* 5–14.

Chambless, D., Foa, E., Groves, G., & Goldstein, A. (1982). Exposure and communications training in the treatment of agoraphobia. *Behaviour Research and Therapy, 20,* 219–231.

Chang, E. C. (Ed.). (2008). *Self-criticism and self-enhancement: Theory, research, and clinical applications.* Washington, DC: American Psychological Association.

Chapman, L. J., & Chapman, J. P. (1969). Illusory correlation (a an) obstacle to the use of valid psychodiagnostic signs. *Journal of Abnormal Psychology, 74,* 193–204.

Chatwin, J., & Tovey, P. (2004). Complementary and alternative medicine (CAM), cancer and group-based action: A critical review of the literature. *European Journal of Cancer Care, 13,* 210–218.

Chow, M. J., Anderson, G. C., Good, M., Dowling, D. A., Shiau, S. H., & Chu, D. M. (2002). A randomized controlled trial of early kangaroo care for preterm infants: effects on temperature, weight, behavior, and acuity. *Journal of Nursing Research, 10,* 129–142.

Christensen, H., & Griffiths, K. M. (2002). The prevention of depression using the internet. *The Medical Journal of Australia, 177,* S122–S125.

Christensen, H., Griffiths, K. M., & Jorn, A. F. (2004). Delivering interventions for depression by using the internet: A randomized controlled trial. *British Medical Journal, 328,* 265–268.

Chu, B. C. (2008). Empirically supported training approaches: The who, what, and how of disseminating psychological interventions. *Clinical Psychology: Science and Practice, 15,* 308–312.

Chung, H., Culpepper, L., De Wester, J. N., Grieco, R. L., Kaye, N. S., Lipkin, M., et al. (2007). Clinical management of bipolar disorder: Role of the primary care provider. *Supplement to the Journal of Family Practice, 56,* 43–56.

Clay, S., Schell, B., Corrigan, P. W., & Ralph, R. O. (Eds.). (2005). On our own, together: Peer programs for people with mental illness. Nashville, TN: Vanderbilt University Press.

Clark, D. A. (2004). *Cognitive-Behavioral therapy for OCD.* New York: Guilford.

Clark, F. (1973). Self-administered desensitization. *Behaviour Research and Therapy, 11,* 335–338.

Clark, A., Kirkby, K. C., Daniels, B. A., & Marks, I. M. (1998). A pilot study of computer-aided vicarious exposure for obsessive-compulsive disorder. *Australian and New Zealand Journal of Psychiatry, 32,* 268–275.

Clark, P. G., Dawson, S. J., Scheiderman-Miller, C., & Post, M. L. (2002). TeleRehab: Stroke teletherapy and management using two-way interaction video. *Neurology Report, 26,* 87–93.

Clarke, G., Lynch, F., Spofford, M., & DeBar, L. (2006). Trends influencing future delivery of mental health services in large healthcare systems. *Clinical Psychology, Science and Practice, 13,* 287–292.

Clum, G. A. (2008). Self-help interventions: Mapping the role of self-administered treatments in mental health. In P. L. Watkins & G. A. Clum (Eds.), *Handbook of self-help therapies* (pp. 41–58). Mahwah, NJ: Erlbaum.

Clum, G. A., & Watkins, P. L. (2008). Self-help therapies: Retrospect and prospect. In P. L. Watkins & G. A. Clum (Eds.), *Handbook of self-help therapies* (pp. 419–436). New York: Rutledge.

Cohen, L. J. (1993). The therapeutic use of reading: A qualitative study. *Journal of Poetry Therapy, 7,* 73–83.

Cohen, P., Crawford, T. N., Johnson, J. G., & Kasen, S. (2005). The Children in the Community Study of developmental course of personality disorder. *Journal of Personality Disorders, 19,* 466–486.

Coid, J. W. (1993). An affective syndrome in psychopaths with borderline personality disorder? *British Journal of Psychiatry, 162,* 641–650.

Colby, K. M. (1995). Clinical computing: A computer program using cognitive therapy to treat depressed patients. *Psychiatric Services, 46,* 1223–1225.

Coon, D. W., Thompson, L. W., & Gallagher-Thompson, G. (2007). Adapting homework for an older adult client with cognitive impairment. *Cognitive and Behavioral Practice, 14,* 252–260.

Cooney, J. (1992). Sexual abuses and offenses. In L. L'Abate, J. A. Farrar, & D. A. Serritella (Eds.), *Handbook of differential treatments for addictions* (pp. 123–150). Boston: Allyn & Bacon.

Cooney, N. L., Kadden, R. M., Litt, M. D., & Getter, H. (1991). Matching alcoholics to coping skills or interactional therapies: Two year-follow-up results. *Journal of Consulting and Clinical Psychology, 59,* 598–601.

Cornes, C. (1990). Interpersonal psychotherapy of depression. In R. Wells and V. Gianetti (Eds.), *Handbook of the brief psychotherapies.* New York: PlenumPress.

Corrigan, P. W., Wassel, A. K., & Rafacz, J. D. (2008). An evidence-based approach to psychiatric rehabilitation. In L. L'Abate (Ed.), *Toward a science of clinical psychology: Laboratory evaluations and interventions* (pp. 283–305). New York: Nova Science.

Cotler, S. B. (1970). Sex differences and generalization of anxiety reduction with auto- mated desensitization and minimal therapist interaction. *Behaviour Research and Therapy, 8,* 273–285.

Craske, M. G., & Barlow, D. H. (2006). *Mastery of your anxiety and worry: Workbook* (2nd ed.). New York: Oxford University Press.

Craske, M. G., & Barlow, D. H. (2007a). *Mastery of your anxiety and panic: Therapist Guide.* New York: Oxford University Press.

Craske, M. G., & Barlow, D. H. (2007b). *Mastery of your anxiety and panic, Workbook for primary care settings.* New York: Oxford University Press.

Craske, M. G., Barlow, D. H., & Meadows, E. (1994). *Therapist's guide for the mastery of your anxiety and panic II & agoraphobia supplement (Map II) program.* New York: Graywind Publications Incorporated

Crawford, J. J., & Pomerinke, K. A. (2003). *Therapy pets: The animal-human healing partnership.* Amherst, NY: Prometheus Books.

Cregor, M. (2008). The building blocks of positive behavior. *Teaching Tolerance, 34,* 18–21.

Crits-Christoph, P., Baranackie, K., Durcias, J. S., Beck, A. T., Carroll, K., Perry, K., et al. (1991). Meta-analysis of therapist effects in psychotherapy outcome studies. *Psychotherapy Research, 1,* 81–91.

Csikszentmihaly, M. (2004). Materialism and the evolution of consciousness. In T. Kasser & A. D. Kanner (Eds.), *Psychology and consumer culture: The struggle for a good life in a materialistic world* (pp. 91–106). Washington, DC: American Psychological Association.

Cucciare, M. A., Weingardt, K. R., & Villafranca, S. (2008). Using blended learning toimplement evidence-based psychotherapies. *Clinical Psychology: Science and Practice, 15,* 299–307.

Cuijpers, P. (1997). Bibliotherapy in unipolar depression: A meta-analysis. *Journal of Behavior Therapy and Experimental Psychiatry, 28,* 139–147.

Cuijpers, P, van Straten, A., & Andersson, G. (2008). Internet-administered cognitive behavioral therapy for health problems: A systematic review. *Journal of Behavioral Medicine, 31,* 169–177.

Cullen, L., & Barlow J. (2002). 'Kiss, cuddle, squeeze': the experiences and meaning of touch among parents of children with autism attending a Touch Therapy Programme. *Journal of Child Health Care, 6,* 171–178.

Cunningham, J. A., Humphreys, K., Koski-Jännes, A., & Cordingley, J. (2005). Internet and paper self-help materials for problem drinking: Is there an additive effect? *Addictive Behaviors, 30,* 1517–1523.

Currie, S. R. (2008). Self-help therapies for insomnia. In P. L. Watkins & G. A. Clum (Eds.), *Handbook of self-help therapies* (pp. 215–241). Mahwah, NJ: Erlbaum.

Curry, S. J., Ludman, E. J., & McClure, J. (2003). Self-administered treatment for smoking cessation. *Journal of Clinical Psychology, 59,* 305–319.

Curry, S. J., Marlatt, G. A., Gordon, J., & Baer, J. S. (1988). A comparison of alternative theoretical approaches to smoking cessation and relapse. *Health Psychology,* 7, 545–556.

Cusinato, M. (2004). Marriage preparation and maintenance. In L. L'Abate (Ed.). *Workbooks in prevention, psychotherapy, and rehabilitation: A resource for clinicians and researchers* (pp. 217–245). Binghamton, New York: Haworth.

Cusinato, M., & L'Abate, L. (in press). *Advances in relational competence theory: With special attention to alexithymia.* New York: Nova Science Publishers.

D'Zurilla, T. J., & Nezu, A. M. (1999). *Problem solving therapy: A social competence approach to clinical intervention* (3rd ed.). New York: Springer.

Daldrup, J. J., Beutler, L. E., Engle, D., & Greenberg, L. (1988). *Focused expressive psychotherapy: Freeing the overcontrolled patient.* New York: Guilford.

Dane, A. V., & Schneider, B. H. (1998). Program integrity in primary and early secondary prevention: Are implementation effects out of control? *Clinical Psychology Review, 18,* 23–45.

Davison, G. C., & Lazarus, A. A. (1995). The dialectics of science and practice. In S. C. Hayes, V. M. Follette, R. M. Dawes, & K. E. Grady (Eds.), *Scientific standards of psychological practice: Issues and recommendations* (pp. 95–120). Reno, NV: Context Press.

Dawes, R. M., Faust, D., & Meehl, P. E. (1989). Clinical versus actuarial judgment. *Science, 243,* 1668–1674.

Day, S. X., & Schneider, P. L. (2002). Psychotherapy using distance technology: Acomparison of face-to-face, video, and audio treatment. *Journal of Counseling Psychology, 49,* 499–503

de Andrés, R., Aillon, N. Bardiot, M., Bourgeois, P., Mertel, S., Nerfin, F., et al. (2006). Impact of the life goals group therapy program for bipolar patients: An open study. *Journal of Affective Disorders, 93,* 253–257.

De Giacomo, P., L'Abate, L., Margari, F., De Giacomo, A., Santamato, W., & Masellis, R. (2008). Sentences with strong psychological impact in psychotherapy: Research in progress. *Journal of Contemporary Psychotherapy, 38,* 65–72.

De Giacomo, P., L'Abate, L., Pennebaker, J. M., & Rumbaugh, D. M. (2008). *Amplifications and applications of Pennebaker's analogic to digital model in health promotion, prevention, and psychotherapy.* Manuscript submitted for publication.

De Giacomo, P., L'Abate, L., Santamato, W., Sgobio, A., Tarquinio, C., De Giacomo, A., et al. (2007). Compass sentences with strong psychological impact in family therapy: Preliminary investigations. *Journal of Family Psychotherapy, 18,* 45–69.

de Graaf, L. E., Gerhards, S. A. H., Evers, S. M. A. A., Arntz, A., Riper, H., Severens, J. L., et al. (2008). Clinical and cost-effectiveness of computerized cognitive behavioural therapy for depression in primary care: Design of a randomized trial. *BioMed Central Public Health, 8,* 1–11.

de Jongh, A., Muris, P., ter Horst, G., & van Zuuren, F. (1995). One-session cognitivetreatment of dental phobia: Preparing dental phobics for treatment by restructuring negative cognitions. *Behaviour Research and Therapy, 33,* 947–954.

DeAngelis, T. (2008). One treatment for emotional disorders? *Monitor on Psychology, 39,* 26–27.

Deckro, G. R., Ballinger, K. M., Hoyt, M., Wilcher, M., Dusek, J., Myers, P., et al. (2002). The evaluation of mind/body intervention to reduce psychological distress and perceived stress in college students. *Journal of American College Health, 50,* 281–287.

Delinsky, S. S., Latner, J. D., & Wilson, G. T. (2006). Binge eating and weight loss in a self-help behavior modification program. *Obesity, 14,* 1244–1249.

Demetrio, D., & Borgonovi, C. (2007). Teaching to remember ourselves: The autobiographical methodology. In L. L'Abate (Ed.), *Low-cost approaches to promote physical and mental health: Theory, research, and practice* (pp. 251–270). New York: Springer.

Den Boer, P. C. A. M., & Raes, C. H. J. M. (1997). *Contact & Relationship*: (1) self-therapy theory manual; (2) manual for practicing cognitive self-therapy; (3) manual for self-assessment of the treatment process. Groningen: Stichting Inde Granaetappel.

Den Boer, P. C. A. M., Wiersma, D., Van den Bosch, R. J. (2004). Why is self-help neglected in the treatment of emotional disorders? A meta-analysis. *Psychological Medicine, 34,* 959–971.

Detweiler-Bedell, J. B., & Whisman, M. A. (2005). A lesson in assigning homework: Therapist, client, and task characteristics in cognitive therapy for depression. *Professional Psychology: Research and Practice, 36,* 219–223.

Devineni, T., & Blanchard, E. B. (2005). A randomized controlled trial of an internet-based treatment for chronic headache. *Behaviour Research and Therapy, 43,* 277–292.

Diagnostic and statistical manual of mental disorders (4th ed.), *Text Revision.* (2000). Washington, DC: American Psychiatric Association.

Diagnostic and statistical manual of mental disorders, 3rd ed., rev. (1987). Washington, DC: American Psychiatric Association.

Dimeff, L. A., & Koerner, K. (2007). *Dialectical behavior therapy in clinical practice: Applications across disorders and settings.* New York: Guilford Press.

Dobson, K. S., & Shaw, B. F. (1988). The use of treatment manuals in cognitive therapy: Experience and issues. *Journal of Consulting and Clinical Psychology, 56,* 673–680.

Dolan, M. S., & Faith, M. S. (2007). Prevention of overweight with young children and families. In J. D. Latner & G. T. Wilson (Eds.), *Self-help approaches for obesity and eating disorders: Research and practice* (pp. 265–288). New York: Guilford.

Doweiko, H. E. (2009). *Concepts of chemical dependency* (7th ed.). Belmont, CA: Brooks/Cole.

Doweiko, H. E. (2008). *Concepts of chemical dependency* (7th ed.). Belmont, CA: Brooks/Cole.

Doweiko, H. E. (2006). *Concepts of chemical dependency* (6th ed.). Belmont, CA: Thomson.

Dulicai, D., & Shelley-Hill, E. (2007). Expressive movement. In L. L'Abate (Ed.), *Low-cost approaches to promote physical and mental health: Theory, research, and practice* (pp. 17–200). New York: Springer.

Duncan, B. L., & Miller, S. D. (2006). Treatment manuals do not improve outcomes. In J. C. Norcorss, L. E. Beutler, & R. F. Levant (Eds.), *Evidence-based practices in mental health: Debate and dialogue on the fundamental questions* (pp. 140–149). Washington, DC: American Psychological Association.

Dworkin, S. F., Turner, J. A., Wilson, L., Massoth, D., Whitney, C., Huggins, K. H., et al. (1994). Brief group cognitive-behavioral intervention for temporomandibular disorders. *Pain, 59,* 175–187.

Eaton, W. W., Drymann, A., Sorenson, A., & McCutcheon, A. (1989). DSM-III Major Depressive Disorder in the community: A latent class analysis of data from the NIMH Epidemiologic Catchment Area Programme. *British Journal of Psychiatry, 155,* 48–54.

Edgar, L. N., Tosberger, Z., & Nowlis, D. (1992). Coping with cancer during the first year after diagnosis: Assessment and intervention. *Cancer, 69,* 817–828.

Ehlers, A., Clark, D. M., Hackmann, A., McManus, F., Fennell, M., Herbert, et al. (2003). A Randomized controlled trial of cognitive therapy, a self-help booklet, and repeated assessments as early interventions for Posttraumatic Stress Disorder. *Archives of General Psychiatry, 60,* 1024–1032.

Ekselius, L., & von Knorring, L. (1999). Changes in personality status during treatment with sertraline or citalopram. *British Journal of Psychiatry, 174,* 444–448.

Elford, R., White, H., Bowering, R., Ghandi, A., Maddiggan, B., St. John, K., et al. (2000). A Randomized, Controlled Trial of Child Psychiatric Assessments Conducted Using Videoconferencing. *Journal of Telemedicine and Telecare, 6* (2), 73–82.

Elgar, F. J., & McGrath, P. J. (2003). Self-administered psychosocial treatments for children and families, *Journal of Clinical Psychology, 59*, 321–339.

Elkin, I., Shea, M. T., Watkins, J. T., Imber, D. S., Sotsky, S. M., Collins, J. F., et al. (1989). National Institute of Mental Health Treatment of Depression Collaborative Research Program. General effectiveness of treatments. *Archives of General Psychiatry, 46*, 971–982; discussion, 983.

Embry, D. D. (2002). The Good Behavior Game: A best practice candidate as a universal behavioral vaccine. *Clinical Child and Family Psychology Review, 5*, 273–287.

Emmelkamp, P. M. G. (2005). Technological innovations in clinical assessment and psychotherapy. *Psychotherapy and Psychosomatics, 74*, 336–343.

Emmelkamp, P. M., Bouman, T. K., & Blaaw, E. (1994). Individualized versus standardized therapy: A comparative evaluation with obsessive-compulsive patients. *Clinical Psychology and Psychotherapy, 1*, 95–100.

Erickson, L., Molina, C. A., Ladd, G. T., Pietrzak, R. H., & Petry, N. M. (2005). Problem and pathological gambling are associated with poorer mental and physical health in older adults. *International Journal of Geriatric Psychiatry, 20*, 754–759.

Ernst, E., Pittler, M. H., & Wilder, B. (2006). *The desktop guide to complementary and alternative medicine: An evidence-based approach*. Philadelphia, PA: Elsevier.

Esterling, B. A., L'Abate, L., Murray, E., & Pennebaker, J. W. (1999). Empirical foundations for writing in prevention and psychotherapy: Mental and physical outcomes. *Clinical Psychology Review, 19*, 79–96.

Faber, D. P., (1997). Jean-Martin Charcot and the epilepsy/hysteria relationship. *Journal of the History of the Neurosciences, 6*, 275–290.

Fabricatore, A. N., & Wadden, T. A. (2006). Obesity. *Annual Review of Clinical Psychology, 2*, 357–377.

Fairburn, C. G. (1995). *Overcoming binge eating*. New York: Guilford Press.

Fairburn, C. G. (1999). *Guided self-help for bulimia nervosa*. Therapist's manual. Oxford, UK: University of Oxford.

Farrar, J. E. (1992a). Excessive exercise. In L. L'Abate, J. A. Farrar, & D. A. Serritella (Eds.), *Handbook of differential treatments for addictions* (pp. 242–252). Boston: Allyn & Bacon.

Farrar, J. E. (1992b). Interpersonal and love relationships. In L. L'Abate, J. A. Farrar, & D. A. Serritella (Eds.), *Handbook of differential treatments for addictions* (pp. 151–164). Boston: Allyn & Bacon.

Farrar, J. E. (1992c). Workaholism. In L. L'Abate, J. A. Farrar, & D. A. Serritella (Eds.), *Handbook of differential treatments for addictions* (pp. 230–241). Boston: Allyn & Bacon.

Farrar, J. E., L'Abate, L., & Serritella, D. A. (1992). The prevention of addictive behaviors. In L. L'Abate, J. A. Farrar, & D. A. Serritella (Eds.), *Handbook of differential treatments for addictions* (pp. 308–328). Boston: Allyn & Bacon.

Farrell, W. (2005). *Why men earn more: The startling truth behind the pay gap—and what women can do about it*. New York: Amacon.

Febbraro, G. A. R., & Clum, G. A. (2008). Self-regulation theory and self-help therapies. In P. L. Watkins & G. A. Clum (Eds.), *Handbook of self-help therapies* (pp. 59–76). Mahwah, NJ: Erlbaum.

Febbraro, G. A. R., Clum, G. A., Roodman, A. A., & Wright, J. H. (1999). The limits of bibliotherapy: A study of the differential effectiveness of self-administered interventions in individuals with panic attacks. *Behavior Therapy, 30*, 209–222.

Feldman, R. (2007). Maternal-infant contact in development: Insights from Kangaroo Care interventions. In L. L'Abate (Ed.), *Low-cost approaches to promote physical and mental health: Theory, research, and practice* (pp. 323–351). New York: Springer.

Feldman, R., Weller, A., Sirota, L., & Eidelman, A. I. (2003). Testing a family intervention hypothesis: The contribution of mother-infant skin-to-skin contact (Kangaroo Care) to family interaction, proximity, and touch. *Journal of Family Psychology, 17*, 94–107.

Fernández-Aranda, F., Núñez, A., Martínez, C., Krug, I., Cappozzo, M., Carrard, I. et al. (2009). Internet-based cognitive-behavioral therapy for bulimia nervosa: A controlled study. *CyberPsychology and Behavior, 12,* 37–41.

Ferriter, M., & Huband, N. (2003). Experiences of parents with a son or daughter suffering from schizophrenia. *Journal of Psychiatric and Mental Health Nursing, 10,* 552–560.

Field, T. M. (1998). Massage therapy effects. *American Psychologist, 53,* 1270–1287.

Field, T. M. (2002). Violence and touch deprivation in adolescents. *Adolescence, 37,* 735–749.

Finch, A. E., Lambert, M. J., & George, B. (2000). Attacking anxiety: A naturalistic study of a multimedia self-help program. *Journal of Clinical Psychology, 56,* 11–21.

Fincham, F. D., & Beach, S. R. H. (2002). Forgiveness: Toward a public health approach to intervention. In J. H. Harvey & A. Wenzel (Eds.), *A clinician's guide to maintaining and enhancing close relationships* (pp. 277–300). Mahwah, NJ: Lawrence Erlbaum Associates.

Finke, M., & Houston, S. J. (2007). Low-cost obesity interventions: The market for foods. In L. L'Abate (Ed.), *Low-cost approaches to promote physical and mental health: Theory, research, and practice* (pp. 73–86). New York: Springer.

Fiorentine, R. (1999). After drug treatment: Are 12-step programs effective in maintaining abstinence? *American Journal of Drug and Alcohol Abuse, 25,* 93–116.

Fiorentine, R., & Hillhouse, M. P. (2000a). Drug treatment and 12-step program participation: The additive effects of integrated recovery activities. *Journal of Substance Abuse Treatment, 18,* 65–74.

Fiorentine, R., & Hillhouse, M. P. (2000b). Exploring the additive effects of drug misuse treatment and 12-step involvement: Does twelve-step ideology matter? *Substance Use and Misuse, 35,* 367–397.

Fisher, D., Beutler, L. E., & Williams, O. B. (1999). STS Clinician Rating Form: Patient assessment and treatment planning. *Journal of Clinical Psychology, 55,* 825–842.

Fitzsimons, G. M., & Bargh, J. A. (2004). Automatic self-regulation. In R. F. Baumeister & K. D. Vohs (Eds.), *Handbook of self-regulation: Research, theory, and applications* (pp. 151–170). New York: Guilford Press.

Floter, S., & Kroger, C. (2007). Self-change: The rule among smokers. In H. Klingemann & L. C. Sobell (Eds.), *Promoting self-change from addictive behaviors: Practical* implications for policy, prevention, and treatment (pp. 101–111). New York: Springer.

Floyd, M., Rohen, N., Shackelford, J. A. M., Hubbard, K. L., Parnell, M. B., Scogin, F., et al. (2006). Two-year follow up of bibliotherapy and individual cognitive therapy for depressed older adults. *Behavior Modification, 30,* 281–294.

Floyd, M., Scogin, F., McKendree-Smith, N. L., Floyd, D. L., & Rokke, P. D. (2004). Cognitive therapy for depression: A comparison of individual psychotherapy and bibliotherapy for depressed older adults. *Behavior Modification, 28,* 297–318.

Foa, E. B., & Tolin, D .F. (2000). Comparison of the PTSD symptom scale—interview version and the clinician-administered PTSD scale. *Journal of Trauma Stress, 13,* 181–191.

Foran, H. M., & O'Leary, K. D. (2008). Alcohol and intimate partner violence: A meta-analytic review. *Clinical Psychology Review, 28,* 1222–1234.

Frances, A. J., Fyer, M. R., & Clarkin, J. F. (1986). Personality and suicide. *Annals of the New York Academy of Sciences, 487,* 281–293.

Frances, R. J., Miller, S. I., & Mack, A. H. (2005). *Clinical textbook of addictive disorders* (3rd ed). New York: Guilford Press.

Franskoviak, P., & Segal, S. P. (2002). Substance use and mental disorder diagnostic profiles in a sample of long-term self-help agency users. *American Journal of Orthopsychiatry, 72,* 232–240.

Frey, D. H., & Raming, H. E. (1979). A taxonomy of counseling goals and methods. *Personnel and Guidance Journal, 57,* 26–33.

Fulton, M. C. (2004). Breaking through defenses. In P. J. Carnes & K. M. Adams (Eds.), *Clinical management of sex addiction* (pp. 31–44). New York: Brunner-Routledge.

Gabby, A. R. (2006). *A-Z guide to drug-herb-vitamin interactions, revised and expanded* (2nd ed.): *Improve your health and avoid side effects when using common medications and natural supplements together*. A. R. Gabby and Healthcare M K. (2001). Cognitive and neuro-behavioral functioning after mild versus moderate traumatic brain injury in older adults. *Journal of the International Neuropsychological Society, 7*, 373–383.

Galanter, M., Hayden, F., Casteñeda, R., & Franco, H. (2005). Group therapy, self-help groups, and network therapy. In R. J. Francis, S. I. Miller, & A. H. Mack (Eds.), *Clinical textbook of addictive disorders* (pp. 502–527). New York: Guilford Press.

Gartner, A., & Reissman, F. (1979). *Self help in the human services*. San Francisco: Jossey-Bass.

Garvin, V., Striegel-Moore, R. H., Kaplan, A., & Wonderlich, S. A. (2001). The potential of professionally developed self-help interventions for the treatment of eating disorders. In R. H. Striegel-Moore & L. Smolak (Eds.), *Eating disorders: Innovative directions in research and practice* (pp. 153–172). Washington, DC: American Psychological Association.

Gatz, M., Crowe, M., Fiske, A., Fung, W., Kelly, C., & Levy, B. (2002). Promoting mental health in later life. In L. A. Jason, & D. S. Glenwick (Eds.), *Innovative strategies for promoting health and mental health across the life span* (pp. 272–297). New York: Springer.

Gaw, K. F., & Beutler, L. E. (1995). Integrating treatment recommendations. In L. E. Beutler & M. Berren (Eds.), *Integrative assessment of adult personality* (pp.280–309). New York: Guilford Press.

Ghosh, A., & Marks, I. M. (1987). Self-treatment of agoraphobia by exposure. *Behavior Therapy, 18*, 3–15.

Gidron, Y., Peri, T., Connolly, J. F., & Shaley, A. Y. (1996). Written disclosure in posttraumatic stress disorder: Is it beneficial for the patient? *Journal of Nervous & Mental Disease, 184*, 505–507.

Gilroy, L. J., Kirkby, K. C., Daniels, B. A., Menzies, R. G., & Montgomery, I. M. (2000). Controlled comparison of computer-aided vicarious exposure versus live exposure in the treatment of spider phobia. *Behavior Therapy, 31*, 733–744.

Giovannucci, E. (2007). Vitamins, minerals, and health. In L. L'Abate (Ed.), *Low-cost approaches to promote physical and mental health: Theory, research, and practice* (pp. 103–118). New York: Springer.

Girodo, M., & Henry, D. R. (1976). Cognitive, physiological, and behavioral componentsof anxiety in flooding. *Canadian Journal of Behavioural Science, 8*, 224–231.

Glasser, D., & Andria, R. (1999). The new face of self-help: Online support for anxiety disorders. *Dissertation Abstracts International: Section B: The Sciences and Engineering, 59*(7-B), 3691.

Goering, P., Durbin, J., Sheldon, C. T., Ochocka, J., Nelson, G., & Krupa, T. (2006). Who uses consumer-run self-help organizations? *American Journal of Orthopsychiatry, 76*, 367–373.

Goldstein, F. C., Levin, H. S., Goldman, W. P., Clark, A. N., & Altonen, T. K. (2001). Cognitive and neuro-behavioral functioning after mild versus moderate traumatic brain injury in older adults. *Journal of the International Neuropsychological Society, 7*, 373–383.

Gordon, T. (1975). *Parent effectiveness training: The tested way to raise children*. New York: New American Library, Inc.

Gorfain, D. S., & MacLeaod, C. M. (Eds.). (2007). *Inhibition in cognition*. Washington, DC: American Psychological Association.

Gottlieb, R. (2008). *The complete mental health directory* (6th ed.) New York: Grey House Publishing.

Gould, R. A., & Clum, G. A. (1993). A meta-analysis of self-help treatment approaches. *Clinical Psychology Review, 13*, 169–186.

Gould, R. A., & Clum, G. A. (1995). SH plus minimal therapist contact in the treatment of panic disorder: A replication and extension. *Behavior Therapy, 26*, 535–546.

Gould, R. A., Clum, G. A., & Shapiro, D. (1993). The use of bibliotherapy in the treatment of panic: A preliminary investigation. *Behavior Therapy, 24*, 241–252.

Grady, B. J. (2002). Comparative cost analysis of an integrated military telemental health-care service. *Telemedicine Journal and e-Health, 8*, 293–300.

Grady, B. J., & Mercer, T. (2005). A retrospective evaluation of telemental healthcare services for remote military populations. *Telemedicine and e-Health, 11*, 551–558.

Gray, N. J., Klein, J. D., Noyce, P. R., Sesselberg, T. S., & Cantrill, J. A. (2005). Health-information-seeking behaviour in adolescence: The place of the internet. *Social Science and Medicine, 60*, 1467–1478.

Green, E. C., & Kreuter, M. W. (1999). *Health promotion planning: An educational and ecological approach.* Mountain View, CA: Mayfield.

Gregory, R. J., Canning, S. S., Lee, T. W., & Wise, J. C. (2004). Cognitive bibliotherapy for depression: A meta-analysis. *Professional Psychology, 35*, 275–280.

Greenberger, D., & Padesky, C. (1995). *Mind over mood: Change how you feel by changing the way you think.* New York: Guilford Press.

Greenwood, C. R., Horton, B. T., & Utley, C. A. (2002). Academic engagement: Current perspectives on research and practice. *School Psychology Review, 31*, 328–349.

Greist, J. H., Marks, I. M., Baer, L., Kobak, K., Wenzel, K., Hirsch, M. et al. (2002). Behaviour therapy for obsessive compulsive disorder guided by a computer or clinician compared with relaxation as a control. *Journal of Clinical Psychiatry, 63*, 138–145.

Griffiths, K. M., & Christensen, H. (2007). Internet-based mental health programs: A powerful tool in the rural medical kit. *Australian Journal of Rural Health, 15*, 81–87.

Grilo, C. M. (2007). Guided self-help for binge-eating disorder. In J. D. Latner & G. T. Wilson (Eds.), *Self-help approaches for obesity and eating disorders: Research and practice* (pp. 73–91). New York: Guilford Press.

Gronwall, D. (1986). Rehabilitation programs for patients with mild head injury: Components, problems, and evaluation. *Journal of Head Trauma Rehabilitation, 1*, 53–63.

Gruenwald, J., Brendler, T., & Jaenicke, C. (2007). *PDR for herbal medicines* (4th ed.). Montvale, NJ: Thompson.

Gulledge, A. K., Gulledge, M. H., & Stahman, R. F. (2003). Romantic physical affection types and relationship satisfaction. *American Journal of Family Therapy, 31*, 233–242.

Gulledge, A. K., Hill, M., Lister, Z., & Sallion, C. (2007). Non-erotic physical affection: It's good for you. In L. L'Abate (Ed.), *Low-cost approaches to promote physical and mental health: Theory, research, and practice* (pp. 371–384). New York: Springer.

Gullotta, T., & Bloom, M. (Eds.). (2003). *Encyclopedia of primary prevention and health promotion.* New York: Kluwer Academic.

Gunderson, J. G., Morey, L. C., Stout, R. L., Skodol, A. E., Shea, M. T., McGlashan, T. H., et al. (2004). Major depressive disorder and borderline personality disorder revisited: Longitudinal interactions. *Journal of Clinical Psychiatry, 65*, 1049–1056.

Gunderson, J. G., Shea, M. T., Skodol, A. E., McGlashan, T. H., Morey, L. C., Stout, R. L., et al. (2000). The Collaborative Longitudinal Personality Disorders Study: Development, aims, design, and sample characteristics. *Journal of Personality Disorders, 14*, 300–315.

Gura, T. (2008). Addicted to starvation. *Scientific American: Mind, 19*, 61–67.

Hacker, H., Lauber, C., & Rossler, W. (2005). Internet forums: A self-help approach for individuals with schizophrenia? *Acta Psychiatrica Scandinavica, 112*, 474–477.

Haddock, C. K., Rowan, A. B., Andrasik, F., Wilson, P. G., Talcott, G. W., & Stein, R. J. (1997). Home-based behavioral treatments for chronic benign headache: A meta-analysis of controlled trials. *Cephalagia, 17*, 113–118.

Haker, H., Lauber, C., & Rössler, W. (2005). Internet forums: A self-help approach for individuals with schizophrenia? *Acta Psychiatrical Scandinavica, 112*, 474–477.

Hamilton, M. (1960). A rating scale for depression. *Journal of Neurological Neurosurgical Psychiatry, 23*, 56–61.

Hamilton, M. (1967). Development of a rating scale for primary depressive illness. *British Journal of Social and Clinical Psychology, 5*, 278–296.

Harcourt, L., Kirkby, K., Daniels, B., & Montgomery, L. (1998). The differential effect of personality on computer-based treatment of agoraphobia. *Comprehensive Psychiatry, 39*, 303–307.

Harris, A. H. S. (2006). Does expressive writing reduce health care utilization? A meta-analysis of randomized trials. *Journal of Consulting and Clinical Psychology, 74*, 243–252.

Harris, S. R., Kemmerling, R. L., & North, M. M. (2002). Brief virtual reality therapy for public speaking anxiety. *Cyberpsychology and Behavior, 5*, 543–550.

Harwood, T. M., & Beutler, L. E., (2008). EVTs, EBPs, ESRs, and RIPs: Inspecting the varieties of research based practices. In L. L'Abate (Ed.), *Toward a science of clinical psychology: Laboratory evaluations and interventions* (pp. 161–176). New York: Nova Science Publishers, Inc.

Harwood, T. M., & Beutler, L. E. (2009). How to assess clients in pretreatment planning. In J. N. Butcher (Ed.), *Oxford handbook of personality assessment*. Oxford: Oxford University Press.

Harwood, T. M., Fraga, E. D., & Beutler, L. E. (2001). Family therapy and the application of systematic treatment selection. *Systemas Familiares, 17*, 95–111.

Harwood, T. M., & Williams, O. B. (2003). Identifying treatment-relevant assessment: Systematic treatment selection. In L. E. Beutler & G. Groth-Marnat (Eds.), *Integrative assessment of adult personality* (2nd ed., pp. 65–81). New York: Guilford Press.

Haug, S., Strauss, B., Gallas, C., & Kordy, H. (2008). New prospects for process research in group therapy: Text-based process variables in psychotherapeutic Internet chat groups. *Psychotherapy Research, 18*, 88–96.

Hecker, J., Losee, M., Fritzler, B., & Fink, C. (1996). Self-directed versus therapist-directed cognitive behavioral treatment for panic disorder. *Journal of Anxiety Disorders, 10*, 253–265.

Hellerich, G. (2001). Madness and self-help culture: A postmodern phenomenon. *Ethical Human Sciences & Services, 3*, 97–106.

Hellstrom, K., & Öst, L. (1995). One-session therapist-directed exposure versus two forms of manual-directed self-exposure in the treatment of spider phobia. *Behaviour Research and Therapy, 33*, 959–965.

Hellstrom, K., Fellenius, J., & Öst, L. (1996). One versus five sessions of applied tensionin the treatment of blood phobia. *Behavior Research and Therapy, 34*, 101–112.

Hembree-Kigin, T., & McNeil, C. B. (1995). *Parent-child interaction therapy*. NewYork: Plenum Publishers.

Henderson, D. K. (1939). *Psychopathic states*. New York: Norton.

Henderson, K. E., & Schwartz, M. E. (2007). Treatment of overweight children: Practical strategies for parents. In J. D. Latner & G. T. Wilson (Eds.), *Self-help approaches for obesity and eating disorders: Research and practice* (pp. 289–309). New York: Guilford.

Hendricks, M. C. P., Nelson, J. K., Cornelius, R. R., & Vingerhoets, J. J. M. (2008). Why crying improves our well-being: An attachment-theory perspective on the functions of human crying. In A. Vingerhoets, I. Nyklicek, & J. Denollet (Eds.), *Emotional regulation: Conceptual and clinical issues* (pp. 87–96). New York: Springer.

Henry, W. P., Schacht, T. E., Strupp, H. H., Butler, S. F., & Binder, J. L. (1993). Effects of training in time-limited dynamic psychotherapy: Mediators of therapists' responses to training. *Journal of Consulting and Clinical Psychology, 61*, 441–447.

Henry, W. P., Strupp, H. H., Butler, S. F., Schacht, T. E., & Binder, J .L. (1993). Effects of training in time-limited dynamic psychotherapy: Changes in therapist behavior. *Journal of Consulting and Clinical Psychology, 61*, 434–440.

Hibbeln, J. R. (2002). Seafood consumption, the DHA content of mothers' milk and prevalence rates of postpartum depression: A cross-national, ecological analysis. *Journal of Affective Disorders, 69*, 15–29.

Higgins, E. T. (2001). Promotion and prevention experiences: Relating emotions to non-emotional motivational states. In J. P. Forgas (Ed.), *Handbook of affect and social cognition* (pp. 186–211). Mahwah, NJ: Lawrence Erlbaum Associates.

Hirai, M., & Clum, G. (2005). An internet-based self-change program for traumatic event related fear, distress, and maladaptive coping. *Journal of Traumatic Stress, 18*, 631–636.

Hirai, M., & Clum, G. A. (2008). Self-help therapies for anxiety disorders. In P. L. Watkins & G. A. Clum (Eds.), *Handbook of self-help therapies* (pp. 77–107). Mahwah, NJ: Erlbaum.

Hodges, J. Q., Keele, C., & Evans, C. J. (2003). Use of self-help services and consumer satisfaction with professional mental health services. *Psychiatric Services, 54,* 1161–1163.

Hogan, C. (2007). Implications of prescriptive approaches for policy, health promotion, epidemiology, and public health. In L. L'Abate (Ed.), *Low-cost approaches to promote physical and mental health: Theory, research, and practice* (pp. 505–519). New York: Springer.

Hogan, R. A., & Kirchner, J. H. (1968). Implosive, eclectic verbal and bibliotherapy in the treatment of the fear of snakes. *Behaviour Research and Therapy, 6,* 167–171.

Hogarty, G. (2002). *Personal therapy for schizophrenia and related disorders: A guide to individualized treatment.* New York: Guilford Press.

Holbrook, T. L., Hoyt, D. B. (2004). The impact of major trauma: Quality-of-life outcomes are worse in women than in men, independent of mechanism and injury severity. *Journal on Trauma, 56,* 284–290.

Holbrook, T. L., Hoyt, D. B., Stein, M. B., & Seiber, W. J. (2002). Gender differences in long-term posttraumatic stress disorder outcomes after major trauma: Women are at higher risk of adverse outcomes than men. *Journal on Trauma, 53,* 882–888.

Holdsworth, N., Paxton, R., Seidel, S., Thomson, D., & Shrubb, S. (1996). Parallel evaluations of new guidance materials for anxiety and depression in primary care.*Journal of Mental Health , 5,* 195–207.

Honos-Webb, L., Endres, L. M., Shaikh, A., Harrick, E. A., Lani, J. A., & Knobloch- Fedders, L. M. (2002). Rewards and risks of exploring negative emotion: An assimilation model account. In S. R. Fussell (Ed.), *The verbal communication of emotions: Interdisciplinary perspectives* (pp. 231–251). Mahwah, NJ: Lawrence Erlbaum Associates.

Housley, J., & Beutler, L. E. (2006). *Treating victims of mass disaster and terrorism.* New York: Hogrefe & Huber Publishers.

Houts, A. C., & Graham, K. (1986). Can religion make you crazy? Impact of client and therapist religious values on clinical judgments. *Journal of Consulting and Clinical Psychology, 54,* 267–271.

Hrabosky, J. I., & Cash, T. F. (2007). Self-help treatment for body-image disturbances. In J. D. Latner & G. T. Wilson (Eds.), *Self-help approaches for obesity and eating disorders: Research and practice* (pp. 118–138). New York: Guilford.

Huband, N., McMurran, M., Evans, C., & Duggan, C. (2007). Social problem-solving plus psychoeducation for adults with personality disorder. *British Journal of Psychiatry, 190,* 307–313.

Hubble, M. A., Duncan, B. L., & Miller, S. D. (1999). (Eds.). *The heart & soul of change: What works in psychotherapy.* Washington, DC: American Psychological Association.

Hughes, B. M. (2007). How should clinical psychologists approach complementary and alternative medicine: Empirical, epistemological, an ethical considerations. *Clinical Psychology Review, 28,* 657–675.

Humphreys, K. (2004). *Circles of recovery: Self-help organizations for addictions.* New York: Cambridge University Press.

Humphreys, K., & Finney, J. W., & Moos, R. H. (1994). Applying a stress and coping framework to research on mutual help organizations. *Journal of Community Psychology, 22,* 312–317.

Humphreys, K., & Moos, R. H. (1996). Reduced substance-abuse-related health care costs among voluntary participants in Alcoholics Anonymous. *Psychiatric Services, 47,* 709–713.

Humphreys, K., & Moos, R. H. (2007). Encouraging post-treatment self-help group involvement to reduce demand for continuing care services: Two year clinical and utilization outcomes. *Alcoholism: Clinical and Experimental Research, 31,* 64–68.

Humphreys, K., Moos, R. H., & Finney, J. W. (1996). Life domains, alcoholics anonymous, and role incumbency in the 3-year course of problem-drinking. *Journal of Nervous and Mental Disease, 184,* 475–481.

Humphreys, K., Phibbs, C. S., & Moos, R. H. (1996). Innovative methodologies for longitudinal evaluation of human service programs. *Evaluation and Program Planning. Special Issue, 19,* 301–308.

Jacobson, N. S., & Truax, P. (1991). Clinical significance: A statistical approach to defining meaningful change in psychotherapy research. *Journal of Consulting and Clinical Psychology, 59,* 12–19.

James, T. B. (2003). *Domestic violence: The 12 things you aren't supposed to know.* Chula Vista, CA: Aventine Press.

Jannoun, L., Murphy, M., Catalan, J., & Gelder, M. (1980). A home-based treatment program for agoraphobia: Replication and controlled evaluation. *Behavior Therapy, 11,* 294–305.

Jarrett, O. S., Hoge, P., Davies, G., Maxwell, D., Yetley, A., & Dickerson, C. (1998). Impact of recess on classroom behavior: Group effects and individual differences. *The Journal of Educational Research, 92,* 121–126.

Jason, L. A., & Glenwick, D. S. (2002). Introduction: An overview of preventive and ecological perspectives. In L. A. Jason, & D. S. Glenwick (Eds.), *Innovative strategies for promoting health and mental health across the life span* (pp. 3–16). New York: Springer.

Joannides, P., & Gross, D. (2009). *The guide to getting it on,* 6th ed. Waldport, OR:Goofy Foot Press.

Jones, N. A., & Mize, K. D. (2007). Touch positively affects development. In L. L'Abate (Ed.), *Low-cost approaches to promote physical and mental health: Theory, research, and practice* (pp. 353–370). New York: Springer.

Jordan, J., Bardé, B., & Zeiher, A. (2006). *Contributions toward evidence-based psychocardiology: A systematic review of the literature.* Washington, DC: American Psychological Association.

Jordan, K., & L'Abate, L. (1995). Programmed writing and therapy with symbiotically enmeshed patients. *American Journal of Psychotherapy, 49,* 225–236.

Jorm, A. T., & Griffiths, K. M. (2006). Population promotion of informal self-help strategies for early intervention against depression and anxiety. *Psychological Medicine, 26,* 3–6.

Jurish, S. E., Blanchard, E. B., Andrasik, F., Teders, S. J., Neff, D. F., & Arena, J. G. (1983). Home versus clinic-based treatment of vascular headache. *Journal of Consulting and Clinical Psychology, 51,* 743–751.

Kacewicz, E., Slatcher, R. B., & Pennebaker, J. W. (2007). Expressive writing: An alternative to traditional methods. In L. L'Abate (Ed.), *Low-cost approaches to promote physical and mental health: Theory, research, and practice* (pp. 271–394). New York: Springer.

Kamholz, B., & Unützer, J. (2007). Depression after hip fracture. *Journal of the American Geriatrics Society, 55,* 126–127.

Karpe, J. A., & Scogin, F. R. (2008). Self-help therapies for depression. In P. L. Watkins & G. A. Clum (Eds.), *Handbook of self-help therapies* (pp. 109–128). Mahwah, NJ: Erlbaum.

Kaskutas, L. A., Ammon, L., Delucchi, K., Room, R., Bond, J., & Weisner, C. (2005). Alcoholics Anonymous careers: Patterns of AA involvement five years after-treatment entry. *Alcoholism Clinical & Experimental Research, 29,* 1983–1990.

Katz, D. L., Yeh, M. C., Kennedy, D., & O'Connell, M. (2007). Diets, health, and weight control: What do we know? In L. L'Abate (Ed.), *Low-cost approaches to promote physical and mental health: Theory, research, and practice* (pp. 47–72). New York: Springer.

Katz, L. Y., Cox, B. J., Gunasekara, S., & Miller, A. L. (2004). Feasibility of dialectical behavior therapy for suicidal adolescent inpatients. *Journal of the American Academy of Child and Adolescent Psychiatry, 43,* 276–282.

Kazantzis, N., & L'Abate, L. (Eds.). (2007). *Handbook of homework assignments in psychotherapy: Theory, research, and prevention.* New York: Springer.

Kazantzis, N., & Lampropoulos, G. K. (2002). Reflecting on homework in psychotherapy: What can we conclude from research and experience? *Psychotherapy in Practice, 58,* 577–585.

Kazantzis, N., Deane, F. P., Ronan, K. E., & L'Abate, L. (Eds.). (2005). *Using homework assignments in cognitive behavior therapy.* New York: Rutledge.

Kazdin, A. E. (2005). *Parent management training: Treatment for oppositional, aggressive, and antisocial behavior in children and adolescents.* New York: Oxford University Press.

Kazdin, A. E. (2008). *The Kazdin method for parenting the defiant child with no pills, notherapy, no contest of wills.* New York: Houghton Mifflin, Co.

Keene, D. W. (2008). Women earn 77% of men and other falsehoods. *Independent Women's Forum*. September, 22, 2008.

Kelly, J. F., McKellar, J. D., & Moos, R. (2003). Major depression in patients with substance use disorders: relationship to 12-step self-help involvement and substance abuse outcomes. *Addiction, 98*, 499–508.

Kelly, R. E. (1975). The post-traumatic syndrome: An iatrogenic disease. *Forensic Science, 6*, 17–24.

Kendall, P. C. (1994). Treating anxiety disorders in youth: Results of a randomized clinical trial. *Journal of Consulting and Clinical Psychology, 62*, 100–101.

Kendall, P. D., Kane, M., Howard, B., & Sigueland, L. (1990). *Cognitive-behavioral treatment of anxious children: Treatment manual*. Available from the author, Department of Psychology, Temple University, Philadelphia, PA 19122.

Kennedy, A., Robinson, A., & Rogers, A. (2003). Incorporating patients' views and experiences of life with IBS in the development of an evidence based self-help guidebook. *Patient Education and Counseling, 50*, 303–310.

Kenwright, M., Marks, I., Graham, C., Franses, A., & Mataix-Cols, D. (2005). Brief scheduled phone support from a clinician to enhance computer-aided SH for obsessive-compulsive disorder: Randomized controlled trial. *Journal of Clinical Psychology, 61*, 1499–1508.

Kessler, R. C. (1995). The national comorbidity survey: Preliminary results and future directions. *International Journal of Methods in Psychiatric Medicine, 5*, 139–151.

Kessler, R. (2008a). Integration of care is about money too: The health and behavior codes as an element of a new financial paradigm. *Family Systems & Health, 26*, 207–216.

Kessler, R. (2008b). The difficulty of making psychology research and clinical practice relevant to medicine: Experiences and observations. *Journal of Clinical Psychology in Medical Settings, 15*, 65–72.

Kimura, D. (1992). Sex differences in the brain. *Scientific American*, September.

Kinder, B. N. (1997). Eating disorders. In S. M. Turner & M. Hersen (Eds.), *Adult psychopathology and diagnosis* (3rd ed). New York: John Wiley and Sons.

Kinsbourne, M. (2005). A continuum of self-consciousness that emerges in phylogeny and ontogeny. In H. S., Terrace, & J. Metcalfe (Eds.), *The missing link in cognition: Origins of self-reflective consciousness* (pp. 142–156). New York: Oxford University Press.

Kirkby, K., Daniels, B., Harcourt, L., & Romano, A. (1999). Behavioral analysis of computer-administered vicarious exposure in agoraphobic subjects: The effect of personality on in-session treatment process. *Comprehensive Psychiatry, 40*, 386–390.

Klein, M. (2007). *The power makers: Steam, electricity, and the men who invented modern America*. New York: Bloomsbury.

Klerman, G. L., Weissman, M. M., Rounsaville, B. J., & Chevron, E. S. (1984). *Interpersonal psychotherapy of depression*. New York: Basic Books.

Klesges, R. C., Mizes, J. S., & Klesges, L. M. (1987). Self-help dieting strategies in college males and females. *International Journal of Eating Disorders, 6*, 409–417.

Klingemann, H., & Klingemann, J. (2007). Hostile and favorable societal climates for self-change: Some lessons for policymakers. In H. Klingemann & L. C. Sobell (Eds.), *Promoting self-change from addictive behaviors: Practical implications for policy, prevention, and treatment* (pp. 187–212). New York: Springer.

Klingemann, H., & Sobell, L. C. (Eds.). (2007). *Promoting self-change from addictive behaviors: Practical implications for policy, prevention, and treatment*. New York: Springer.

Knudson, B., & Boyle, A. (2002). Parents' experiences of caring for sons and daughters with schizophrenia: A qualititative analysis of coping. *European Journal of Psychotherapy, Counseling & Health, 5*, 169–183.

Koch, J. L. A. (1981). *Die psychopathischen minderwertigkeiten*. Ravensburg, Germany: Dorn.

Kosten, R. A., Kosten, T. R., & Rounsaville, B. J. (1989). Personality disorders in opiate addicts show prognostic specificity. *Journal of Substance Abuse Treatment, 6*, 163–168.

Kretschmer, E. (1922). *Korperbau und charakter*. Berlin, Germany: Springer.

Kreulen, G. J., & Braden, C. J. (2004). Model test of the relationship between self-help-promoting nursing interventions and self-care and health status outcomes. *Research in Nursing & Health*, 27, 97–109.

Kushner, M. G., Donahue, C., Sletten, S., Thuras, P., Abrams, K., Peterson, J., et al. (2006). Cognitive behavioral treatment of comorbid anxiety disorder in alcoholism treatment patients: Presentation of a prototype program and future directions. *Journal of Mental Health*, 15, 697–707.

Kypri, K., & Cunningham, J. A. (2008). Self-help therapies for problem-drinking. In P. L. Watkins & G. A. Clum (Eds.), *Handbook of self-help therapies* (pp. 243–266). Mahwah, NJ: Erlbaum.

L'Abate, L. (in press). Bibliography of secondary sources for relational competence theory. In M. Capitelli, P. De Giacomo, L. L'Abate, & S. Longo (Eds.), *Mind, science, and creativity: The Bari symposium* (pp. 000–000). New York: Nova Science Publishers.

L'Abate, L. (2010). *Sourcebook of interactive practice exercises in mental health*. New York: Springer-Science.

L'Abate, L. (2009a). A structured, theory-derived interview for intimate relationships. *The Family Psychologist*, 25, 12–14.

L'Abate, L. (2009b). Hurt feelings: The last taboo for researchers and clinicians? In A. L. Vangelisti (Ed.), *Feeling hurt in close relationships* (pp. 479–498). New York: Cambridge University Press.

L'Abate, L. (2009c). The Drama Triangle: An attempt to resurrect a neglected pathogenic model in family theory and practice. *American Journal of Family Therapy*, 37, 1–11.

L'Abate, L. (2009d). *The Praeger handbook of play across the life cycle: Fun from infancy to old age*. Westport, CT: Praeger.

L'Abate, L. (2008a). Proposal for including distance writing in couple therapy. *Journal of Couple & Relationship Therapy*, 7, 337–362.

L'Abate, L. (Ed.) (2008b). *Toward a science of clinical psychology: Laboratory evaluations and interventions*. New York: Nova Science.

L'Abate, L. (2008c). Working at a distance from participants: Writing and nonverbal media. In L. L'Abate (Ed.), *Toward a science of clinical psychology: Laboratory evaluations and interventions* (pp. 355–383). New York: Nova Science.

L'Abate, L. (2007a). A completely preposterous proposal: The dictionary as an initial vehicle of behavior change in the family. *The Family Psychologist*, 23, 39–43.

L'Abate, L. (2007b). Animal companions. In L. L'Abate (Ed.), *Low-cost approaches to promote physical and mental health: Theory, research, and practice* (pp. 473–484). New York: Springer-Science.

L'Abate, L. (Ed.) (2007c). *Low-cost approaches to promote physical and mental health: Theory, research, and practice*. New York: Springer-Science.

L'Abate, L. (2005). *Personality in intimate relationships: Socialization and psycho-pathology*. New York: Springer-Science.

L'Abate, L. (2004a). *A guide to self-help mental health practice exercises for clinicians and researchers*. Binghamton, NY: Haworth.

L'Abate, L. (Ed.) (2004b). *Using practice exercises in prevention, psychotherapy, and rehabilitation: A resource for clinicians and researchers*. Binghamton, NY: Haworth.

L'Abate, L. (2003a). *Family psychology III: Theory-building, theory-testing, and psychological interventions*. Lanham, MD: University Press of America.

L'Abate, L. (2003b). Treatment through writing: A unique new direction. In T. L. Sexton, G. Weeks, & M. Robbins (Eds.), *The handbook of family therapy* (pp. 397–409). New York: Brunner-Routledge.

L'Abate, L. (2002). *Beyond psychotherapy: Programmed writing and structured computer-assisted interventions*. Westport, CT: Ablex.

L'Abate, L. (2001a). Distance writing and computer-assisted interventions in the delivery of mental health services. In L. L'Abate (Ed.), *Distance writing and computer-assisted interventions in psychiatry and mental health* (pp. 215–226). Westport, CT: Ablex.

L'Abate, L. (2001b). Hugging, holding, huddling, and cuddling (3HC): A task prescription in couples and family therapy. *The Journal of Clinical Activities, Assignments, & Handouts in Psychotherapy Practice, 1*, 5–18.

L'Abate, L. (1992a). Excessive spending. In L. L'Abate, J. A. Farrar, & D. A. Serritella (Eds.), *Handbook of differential treatments for addictions* (pp. 253–270). Boston: Allyn & Bacon.

L'Abate, L. (1992b). Introduction. In L. L'Abate, J. A. Farrar, & D. A. Serritella (Eds.), *Handbook of differential treatments for addictions* (pp. 1–4). Boston: Allyn & Bacon.

L'Abate, L. (1992c). Guidelines for treatment. In L. L'Abate, J. A. Farrar, & D. A. Serritella (Eds.), *Handbook of differential treatments for addictions* (pp. 42–60). Boston: Allyn & Bacon.

L'Abate, L. (1992d). Major therapeutic issues. In L. L'Abate, J. A. Farrar, & D. A. Serritella (Eds.), *Handbook of differential treatments for addictions* (pp. 5–22). Boston: Allyn & Bacon.

L'Abate, L. (1992e). *Programmed writing: A self-administered approach for interventions with individuals, couples, and families*. Pacific Grove, CA: Brooks/Cole.

L'Abate, L. (1990). *Building family competence: Primary and secondary prevention strategies*. Newbury Park, CA: Sage.

L'Abate, L. (1986). *Systematic family therapy*. New York: Brunner/Mazel.

L'Abate, L. (1977). *Enrichment: Structured interventions with couples, families, and groups*. Washington, DC: University Press of America.

L'Abate, L. (1976). *Understanding and helping the individual in the family*. New York: Grune & Stratton.

L'Abate, L, & Bliwise, N. G. (Eds.) (2009). *Handbook of technology in psychology, psychiatry, and mental health*. Book proposal submitted for publication.

L'Abate, L., & Harwood, T. M. (2009). Toward a technology for clinical psychology: The future is now. Manuscript submitted for publication.

L'Abate, L., & Goldstein, J. (2007). Workbooks to promote mental health and life-long learning. In L. L'Abate (Ed.), *Low-cost approaches to promote physical and mental health: Theory, research, and practice* (pp. 285–303). New York: Springer-Science.

L'Abate, L., & Cusinato, M. (2007). Linking theory with practice: Theory-derived interventions in prevention and family therapy. *The Family Journal: Counseling and Therapy with Couples and Families, 15*, 318–327.

L'Abate. L., & De Giacomo, P. (2003). *Improving intimate relationships: Integration of theoretical models with preventions and psychotherapy applications*. Westport, CT: Praeger.

L'Abate, L., & Harrison, M. G. (1992). Treating co-dependency. In L. L'Abate, J. A. Farrar, & D. A. Serritella (Eds.), *Handbook of differential treatments for addictions* (pp. 286–307). Boston: Allyn & Bacon.

L'Abate, L., & Weinstein, S. E. (1987). *Structured enrichment programs for couples and families*. New York: Brunner/Mazel.

L'Abate, L., & Young, L. (1987). *Casebook of structured enrichment programs for couples and families*. New York: Brunner/Mazel.

L'Abate, L., & McHenry, S. (1983). *Handbook of marital interventions*. New York: Grune & Stratton.

L'Abate, L., L'Abate, B. L., & Maino, E. (2005). A review of 25 years of part-time professional practice: Workbooks and length of psychotherapy. *American Journal of Family Therapy, 33*, 19–31.

L'Abate, L., Hewitt, D. W., & Samples, G. T. (1992). Religious fanaticism. In L. L'Abate, J. A. Farrar, & D. A. Serritella (Eds.), *Handbook of differential treatments for addictions* (pp. 271–285). Boston: Allyn & Bacon.

L'Abate, L., Farrar, J. E., & Serritella, D. A. (Eds.) (1992). *Handbook of differential treatments for addictions*. Boston: Allyn & Bacon.

L'Abate, L., Ganahl, G., & Hansen, J. C. (1986). *Methods of family therapy*. Englewood Cliffs, NJ: Prentice-Hall.

L'Abate, L., Cusinato, M., Maino, E., Colesso, W., & Scilletta, C. (2010). *Relational competence theory: Research and mental health applications*. New York: Springer-Science.

Lackner, J. M., Morley, S., Dowzer, C., Mesmer, C., & Hamilton, S. (2004). Psychological treatments for irritable bowel syndrome: A systematic review and meta-analysis. *Journal of Consulting and Clinical Psychology, 72*, 1100–1113.

LaGow, B. (2007). PDR drug guide for mental health professionals, (3rd ed.). Montvale, NJ: Thompson.

Laird, J. D., & Strout, S. (2007). Emotional behaviors as emotional stimuli. In J. A. Coan & J. B. Allen (Eds.), *Handbook of emotion elicitation and assessment* (pp. 54–64). New York: Oxford University Press.

Laitinen, I., Ettorre, E., & Sutton, C. (2006). Empowering depressed women: Changes in "individual" and "social" feelings in guided self-help groups in Finland. *European Journal of Psychotherapy and Counseling, 8*, 305–320.

Lambert, M. J. (1992). Psychotherapy outcome research: Implications for integrative andeclectic therapists. In J. C. Norcross & M. R. Goldfried (Eds.), *Handbook of Psychotherapy Integration* (pp. 94–129). New York: Basic Books.

Lambert, M., & Bergin, A. E. (1994). The effectiveness of psychotherapy. In A. E. Bergin & S. L. Garfield (Eds.), *Handbook of Psychotherapy and Behavior Change* (4th ed.) pp. 143–189. New York: John Wiley.

Lambert, M. J. & Ogles, B. M. (1988). Treatment manuals: Problems or promise. *Journal of Integrative and Eclectic Psychotherapy, 7*, 187–204.

Lambert, M. J., & Ogles, B. J. (2004). The efficacy and effectiveness of psychotherapy. In M. J. Lambert (Ed.). *Bergin and garfield's handbook of psychotherapy and behavior change* (5th ed., pp. 227–306). New York: John Wiley & Sons, Inc.

Lambert, M. J., & Whipple, J. L. (2008). Measuring and improving psychotherapy outcome: Laboratory methods in routine clinical practice. In L. L'Abate (Ed.), *Toward a science of clinical psychology: Laboratory evaluations and interventions* (pp. 177–196). New York: Nova Science.

Lancaster, T., & Stead, L. F. (2005). Self-help interventions for smoking cessation. *Cochrane Database of Systematic Reviews, 3*. Art. No.: CD001118.

Landreville, P., Landry, J., Baillargeon, L., Guérette, A., & Matteau, E. (2001). Older adults' acceptance of psychological and pharmacological treatments for depression. *Journal of Gerontology: Psychological Sciences, 56B*, 285–291.

Lang, P. J., Malamed, B. G., & Hart, J. A. (1970). A psychophysical analysis of fearModification using an automated desensitization procedure. *Journal of AbnormalPsychology, 76*, 220–234.

Lange, A., Rietdijk, D., Hudcovicova, M., van de Ven, J. P., Schrieken, B., & Emmelkamp, P. (2003). Interplay: A controlled randomized trial of the standardized treatment of posttraumatic stress through the Internet. *Journal of Consulting & Clinical Psychology, 71*, 901–909.

Latner, J. D. (2001). Self-help in the long-term treatment of obesity. *Obesity Reviews, 2*, 87–97.

Latner, J. D., & Wilson, G. T. (2007). Continuing care and self-help in the treatment of obesity. In J. D. Latner & G. T. Wilson (Eds.), *Self-help approaches for obesity and eating disorders: Research and practice* (pp. 223–239). New York: Guilford Press.

Latner, J. D., Wilson, G. T., Stunkard, A. J., & Jackson, M. L. (2002). Self-help and long-term behavior therapy for obesity. *Behaviour Research and Therapy, 40*, 805–812.

Lazarus, A. A. (1976). *Multimodal behavior therapy*. New York: Springer.

Learmonth, D., Trosh, J., Rai, S., Sewell, J., & Cavanagh, K. (2008). The role of computer-aided psychotherapy within an NHS CBT specialist service. *Counseling and Psychotherapy Research, 8*, 117–123.

Lembke, A., Miklowitz, D. J., Otto, M. W., Zhang, H., Wisniewski, S. R., Sachs, G. S., et al. (2004). Psychosocial service utilization by patients with bipolar disorders: Data from the first 500 participants in the systematic treatment enhancement program. *Journal of Psychiatric Practice, 10*, 81–87.

Lepore, S. J., & Greenberg, M. A. (2002). Mending broken hearts: Effects of expressive writing on mood, cognition processing, social adjustment, and health following a relationship breakup. *Psychology and Health, 17*, 547–560.

Lepore, S. J., & Smyth, J. M. (Eds.). (2002). *The writing cure: How expressive writing promotes health and emotional well-being*. Washington, DC: American Psychological Association.

Levendusky, P. G. (2000). Dialectical behavior therapy: So far so soon. *Clinical Psychology: Science and Practice, 7*, 99–100.

Levin, H. S., Mattis, S., Ruff, R. M., Eisenberg, H. M., Marshall, L. F., Tabaddor, K., et al. (1987). Neurobehavioral outcome following minor head injury: A three center study. *Journal of Neurosurgery, 66*, 234–243.

Levine, M., & Calvanio, R. (2007). Recording of personal information as an intervention and as electronic health support. In L. L'Abate (Ed.), *Low-cost approaches to promote physical and mental health: Theory, research, and practice* (pp. 227–250). New York: Springer.

Levy, L. H. (2000). Self-help groups In J. Rappaport & E. Seidman (Eds.), *Handbook of community psychology* (591–613). Dordrecht, NE: Kluwer Academic.

Lewinsohn, P. M., Munoz, R. F., Youngren, M. A., & Zeiss, A. M. (1986). *Control your depression*. New York: Prentice Hall.

Lewis, J. E. (1992). Treating the alcohol-effected family. In L. L'Abate, J. A. Farrar, & D. A. Serritella (Eds.), *Handbook of differential treatments for addictions* (pp. 61–83). Boston: Allyn & Bacon.

Lewis, T., Amini, F., & Lannon, R. (2000). *A general theory of love*. New York: Vantage Books.

Lidren, D. M., Watkins, P. L., Gound, R. A., Clum, R. A., Asterino, M., & Tulloch, H. L. (1994). A comparison of bibliotherapy and group therapy in the treatment of panic disorder. *Journal of Consulting and Clinical Psychology, 62*, 865–869.

Lilienfeld, S. O. (2007). Psychosocial treatments that cause harm. *Perspectives on Psychological Science, 2*, 53–70.

Lindren, D. M., Watkins, P. L., Gould, R. A., Clum, R. A., Asterino, M., & Tulloch, H. L. (1994). A comparison of bibliotherapy and group therapy in the treatment of panic disorder. *Journal of Consulting and Clinical Psychology, 62*, 865–869.

Linehan, M. M. (1993a). *Cognitive-behavioral treatment of borderline personality disorder*. New York: Guilford Press.

Linehan, M. M. (1993b). *Skills training manual for treating borderline personality disorder*. New York: Guilford Press.

Linehan, M. M. (2000). The empirical basis of dialectical behavior therapy: Development of new treatments versus evaluation of existing treatments. *Clinical Psychology: Science and Practice, 7*, 113–119.

Linehan, M. M.,& Dimeff, L. A. (1997). *Dialectical behavior therapy for substance abuse treatment manual*. Seattle, WA: University of Washington.

Linehan, M. M., Armstrong, H. E., Suarez, A., Allmon, D., & Heard, H. L. (1991). Cognitive-behavioral treatment of chronically parasuicidal borderline patients. *Archives of General Psychiatry, 48*, 1060–1064.

Linehan, M. M., Comtois, K. A., Murray, A. M., Brown, M. Z., Gallop, R. J., & Heard, H. L., (2006). Two-year randomized controlled trial and follow-up of dialectical behavior therapy vs therapy by experts for suicidal behaviors and borderline personality disorder. *Archives of General Psychiatry, 63*, 757–766.

Linehan, M. M., Dimeff, L. A., Reynolds, S. K., Comtois, K. A., Welch, S. S., Heagerty, P., et al. (2002). Dialectical behavior therapy versus comprehensive validation therapy plus 12-step for the treatment of opioid dependent women meeting criteria for borderline personality disorder. *Drug and Alcohol Dependence, 67*, 13–26.

Linehan, M. M., Rizvi, S. L., Welch. S. S., & Page, B. (2002). Psychiatric aspects of suicidal behaviour: Personality Disorders. In K. Hawton & K. van Heeringen (Eds.), *The international handbook of suicide and attempted suicide* (pp. 147–178). Sussex: Wiley.

Linehan, M. M., Tutek, D. A., & Dimeff, L. A. (1996). *Comprehensive Validation Therapy for substance abusers*. Seattle, WA: University of Washington.

Lipsey, M. W., & Wilson, D. B. (1993). The efficacy of psychological, educational, and behavioral treatment: Confirmation from meta-analyses. *American Psychologist, 48*, 1181–1209.

Litz, B. T., Engel, C. C., Bryant, R. A., & Papa, A. (2007). A randomized, controlled proof-of-concept trial of an internet-based, therapist-assisted self-management treatment for posttraumatic stress disorder. *American Journal of Psychiatry, 164*, 1676–1683.

Litz, B. T., Williams, L., Wang, J., Bryant, R., & Engle, C. C. (2004). A therapist-assisted internet self-help program for traumatic stress. *Professional Psychology: Research and Practice, 35*, 628–634.

Ljotsson, B., Lundin, C., Mitsell, K., Carlbring, P., Ramklint, M., & Ghaderi, A. (2007). Remote treatment of bulimia nervosa and binge eating disorder: A randomized trial of internet-assisted cognitive behavioural therapy. *Behaviour Research and Therapy, 45*, 649–661.

Loeb, K. L., Wilson, G. T., Gilbert, J. S., & Labouvie, E. (2000). Guided and unguidedself-help for binge eating. *Behavior Research and Therapy, 38*, 259–272.

Loo, J. M. Y., Raylu, N., & Oei, T. P. S. (2008). Gambling among the Chinese: A comprehensive review. *Clinical Psychology Review, 28*, 1152–1166.

Lorig, K. R., & Holman, H. (1993). Arthritis self-management interventions. *Medical Care, 42*, 346–354.

Lorig, K. R., Holman, H., Sobel, D., Laurent, D., Gonzalez, V., & Minor, M. (2006). *Living a healthy life with chronic conditions: Self-management of heart disease, arthritis, diabetes, asthma, bronchitis, emphysema, and others* (3rd ed.). Boulder, CO: Bull Publishing Company.

Lorig, K. R., Ritter, P. L., Laurent, D. D., & Fries, J. F. (2004). Long-term randomized controlled trials of tailored-print and small-group arthritis self-management interventions. *Medical Care, 42*, 346–354.

Lovibond, S. H., & Lovibond, P. F. (1995). *Manual for the depression, anxiety, and stress scales* (2nd ed.). Sydney: Psychological Foundation of Australia.

Luborsky, L. (1984). *Principles of psychoanalytic psychotherapy: A manual for supportive-expressive treatment*. New York: Basic Books.

Luborsky, L., & DeRubeis, R. J. (1984). The use of psychotherapy treatment manuals: A small revolution in psychotherapy research style. *Clinical Psychology Review, 4*, 5–14.

Lumley, M. A., & Provenzano, K. M. (2003). Stress management through written emotional disclosure improves academic performance among college students with physical symptoms. *Journal of Educational Psychology, 95*, 641–649.

Lundy, B. L., Jones, N. A., Field, T., Nearing, G., Davalos, M., & Pietro, P. A. (1999). Prenatal depression effects on neonates. *Infant Behavior & Development, 22*, 119–129.

Lynch, T. R., & Cheavens, J. S. (in press). Dialectical behavior therapy for depression with co-morbid personality disorder: An extension of standard DBT with a special emphasis on the treatment of older adults. In L. A. Dimeff & K. Koerner (Eds.), *Real world adaptations of DBT*. New York: Guilford Press.

Lynch, T. R., & Cheavens, J. S. (2008). Dialectical Behavior Therapy for comorbid personality disorders. *Journal of Clinical Psychology: In Session, 64*, 154–167.

Mackrill, T. (2008). Solicited diary studies of psychotherapy in qualitative research – pros and cons. *European Journal of Psychotherapy, 10*, 5–18.

Maddi, S. R. (1980). *Personality theories: A comparative analysis* (4th ed.). Homewood, IL: The Dorsey Press.

Magura, S., Cleland, C., Vogel, H. S., Knight, E. L., & Laudet, A. B. (2007). Effects of "dual focus" mutual aid on self-efficacy for recovery and quality of life. *Administrative Policy on Mental Health Services Research, 34*, 1–12.

Magura, S., Knight, E. L., Vogel, H. S., Mahmood, D., Laudet, A. B., & Rosenblum, A. (2003). Mediators of effectiveness in dual-focus self-help groups. *The American Journal of Drug and Alcohol Abuse, 29*, 301–322.

Magura, S., Laudet, A. B., Mahmood, D., Rosenblum, A., Vogel, H. S., & Knight, E. L. (2003). Role of self-help processes in achieving abstinence among dually diagnosed persons. *Addictive Behaviors, 28*, 399–413.

Mahalik, J. R., & Kivlighan, D. M. (1988). Self-help treatment for depression: Who succeeds? *Journal of Counseling Psychology, 35*(3), 237–242.

Maheu, M. M., Pulier, M. L., Wilhelm, F. H., MacMenarim, J. P., & Brown-Connolly, N. E. (2005). *The mental health professional and the new technologies: A handbook for practice today*. Mahwah, NJ: Lawrence Erlbaum Associates.

Mains, J. A., & Scogin, F. R. (2003). The effectiveness of self-administered treatments: Apractice-friendly review of the research. *Journal of Clinical Psychology, 59*, 237–246.

Maino, E. (2004). Intimacy in couples: Evaluating a workbook. In L. L'Abate (Ed.). *Workbooks in prevention, psychotherapy, and rehabilitation: A resource for clinicians and researchers* (pp. 265–280). Binghamton, NY: Haworth.

Maino, E., Pasinato, S., Fara, D., Tampone, U., & Molteni, M. (2004). Couples with a handicapped child: Experiencing intimacy. In L. L'Abate (Ed.), *Workbooks in prevention, psychotherapy, and rehabilitation: A resource for clinicians and researchers* (pp. 327–347). Binghamton, NY: Haworth.

Malatesta, V. J. (1995, May). Technological behavior therapy for obsessive-compulsive disorder: The need for adequate case formulation. *Behavior Therapist, 2*, 88–89.

Malik, M. M., Beutler, L. E., Alimohamed, S., Galagher-Thompson, D., Thompson, L. (2003). Are all cognitive therapies alike? A comparison of cognitive and non-cognitive therapy process and implications for the application of empirically supported treatments. *Journal of Consulting and Clinical Psychology, 71*, 150–158.

Marcus, B. H., Williams, D. M., & Whitely, J. A. (2007). Self-help strategies for promoting and maintaining physical activity. In J. D. Latner & G. T. Wilson (Eds.), *Self-help approaches for obesity and eating disorders: Research and practice* (pp. 55–72). New York: Guilford.

Marks, T. M. (1991). Self-administered behavioural treatment. *Behavioural Psychotherapy, 19*, 42–46.

Marks, I. (2004). Psychiatry in the future. *Psychiatric Bulletin, 28*, 319–320.

Marks, I. M., Baer, L., Greist, J. H., Park, J., Bachofen, M., Nakagawa, A., et al. (1998). Home self–assessment of obsessive–compulsive disorder: Use of a manual and a computer–conducted telephone interview: Two U.K.-U.S. studies. *British Journal of Psychiatry, 172*, 406–412.

Marks, I. M., Cavanagh, K., & Gega, L. (2007). *Hands-on help: Computer-aided psychotherapy*. New York: Psychology Press.

Marks, I., Kenwright, M., McDonough, M., Whittaker, M., O'Brien, T., & Mataix-Cols, D. (2004). Saving clinicians' time by delegating routine aspects of therapy to a computer: A randomized controlled trial in panic/phobia disorder. *Psychological Medicine, 34*, 9–17.

Mars, R. W. (1995). A meta-analysis of bibliotherapy studies. *American Journal of Community Psychology, 23*, 843–870.

Martinez, R., Whitfield, G., Dafters, R., & Williams, C. (2008). Can people read self-help manuals for depression? A challenge for the stepped care model and book prescription schemes. *Behavioral and Cognitive Psychotherapy, 36*, 89–97.

Marx, L., & Mazlich, B. (Eds.). (2007). *A culture of improvement: Technology and the western millennium*. Cambridge, MA: MIT Press.

Masheb, R. M., & Grilo, C. M. (2008). Examination of predictors and moderators for self-help treatments of binge-eating disorder. *Journal of Consulting and Clinical Psychology, 76*, 900–904.

Mathews, A., Teasdale, J., Munby, M., Johnston, D., & Shaw, P. A. (1977). A home-based treatment program for agoraphobia. *Behavior Therapy, 8*, 915–924.

Maurin, J. G., & Boyd, C. B. (1990). Burden of mental illness on the family: A critical review. *Archives of Psychiatric Nursing, 4*, 99–107.

McCray, G. M. (1978). Excessive masturbation of childhood: A symptom of tactile deprivation? *Pediatrics, 62*, 277–279.

McFadden, L., Seidman, E., & Rappaport, J. (1992). A comparison of exposed theories of self-and mutual-help: Implications for mental health professionals. *Professional Psychology: Research and Practice, 23*, 515–520.

McGrady, A. (2007). Relaxation and meditation. In L. L'Abate (Ed.), *Low-cost approaches to promote physical and mental health: Theory, research, and practice* (pp. 161–176). New York: Springer.

McIntosh, V., Jordan, J. Carter, J. D., Latner, J. D., & Wallace, A. (2007). Appetite-focused cognitive-behavioral therapy for binge eating. In J. D. Latner & G. T. Wilson (Eds.), *Self-help approaches for obesity and eating disorders: Research and practice* (pp. 325–346). New York: Guilford.

McKay, M., Wood, J. C., & Brantley, J. (2007). *Dialectical behavior therapy workbook: Practical DBT exercises for learning mindfulness, interpersonal effectiveness, emotion regulation, and distress tolerance* (New Harbinger self-help workbook). Oakland, CA: New Harbinger Publications, Inc.

McKendree-Smith, N. L., Floyd, M., & Scogin, F. R. (2003). Self-administered treatments for depression: A review. *Journal of Clinical Psychology, 59,* 275–288.

McKinnon, R., & Yodofsky, C. (1986). *The psychiatric evaluation in clinical practice.* Philadelphia: Lippincott.

McMahan, O., & Arias, J. (2004). Workbooks and psychotherapy with incarcerated felons: Replication of research in progress. In L. L'Abate (Ed.), *Workbooks in prevention, psychotherapy, and rehabilitation: A resource for clinicians and researchers* (pp. 205–213). Binghamton, NY: Haworth.

McMurran, M., Egan, V., Richardson, C., & Ahmadi, S. (1999). Social Problem-Solving in mentally disordered offenders: A brief report. *Criminal Behavior and Mental Health, 9,* 315–322.

McMurran, M., Fyffe, S., McCarthy, L., Duggan, C., & Latham, A. (2001). "Stop & Think!" Social Problem-Solving therapy with personality disordered offenders. *Criminal Behavior and Mental Health, 11,* 273–285.

McNamee, G., O'Sullivan, G., Lelliott, P., & Marks, I. (1989). Telephone-guided treatment for housebound agoraphobics with panic disorder: Exposure vs.relaxation. *Behavior Therapy, 20,* 491–497.

McWilliams, N., & Weinberger, J. (2003). Psychodynamic psychotherapy. In G. Stricker and T. A. Widiger, (Eds.), *Handbook of psychology* (Vol. 8), *Clinical Psychology.* New York: John Wiley & Sons, Inc.

Mealey, L. (2000). *Sex differences: Developmental and evolutionary strategies.* New York: Academic Press.

Meehl, P. E. (1960). The cognitive activity of the clinician. *American Psychologist, 15,* 19–27.

Meichenbaum, D. (1996). *Stress inoculation training for coping with stressors. The Clinical Psychologist, 49,* 4–7.

Meichenbaum, D. (1994). *A clinical handbook/practical therapist manual for assessing and treating adults with post traumatic stress disorder.* Waterloo, Ontario: Institute Press.

Meichenbaum, D. (1985). *Stress Inoculation Training.* New York: Pergamon Press.

Meissen, G., Warren, M., Nansel, T., & Goodman, S. (2002). Self-help group leaders as community helpers: An impact assessment. *Journal of Rural Community Psychology, E5.*

Mellor, D., Davison, T., McCabe, M., George, K., Moore, K., & Ski, C. (2006). Satisfaction with general practitioner treatment of depression among residents of aged care facilities. *Journal of Aging and Health, 18,* 435–457.

Menchola, M., Arkowitz, H. S., & Burke, B. L. (2007). Efficacy of self-administered treatments for depression and anxiety. *Professional Psychology: Research and Practice, 38,* 421–429.

Meyer, D. (2007). Online self-help: Developing a student-focused website for depression. *Counseling and Psychotherapy Research, 7,* 151–156.

Miklowitz, D. J., Axelson, D. A., Birmaher, B., George, E. L., Taylor, D. O., Schneck, C. D., et al. (2008). Family-focused treatment for adolescents with bipolar disorder: Results of a 2-rear randomized trial. *Arch Gen Psychiatry. 65,* 1053–1061.

Miklowitz, D. J., Otto, M. W., Frank, E., Reilly-Harrington, N. A., Wisniewski, S. R., Kogan, J. N., et al. (2007). Psychosocial treatments for bipolar depression: A 1-year randomized trial from the systematic treatment enhancement program. *Archives of General Psychiatry, 64,* 419–427.

Miklowitz, D. J., Otto, M. W., Wisniewski, S. R., Araga, M., Frank, E., Reilly-Harrington, N. A., et al. (2006). Psychotherapy, symptom outcomes, and role functioning over one year among patients with bipolar disorder. *Psychiatric Services, 57*, 959–965.

Miller, A. L., Rathus, J. H., & Linehan, M. M. (2007). *Dialectical behaviour theraphy with suicidal adolescents*. New York: Guilford Press.

Miller, A. L., Rathus, J. H., & Linehan, M. M. Wetzler, S., & Leigh, E. (1997). Dialectical behaviour theraphy adapted for suicidal adolescents. *Journal of Practical Psychiatry & Behavioral Health, 3*, 78–86.

Milsom, V. A., Perri, M. G., & Rejeski, W. J. (2007). Guided group support and the long-term management of obesity. In J. D. Latner & G. T. Wilson (Eds.), *Self-help approaches for obesity and eating disorders: Research and practice* (pp. 205–222). New York: Guilford.

Minden, J. A., & Jason, L. A. (2002). Preventing chronic health problems. In L. A. Jason & D. S. Glenwick (Eds.), *Innovative strategies for promoting health and mental health across the life span* (pp. 227–243). New York: Springer.

Minderhoud, J. M., Boelens, M. E., Huizenga, J., & Saan, R. J. (1980). Treatment of minor head injuries. *Clinical Neurology and Neurosurgery, 82*, 127–140.

Miotto, P., de Coppi, M., Frezza, M., & Preti, A. (2003). Eating disorders and suicide risk factors in adolescents: An Italian community-based study. *Journal of Nervous & Mental Disease, 191*, 437–443.

Mitchell, B. A. (2006). *The boomerang age: Transitions to adulthood in families*. New Brunswick, NJ: Aldine.

Mittenberg, W., Canyock, E. M., Condit, D., & Patton, C. (2001). Treatment of post-concussion syndrome following mild head injury. *Journal of Clinical and Experimental Neuropsychology, 23*, 829–836.

Modestin, J., Abrecht, I., Tschaggelar, W., & Hoffman, H. (1997). Diagnosing borderline: A contribution to the question of its conceptual validity. *Archives Psychiatrica Nevenkra, 233*, 359–370.

Mohr, D. C., Vella, L., Hart, S., Heckman, T., & Simon, G. (2008). The effect of telephone-administered psychotherapy on symptoms of depression and attrition:A meta-analysis. *Clinical Psychology: Science and Practice, 15*, 243–253.

Mond, J. M., Marks, P., Hay, P. J., Rodgers, B., Kelly, C., Owen, C., et al. (2007). Mental Health literacy and eating-disordered behavior: Beliefs of adolescent girls concerning the treatment of and treatment-seeking for bulimia nervosa. *Journal of Youth and Adolescence, 36*, 753–762.

Moore, J. E., Von Korff, M., Cherkin, D., Saunders, K., & Lorig, K. (2000). A randomized trial of a cognitive-behavioral program for enhancing back pain self care in a primary care setting. *Pain, 88*, 145–153.

Moos, R., Finney, J., Ouimette, P. C., & Suchinsky, R. (1999). A comparative evaluation of substance abuse treatment: I. Treatment orientation, amount of care, and 1-year outcomes. *Alcoholism: Clinical and Experimental Research, 23*, 529–536.

Morgan, S. R. (1976). Bibliotherapy: A broader concept. *Journal of Clinical Child Psychology, 5*, 39.

Morgenstern, J., Labouvie, E., McCray, B. S., Kahler, C. W., & Frey, R. M. (1997). Affiliation with alcoholics anonymous after treatment: A study of its therapeutic effects and mechanisms of action. *Journal of Consulting and Clinical Psychology, 65*, 768–777.

Morley, S., Shapiro, D. A., & Biggs, J. (2004). Developing a treatment manual for attention management in chronic pain. *Cognitive Behavior Therapy, 33*, 1–11.

Morrison, T., Waller, G., Meyer, C., Burditt, E., et al. (2003). Social comparisons in eating disorders. *Journal of Nervous & Mental Disease, 191*, 553–555.

Moss, M. K., & Arend, R. A. (1977). Self-directed contact desensitization. *Journal of Consulting and Clinical Psychology, 45*, 730–738.

Moufakkir, O. (2006). An analysis of elderly gamers' trip characteristics and gambling behavior: Comparing the elderly with their younger counterparts. *UNLV Gaming Research and Review Journal, 10*, 63–75.

Mrazek, P. J., & Haggerty, R. J. (Eds.). (1994). *Reducing risks for mental disorders: Frontiers for preventive intervention research*. Washington, DC: National Academic Press.

Muehlenkamp, J. L. (2006). Empirically supported treatments and general therapy guidelines for non-suicidal self-injury. *Journal of Mental Health Counseling, 28*, 166–185.

Murray, L. (2006). *PDR for nonprescription drugs, dietary supplements, and herbs: The definitive guide to OTC medications*. Montvale, NJ: Thompson.

Musto, D. G. (1991). Opium, cocaine and marijuana in American history. *Scientific American, 265*, 40–47.

National Institute for Clinical Excellence (2004). *Clinical Guideline 23 Depression: Management of Depression in Primary and Secondary Care*. From http://guidance.nice.org.uk/page.aspx?.=236667

Nelson, J. N. (2008). Crying in psychotherapy: Its meaning, assessment, and management based on attachment theory. In A. Vingerhoets, I. Nyklicek, & J. Denollet (Eds.), *Emotional regulation: Conceptual and clinical issues* (pp. 202–214). New York: Springer

Nelson, E., Barnard, M., & Ermer, D. (2000). A comparison of two Tele-KidCare interventions (cognitive behavioral therapy or pharmacological treatment) to current community services for childhood depression. *Telemedicine Journal, 6*(1), 129.

Neufeldt, S. N., Iversen, J. N., & Juntenen, C. L. (1995). *Supervision strategies for the first practicum*. Alexandria, VA: American Counseling Association.

Neumann, J. K. (1981). Self-help depression treatment: An evaluation of an audio cassette program with hospitalized residents. *The Behavior Therapist, 4*, 15–16.

Newman, M. G. (2000). Recommendations for a cost offset model of psychotherapy allocation using generalized anxiety disorder as an example. *Journal of Consulting and Clinical Psychology, 68*, 549–555.

Newman, M. G., Erickson, T., Przeworski, A., & Dzus, E. (2003). Self-help and minimal contact therapies for anxiety disorders: Is human contact necessary for therapeutic efficacy? *Journal of Clinical Psychology, 59*, 251–274.

Nicholas, J., Oliver, K., Lee, K., & O'Brien, M. (2004). Help-seeking behaviour and the internet: An investigation among Australian adolescents. *Australian e-Journal for the Advancement of Mental Health, 3*, 1–8.

Nielsen, A. (2005). Gender pay gap is feminist fiction. *Independent Women's Forum*, April 15, 2005.

Nisbett, R., & Ross, L. (1980). *Human inference*. Englewood Cliffs, NJ: Prentice-Hall.

Nock, M. K., & Prinstein, M. J. (2004). A functional approach to the assessment of self-mutilative behavior. *Journal of Consulting and Clinical Psychology, 72*, 885–890.

Nock, M. K., & Prinstein, M. J. (2005). Contextual features and behavioral functions of self-mutilation among adolescents. *Journal of Abnormal Psychology, 114*, 140–146.

Nock, M. K., Joiner, T. E., Gordon, K., Lloyd-Richardson, E., & Prinstein, M. J. (2006). Non-suicidal self-injury among adolescents: Diagnostic correlates and relation to suicide attempts. *Psychiatry Research, 144*, 65–72.

Nock, M. K., Teper, R., & Hollander, M. (2007). Psychological treatment of self-injury among adolescents. *Journal of Clinical Psychology: In Session, 63*, 1081–1089.

Norcross, J. C. (2000). Here comes the self-help revolution in mental health. *Psychotherapy: Theory, Research, Practice, and Training, 37*, 370–377.

Norcross, J. C. (2006). Integrating self-help into psychotherapy: 16 practical suggestions. *Professional Psychology: Research and Practice, 37*, 683–693.

Norcross, J. C., & Prochaska, J. O. (1988). A study of eclectic (and integrative) views revisited. *Professional Psychology: Research and Practice, 19*, 170–174.

Norcross, J. C., & Prochaska, J. O. (1982). A national survey of clinical psychologists: views on training, career choice, and APA. *Clinical Psychologist, 35*, 1–6.

Norcross, J. C., Santrock, J. W., Campbell, L. F., Smith, T. S., Sommer, R., & Zuckerman, E. L. (2003). *Authoritative guide to self-help resources in mental health*. New York: Guilford Press.

Norcross, J. C., Santrock, J. W., Campbell, L. F., Smith, T. P., Sommer, R., & Zuckerman, E. L. (2000). *Authoritative guide to self-help resources in mental health*. New York: Guildford Press.

North, M. M., North, S. M., & and Coble, J. R. (1997). Virtual Reality Therapy: An effective treatment for the fear of public speaking, *International Journal of Virtual Reality, 3*, 2–8.

North, M. M., North, S. M., & Burwick, C. B. (2008). Virtual reality therapy: A vision for a new paradigm. In L. L'Abate (Ed.), *Toward a science of clinical psychology: Laboratory evaluations and interventions* (pp. 307–320). Hauppauge, NY: Nova Science.

Nowlin, N. S. (1983). Anorexia nervosa in twins: Case report and review. *Journal of Clinical Psychiatry, 44*, 101–105.

O'Brien, T. P., & Kelley, J. E. (1980). A comparison of self-directed and therapist-directed practice for fear reduction. *Behavior Research and Therapy, 18*, 573–579.

Ohman, A. (2000). Fear and anxiety: Evolutionary, cognitive, and clinical perspectives. In M. Lewis & J. M. Haviland-Jones (Eds.), *Handbook of emotions* (2nd ed., pp. 573–593). New York: Guilford Press.

Ohman, A. (1993). Fear and anxiety as emotional phenomena: Clinical phenomenology, evolutionary perspectives, and information-processing mechanisms. In M. Lewis & J. M. Haviland (Eds.), *Handbook of emotions* (pp. 511–536). New York: Guilford Press.

Oldridge, M. L., & Hughes, I. C. T. (1992). Psychological well-being in families with a member suffering from schizophrenia. *British Journal of Psychiatry, 161*, 249–251.

Ollendick, T. H., & King, N. J. (2006). Empirically supported treatments typically produce outcomes superior to non-empirically supported treatments. In J. C. Norcorss, L. E. Beutler, & R. F. Levant (Eds.), *Evidence-based practices in mental health: Debate and dialogue on the fundamental questions* (pp. 308–317). Washington, DC: American Psychological Association.

Oncken, C. A., & George, T. P. (2005). Tobacco. In H. R. Kranzler & D. A. Ciraulo (Eds.), *Clinical manual of addiction psychopharmacology*. Washington, DC: American Psychiatric Publishing.

Osgood-Hynes, D. J., Greist, J. H., Marks, I. M., Baer, L., Henemen, S. W., Wenzel, K. W. et al. (1998). Self-administered psychotherapy for depression using a telephone-accessed computer system plus booklets: An open U.S.-U.K. study. *Journal of Clinical Psychiatry, 59*, 358–365.

Öst, L. (1996). One-session group treatment of spider phobia. *Behavior Research and Therapy, 34*, 707–715.

Öst, L., Brandenberg, M., & Alm, T. (1997). One versus five sessions of exposure in the treatment of flying phobia. *Behaviour Research and Therapy, 35*, 987–996.

Öst, L., Ferebee, I., & Furmark, T. (1997). One session group therapy of spider phobia: Direct versus indirect treatments. *Behaviour Research and Therapy, 35*, 721–732.

Öst, L., Salkovskis, P. M., & Hellstrom, K. (1991). One session therapist-directedexposure versus self-exposure in the treatment of spider phobia. *Behavior Therapy, 22*, 407–422.

Öst, L., Stridh, B., & Wolf, M. (1998). A clinical study of spider phobia: Prediction of outcome after self-help and therapist-directed treatments. *Behaviour Research and Therapy, 36*, 17–35.

Öst, L., Hellstrom, K., & Kaver, A. (1992). One versus five sessions of exposure in the treatment of injection phobia. *Behavior Therapy, 23*, 263–282.

Palmer, R. L., Birchall, H., McGrain, L., & Sullivan, V. (2002). Self-help for bulimic disorders: A randomized controlled trial comparing minimal guidance with face-to-face or telephone guidance. *British Journal of Psychiatry, 18*, 230–235.

Patkar, A. A., Vergare, M. J., Batka, V., Weinstein, S. P., & Leone, F. T. (2003). Tobacco smoking: Current concepts in etiology and treatment. *Psychiatry, 66*, 183–199.

Parker, J., & Guest, D. (2002). The integration of psychotherapy in 12-step programs in sexual addiction treatment. In P. J. Carnes & K. M. Adams (Eds.), *Clinical management of sex addiction.* (pp. 115–124). New York: Brunner-Routledge.

Paul, G. (2007). Psychotherapy outcome can be studied scientifically. In S. O. Lilienfeld & W. T. O'Donohue (Eds.), *The great ideas of clinical science: 17 principles that every mental health professional should understand* (pp. 119–147). New York: Rutledge.

Pennebaker, J. W. (2001). Explorations into the health benefits of disclosure: Inhibitory, cognitive, and social processes. In L. L'Abate (Ed.), *Distance writing and computer-assisted interventions in psychiatry and mental health* (pp. 33–44). Westport, CT: Ablex.

Pennebaker, J. W., & Chung, C. K. (2007). Expressive writing, emotional upheavals, and health. In H. Friedman & B. Silver (Eds.), *Handbook of health psychology* (pp. 263–284). New York: Oxford University Press.

Pennebaker, J. W., & Francis, M. E. (1996). *Linguistic inquiry and work count: LIWC*. Mahawah, NJ: Erlbaum.

Persons, J. B. (1991). Psychotherapy outcome studies don't accurately represent current models of psychotherapy: A proposed remedy. *American Psychologist, 46*, 99–106.

Pesamaa, L., Ebeling, H., Kuusimäki, M-L., Winblad, I., Isohanni, M., & Moilanen, I. (2004) Videoconferencing in child and adolescent telepsychiatry: a systematic review of the literature. *Journal of Telemedicine and Telecare, 10*, 187–192.

Peters, M., Abu-Saad, H. H., Vydelingum, V., Dowson, A., & Murphy, M. (2004). Migraine and chronic daily headache management: A qualitative study of patient's perceptions. *Scandinavian Journal of Caring Science, 18*, 294–303.

Peterson, C. B., Mitchell, J. E., Engbloom, S., Nugent, S., Pederson Mussel, M., & Miller, J. (1998). Group cognitive-behavioral treatment of binge eating disorder: A comparison of therapist-led versus self-help formats. *International Journal of Eating Disorders, 24*, 125–136.

Peterson, C. B., Mitchell, J. E., Engbloom, S., Nugent, S., Mussell, M. P., Crow, S. J., et al. (2001). Self-help versus therapist-led group cognitive-behavioral treatment of binge eating disorder at follow-up. *International Journal of Eating Disorders, 30*, 363–374.

Petry, N. M. (2005). Terminology, prevalence rates, and types of gambling. In N. M. Petry (Ed.), *Pathological gambling: Etiology, comorbidity, and treatment*. (pp. 9–33). Washington, DC: Springer Publishing Co.

Pezzot-Pearce, T. O., LeBow, M. C., & Pearce, J. W. (1982). Increasing cost-effectiveness in obesity treatment through the use of self-help behavioral manuals and decreased therapist contact. *Journal of Consulting and Clinical Psychology, 50*, 448–449.

Phelan, T. W. (1996). *1-2-3 Magic: Effective discipline for children 2–12*. New York: Child Management, Inc.

Phillips, K. A., & Nierenberg, A. A. (1994). The assessment and treatment of refractory depression. *Journal of Clinical Psychiatry, 55*, 20–26.

Phillips, R. E., Johnson, G. D., & Geyer, A. (1972). Self-administered systematic desensitization. *Behavior Research and Therapy, 10*, 93–96.

Phipps, A., Edelman, S., Perkins, D., Barisic, M., Deane, F., & Gould, G. (2003). *The good mood guide: A self-help manual for depression*. Wollongong, NSW, Australia: Lifeline South Coast.

Poldrugo, F., & Forti, B. (1988). Personality disorders and alcoholism treatment outcome. *Drug and Alcohol Dependence, 21*, 171–176.

Polivy, J. (2007). The natural course and outcome of eating disorders and obesity. In H. Klingemann & L. C. Sobell (Eds.), *Promoting self-change from addictive behaviors: Practical implications for policy, prevention, and treatment* (pp. 119–126). New York: Springer.

Pool, R. (1994). *Eve's rib: Searching for the biological roots of sex differences*. New York: Crown Publishers.

Post, S. G. (Ed.). (2007). *Altruism & health: Perspectives from empirical research*. New York: Oxford University Press.

Potenza, M. N., & Griffiths, M. D. (2004). Prevention efforts and the role of the clinician. In J. E. Grant & M. N. Potenza (Eds.), *Pathological gambling: A clinical guide to treatment* (pp. 145–158). Washington, DC: American Psychiatric Publishing, Inc.

Potts, R. G. (1998). Spirituality, religion, and the experience of illness. In P. Camic & S. Knight (Eds.), *Clinical handbook of health psychology* (pp. 495–522). Seattle, WA: Hogrefe & Huber.

Prasad, V., & Owens, D. (2001). Using the internet as a source of self-help for people who self-harm. *Psychiatric Bulletin, 25*, 222–225.

President's New Freedom Commission on Mental Health (2003). *Achieving the promise: Transforming mental healthcare in America. Executive summary*. Rockville, MD: DHHS Publication No. SMA-03-3831.

Price, P. (2004). *The cyclothymia workbook: Learn how to manage your mood swings and lead a balanced life*. Oakland, CA: New Harbinger Publications.

Prochaska, J. O., & DiClemente, C. C. (1984). *The transtheoretical approach:crossing traditional boundaries of therapy*. Homewood, IL: Dow Jones-Irwin

Prochaska, J. O., DiClemente, C. C., & Norcross, J. C. (1992). In search of how people change. *American Psychologist, 47*, 1102–1104.

Proudfoot, J. G. (2004). Computer-based treatment for anxiety and depression: Is it feasible? Is it effective? *Neuroscience and Biobehavioral Reviews, 28*, 353–363.

Proudfoot, J. G., Goldberg, D., Mann, A., Everitt, B., Marks, I., & Gray, J. A. (2003). Computerized, interactive, multimedia cognitive-behavioural program for anxiety and depression in general practice. *Psychological Medicine, 33*, 217–227.

Puhl, R. M., & Brownell, K. D. (2007). Strategies for coping with the stigma of obesity. In J. D. Latner & G. T. Wilson (Eds.), *Self-help approaches for obesity and eating disorders: Research and practice* (pp. 347–362). New York: Guilford.

Pulier, M., Mount, T., McMenamin, J., & Maheu, M. (2007). Computers and the Internet. In L. L'Abate (Ed.), *Low-cost approaches to promote physical and mental health: Theory, research, and practice* (pp. 303–321). New York: Springer.

Rahman, Q., Andersson, D., & Govier, E., (2005). A specific sexual orientation-related difference in navigation strategy. *Behavioral Neuroscience, 119*, 311–316.

Ranew, L., & Serritella, D. A. (1992). Substance abuse and addiction. In L. L'Abate, J. A. Farrar, & D. A. Serritella (Eds.), *Handbook of differential treatments for addictions* (pp. 84–96). Boston: Allyn & Bacon.

Rapee, R. M. (1998). *Overcoming shyness and social phobia: A step-by-step guide*. Lifestyle Press.

Rapee, R. M., Abbott, M. J., Baillie, A., & Gaston, J. (2007). Treatment of social phobia through pure self-help and therapist-augmented self-help. *British Journal of Psychiatry, 191*, 246–252.

Rathus, J. H., & Miller, A. L. (2002). Dialectical behavior therapy adapted for suicidal adolescents. *Suicide and Life-Threatening Behavior, 32*, 146–157.

Raylu, N., Oei, T. P. S., & Loo, J. (2008). The current status and future direction of self-help treatments for problem gamblers. *Clinical Psychology Review, 28*, 1372–1385.

Reed, R., McMahan, O., & L'Abate, L. (2001). Workbooks and psychotherapy with incarcerated felons. In L. L'Abate (Ed.), *Distance writing and computer-assisted interventions in psychiatry and mental health* (pp. 157–167). Westport, CT: Ablex.

Rehm, L. P. (2008). How far have we come in teletherapy? Comment on "Telephone-Administered Psychotherapy". *Clinical Psychology: Science and Practice, 15*,259–261.

Relander, M., Troupp, H., & Bjorkesten, G. (1972). Controlled trial of treatment for cerebral concussion. *British Medical Journal, 4*, 777–779.

Rhodes, J. E. (1998). Family, friends, and community: The role of social support in promoting health. In P. Camic & S. Knight (Eds.), *Clinical handbook of health psychology* (pp. 481–493). Seattle, WA: Hogrefe & Huber.

Riper, H., Kramer, J., Smit, F., Conijn, B., Schippers, G., & Cuipers, P. (2007). Web- based self-help for problem drinkers: A pragmatic randomized trial. *Addiction, 103*, 218–227.

Ritchie, E. C., Watson, P. J., & Friedman, M. J. (2006). *Interventions following mass violence and disasters: Strategies for mental health practice*. New York: Guilford Press.

Ritterband, L. M., Cox, D. J., Walker, L. S., Kovatchev, B., McKnight, L., Patel, K., et al. (2003a). An internet intervention as adjunctive therapy for pediatric encopresis. *Journal of Consulting & Clinical Psychology, 71*, 910–917.

Ritterband, L. M., Gonder-Frederick, L. A., Cox, D. J., Clifton, A. D., West, R. W., & Borowitz, S. M. (2003b). Internet interventions: In review, in use, and into the future. *Professional Psychology: Research and Practice, 34*, 527–534.

Rivas-Vasquez, R. A. (2002). Current treatments for bipolar disorder: A review and update for psychologists. *Professional Psychology: Research and Practice, 33*, 212–233.

Robins, L. N. (1993). Vietnam veterans' rapid recovery from heroin addiction: A fluke or normal expectation? *Addiction, 88*, 1041–1054.

Robinson, L. A., Berman, J. S., & Neimeyer, R. A. (1990). Psychotherapy for the treatment of depression: A comprehensive review of controlled outcome research. *Psychological Bulletin, 108*, 30–49.

Roemer, L., Salter, K., Raffa, S. D., & Orsillo, S. M. (2005). Fear and avoidance of internal experience in GAD: Preliminary tests of a conceptual model. *Cognitive Therapy & Research, 29*, 71–88.

Rogers, C. R. (1951). *Client-centered Therapy: Its Current Practice, Implications and Theory.* Cambridge, MA: The Riverside Press.

Rohrmann, S., Hopp, H., & Quirin, M. (2008). Gender differences in psychophysiological responses to disgust. *Journal of Psychophysiology, 22,* 65–75.

Romero, C. (2008). Writing wrongs: Promoting forgiveness through expressive writing. *Journal of Social and Personal Relationships, 25,* 625–642.

Root, L. M., & McCullough, M. E. (2007). Low-cost interventions for promoting forgiveness. In L. L'Abate (Ed.), *Low-cost approaches to promote physical and mental health: Theory, research, and practice* (pp. 414–434). New York: Springer.

Rosen, G. M. (1987). SH treatment books and the commercialization of psychotherapy. *American Psychologist, 42,* 46–51.

Rosen, G. M., Berrera, M., Jr., & Glasgow, R. E. (2008). Good intentions are not enough: Reflections on past and future efforts to advance self-help. In P. L. Watkins & G. A. Clum (Eds.), *Handbook of self-help therapies* (pp. 25–39). Mahwah, NJ: Lawrence Erlbaum Associates.

Rosen, G. M., Glasgow, R. E., & Barrera, M., Jr. (1976). A controlled study to assess the clinical efficacy of totally self-administered systemic desensitization. *Journal of Consulting and Clinical Psychology, 44,* 208–217.

Rosen, G. M., Glasgow, R. E., & Moore, T. E. (2003). Self-help therapy: The science and business of giving psychology away. In S. O. Lillienfield & S. J. Lynn (Eds.), *Science and pseudoscience in clinical psychology* (pp. 399–424). New York: Guilford Press.

Rouget, P., Carrard, I., & Archinard, M. (2005). Self-treatment for bulimia on the internet:first results in Switzerland. *Revue Médicale Suisse, 1,* 359–361.

Rumpf, H. J., Bischof, G., & John, U. (2007). Remission without formal help: New directions in studies using survey data. In H. Klingemann & L. C. Sobell (Eds.), *Promoting self-change from addictive behaviors: Practical implications for policy, prevention, and treatment* (pp. 73–101). New York: Springer.

Safran, J. D., & Muran J. C. (2000). *Negotiating the therapeutic alliance: A relational treatment guide.* New York: Guilford Press.

Sajatovic, M. (2002). Treatment of bipolar disorder in older adults. *International Journal of Geriatric Psychiatry, 17,* 865–873.

Salerno, S. (2005). *SHAM: How the* self-help *movement made America helpless.* New York: Crown.

Salmon, M. P. (2001). Effects of physical exercise on anxiety, depression, and sensitivity to stress. *Clinical Psychology Review, 21,* 33–61.

Salzer, M. S., Rappaport, J., & Segre, L. (2001). Mental health professionals' support of self-help groups. *Journal of Community & Applied Social Psychology, 11,* 1–10.

Sanders, A. K., Blanchard, E. G., & Sykes, M. A. (2007). Preliminary study of a self-administered treatment for irritable bowel syndrome: Comparison to a wait list control group. *Applied Psychophysiological Biofeedback, 32,* 111–119.

Sarafino, F. P. (1994). *Health psychology: Biosocial interventions.* New York: Wiley.

Sarason, I. G., Levine, H. M., Basham, R. B., & Sarason, B. R. (1983). Assessing social support: The Social Support Questionnaire. *Journal of Personality and Social Psychology, 44,* 127–139.

Savin, D., Garry, M. T., Zuccaro, P., & Novins, D. (2006). Telepsychiatry for treating rural American Indian youth. *Journal of the Academy of Child and Adolescent Psychiatry, 45,* 484–488.

Schare, M. L., & Konstas, D. D. (2008). Self-help therapies for cigarette smoking cessation. In P. L. Watkins & G. A. Clum (Eds.), *Handbook of self-help therapies* (pp. 267–287). Mahwah, NJ: Erlbaum.

Scheel, K. R. (2000). The empirical basis of Dialectical Behavior Therapy: Summary, critique, and implications. *Clinical Psychology: Science and Practice, 7,* 68–86.

Schlafly, P. (2003). *Feminist fantasies.* Dallas: Spencer Publishing Company.

Schmidt, U., & Grover, M. (2007). Computer-based intervention for bulimia nervosa and binge eating. In J. D. Latner & G. T. Wilson (Eds.), *Self-help approaches for obesity and eating disorders: Research and practice* (pp. 166–176). New York: Guilford.

Schmitz, J. M., & Delaune, K. A. (2005). Nicotine. In J. H. Lowinson, P. Ruiz, R. B. Millman, & J. G. Langrod (Eds.), *Substance abuse: A comprehensive textbook* (4th ed.), New York: Lippincott, Williams, & Wilkins.

Schneider, J. P. (2004). Understanding and diagnosing sex addiction. In R. H. Coombs (Ed.), *Handbook of addictive disorders: A practical guide to diagnosis and treatment* (pp. 197–232). Hoboken, NJ: John Wiley & Sons, Inc.

Schneider, K. (1923). *Die psychopathischen personlichkeiten*. Berlin, Germany: Springer.

Schoenberg, M. R., Ruwe, W. D., Dawson, K., McDonald, N. B., Houston, B., & Forducey, P. G. (2008). Comparison of functional outcomes and treatment cost between a computer-based cognitive rehabilitation teletherapy program and a face-to-face rehabilitation program. *Professional Psychology: Research and Practice, 39*, 169–175.

Schopp, L., Johnstone, B., & Merrell, D. (2000). Telehealth and neuropsychological assessment: New opportunities for psychologists. *Professional Psychology: Research and Practice, 31*, 179–183.

Schuckit, M. A. (2006). *Drug and alcohol abuse: A clinical guide to diagnosis and treatment* (6th ed.). New York: Springer.

Schuckit, M. A. (2005). Alcohol related disorders. In B. J. Sadock & V. A. Sadock (Eds.), *Comprehensive textbook of psychiatry* 8th ed.). Baltimore: Williams & Wilkins.

Schulte, D., Kunzel, R., Pepping, G., & Schulte-Bahrenberg, T. (1992). Tailor-made versus standardized therapy of phobic patients. *Advances in Behaviour Research and Therapy, 14*, 67–92.

Schultz, S. K. (2007). Depression in the older adult: The challenge of medical co-morbidity. *American Journal of Psychiatry, 164*, 847–848.

Schwartz, C. (2007). Altruism and subjective well-being: Conceptual model and empirical support. In S. G. Post (Ed.), *Altruism and health: Perspectives from empirical research* (pp. 33–42). New York: Oxford University Press.

Schwartz, M. F., & Southern, S. (2000). Compulsive cybersex: The new tea room. *Sexual Addiction & Compulsivity, 7*, 127–144.

Scogin, F. R. (2003). Introduction: The status of self-administered treatments. *Journal of Clinical Psychology, 59*, 247–249.

Scogin, F. R., Bynum, J., Stephens, G., & Calhoon, S. (1990). Efficacy of self-administered treatment programs: Meta-analytic review. *Professional Psychology: Research and Practice, 1*, 42–47.

Scogin, F. R., Floyd, M., Jamison, C., Ackerson, J., Landreville, P., & Bissonnette, L. (1996). Negative outcomes: What is the evidence on self-administered treatments? *Journal of Consulting and Clinical Psychology, 64*(5), 1086–1089.

Scogin, F., Hamblin, D., & Beutler, L. (1987). Bibliotherapy for depressed older adults: A self-help alternative. *The Gerontologist, 27*, 383–387.

Scogin, F. R., Hanson, A., & Welsh, D. (2003). Self-administered treatment stepped-caremodels of depression treatment. *Journal of Clinical Psychology, 59*, 341–349.

Scogin, F., Jamison, C., & Gochneaur, K. (1989). Comparative efficacy of cognitive and behavioral bibliotherapy for mildly and moderately depressed older adults.*Journal of Consulting and Clinical Psychology, 57*, 403–407.

Seale, C., Zieband, S., & Charteris-Black, J. (2006). Gender, cancer experience, and internet use: A comparative keyword analysis of interviews and online cancer support groups. *Social Science and Medicine, 62*, 2577–2590.

Segal, S. P. (2005). Self-help mental health agencies. In S. A. Kirk (Ed.), *Mental disorders in the social environment: Critical perspectives* (pp. 201–213). New York: Columbia University Press.

Segal, S. P., Gomory, T., & Silverman, C. J. (1998). Health status of homeless and marginally housed users of mental health self-help agencies. *Health & Social Work, 23*, 45–52.

Segal, Z. V., Williams, M. G., & Teasdale, J. D. (2002). *Mindfulness-based cognitive therapy for depression: A new approach to preventing relapse*. New York: Guilford Press.

Seivewright, H., Tyrer, P., & Johnson, T. (2002). Change in personality status in neurotic disorders. *The Lancet, 359*, 2253–2254.

Seivewright, H., Tyrer, P., & Johnson, T. (2004). Persistent social dysfunction in anxious and depressed patients with personality disorder. *Acta Psychiatrica Scandinavica, 109*, 104–109.

Seivewright, H., Tyrer, P., Ferguson, B., Murphy, S., North, B., & Johnson, T. (2000). Longitudinal study of the influence of life events and personality status on diagnostic change in three neurotic disorders. *Depression and Anxiety, 11*, 105–113.

Seligman, M. E. P., Steen, T. A., Park, N., & Peterson, C. (2005). Positive psychology progress: Empirical validation of approaches. *American Psychologist, 60*, 410–421.

Selmi, P. M., Klein, M. H., Greist, J. H., Sorrell, S. P., & Erdman, H. P. (1990). Computer-administered cognitive-behavioral therapy for depression. *American Journal of Psychiatry, 147*, 51–56.

Sentell, T. L., & Skumway, M. A. (2003). Low literacy and mental illness in a nationally representative sample. *Journal of Nervous & Mental Disease, 191*, 459–552.

Serritella, D. A. (1992a). Domestic violence as addiction. In L. L'Abate, J. A. Farrar, & D. A. Serritella (Eds.), *Handbook of differential treatments for addictions* (pp. 113–122). Boston: Allyn & Bacon.

Serritella, D. A. (1992b). Tobacco addiction. In L. L'Abate, J. A. Farrar, & D. A. Serritella (Eds.), *Handbook of differential treatments for addictions* (pp. 97–112). Boston: Allyn & Bacon.

Shadish, W. R., Matt, G. E., Navarro, A. M., & Phillips, G. (2000). The effects of psychological therapies under clinically representative conditions: A meta-analysis. *Psychological Bulletin, 126*, 512–529.

Shaffer, H. J. (2007). Considering the unimaginable: Challenges to accepting self-change or natural recovery from addition. In H. Klingemann & L. C. Sobell (Eds.), *Promoting self-change from addictive behaviors: Practical implications for policy, prevention, and treatment* (pp. ix–xiii). New York: Springer.

Shaked, N. (2005). Psychology self-help books: A comprehensive analysis and content evaluation. *Dissertation Abstract International, Section A. Humanities and Social Science, 66*, No. 895.

Shaw, A., Thompson, E. A., & Sharp, D. J. (2006). Expectations of patients and parents of patients with asthma regarding access to complementary therapy information and services via the NHS: A qualitative study. *Health Expectations, 9*, 343–358.

Shaw, B. F. (1983, July). *Training therapists for the treatment of depression: Collaborative study*. Paper presented at the meeting for the Society for Psychotherapy Research, Sheffield, England.

Shea, M. T., & Yen, S. (2003). Stability as a distinction between Axis I and Axis II disorders. *Journal of Personality Disorders, 17*, 373–386

Shechtman, Z. (1999). Bibliotherapy: An indirect approach to treatment of childhood aggression. *Child Psychiatry & Human Development, 30*, 39–53.

Sias, P. M., & Bartoo, H. (2007). Friendship, social support, and health. In L. L'Abate (Ed.), *Low-cost approaches to promote physical and mental health: Theory, research, and practice* (pp. 455–471). New York: Springer.

Silverman, W. H. (1996). Cookbooks, manuals, and paint-by-numbers: Psychotherapy in the 90's. *Psychotherapy, 33*, 207–215.

Singh, H. (2003). Building effective blended learning programs. *Educational Technology, 43*, 51–54.

Skodol, A. E., Gunderson, J. G., Shea, M. T., McGlashan, T. H., Morey, L. C., Sanislow, C. A., et al. (2005). The collaborative longitudinal personality disorders study (CLPS): Overview and implications. *Journal of Personality Disorders, 19*, 487–504.

Skodol, A. E., Pagano, M. E., Bender, D. S., Shea, M. T., Gunderson, J. G., Yen, S., et al. (2005). Stability of functional impairment in patients with schizotypal, borderline, avoidant, or obsessive-compulsive personality disorder over two years. *Psychological Medicine, 35*, 443–451.

Skultety, K. M., & Zeiss, A. (2006). The treatment of depression in older adults in the primary care setting: An evidence-based review. *Health Psychology, 25*, 665–674.

Smart, R. G. (2007). Natural recovery or recovery without treatment from alcohol and drug problems as seen from survey data. In H. Klingemann & L. C. Sobell (Eds.), *Promoting self-change
from addictive behaviors: Practical implications for policy, prevention, and treatment* (pp.
59–71). New York: Springer.

Smith, A. W., & Baum, A. (2003). The influence of psychological factors or restorative function
in health and illness. In J. Suls & K. A. Wallston (Eds.), *Social psychological foundations of
health and illness* (pp. 432–457). Malden, MA: Blackwell.

Smith, K. L., Kirkby, K. C., Montgomery, I. M., & Daniels, B. A. (1997). Computer-delivered
modeling of exposure for spider phobia: Relevant versus irrelevant exposure. *Journal of Anxiety
Disorders, 11*, 489–497.

Smyth, J., & Helm, R. (2003). Focused expressive writing as self-help for stress and trauma.
Journal of Clinical Psychology/In Session: Psychotherapy in Practice, 59, 227–235.

Smyth, J. M., & L'Abate, L. (2001). A meta-analytic evaluation of workbook effectiveness in
physical and mental health. In L. L'Abate (Ed.), *Distance writing and computer-assisted
interventions in psychiatry and mental health* (pp. 77–90). Westport, CT: Ablex.

Smyth, J. M., Nazatian, D., & Arigo, D. (2008). Expressive writing in the clinical conterxt. In
A. Vingerhoets, I. Nyklicek, & J. Denollet(Eds.), *Emotional regulation: Conceptual and
clinical issues* (pp. 215–233). New York: Springer.

Snowdon, D. (2001). *Aging with grace: What the nun study teaches us about leading longer,
healthier, and more meaningful lives.* New York: Bantam Books.

Snyder, C. R., & Ingram, R. E. (2000). (Eds.). *Handbook of psychological change: Psychotherapy
processes & practice for the 21st century.* New York: Wiley.

Sobell, L. C. (2007 not 2008). The phenomenon of self-change: Overview and key issues. In
H. Klingemann & L. C. Sobell (Eds.), *Promoting self-change from addictive behav-
iors: Practical implications for policy, prevention, andtreatment* (pp. 1–30). New York:
Springer.

Sobell, L. C., & Sobell, M. B. (2007). Promoting self-change; Taking the treatment to the community. In H. Klingemann & L. C. Sobell (Eds.), *Promoting self-change from addictive behaviors: Practical implications for policy, prevention, and treatment* (pp. 163–186). New York:
Springer.

Sobell, M. B. (2007). One way to leave your lover: The role of treatment in changing addictive
behaviors. In H. Klingemann & L. C. Sobell (Eds.), *Promoting self-change from addictive
behaviors: Practical implications for policy, prevention, and treatment* (pp. 151–162). New
York: Springer.

Solano, L., Bonadies, M., & Di Trani, M. (2008). Writing for all, for some or for no one? Some
thoughts on the applications and evaluations of the writing technique. In A. Vingerhoets,
I. Nyklicek, & J. Denollet (Eds.), *Emotional regulation: Conceptual and clinical issues*
(pp. 234–246). New York: Springer.

Solano, L., Bonadies, M., & Di Trani, M. (2008). Writing for all, for some or for no one? Some
thoughts on the applications and evaluations of the writing technique. In A. Vingerhoets,
I. Nyklicek, & J. Denollet (Eds.), *Emotional regulation: Conceptual and clinical issues*
(pp. 234–246). New York: Springer.

Sommers, C. H. (2000). *The war against boys: How misguided feminism is harming our young
men.* New York: Simon & Schuster.

Sommers, C. H. (1995). *Who stole feminism?: How women have betrayed women.* New York:
Simon & Schuster.

Spanos, N. P. (1996). *Multiple identities and false memories: A sociocognitive perspective.*
Washington, DC: American Psychological Association.

Sperry, L., Hoffman, L., Cox, R. H., & Cox, B. E. (2007). Spirituality. In L. L'Abate (Ed.),
Low-cost approaches to promote physical and mental health: Theory, research, and practice
(pp. 435–451). New York: Springer.

Spielberger, C. D., Gorsuch, R. L., Lushene, R. E. (1970). *STAI manual for the state-trait anxiety
inventory.* Palo Alto: Consulting Psychologist Press.

Stant, A. D., Ten Vergert, E. M., den Boer, P. C. A. M., & Wiersma, D. (2008). Cost-effectiveness of cognitive self-therapy in participants with depression and anxiety disorders. *Acta Psychiatrica Scandinavica, 117*, 57–66.

Stathopoulous, G., Powers, M. B., Berry, A. C., Smits, A. J., & Otto, M. W. (2006). Exercise interventions for mental health: A quantitative and qualitative review. *Clinical Psychology Science and Practice, 13*, 179–193.

Stefano, S. C., Bacaltchuk, J., Blay, S. L., & Hay, P. (2006). Self-help treatments for disorders of recurrent binge eating: A systematic review. *Acta Psychiatrica Scandinavia, 113*, 452–459.

Stegge, H., & Terwogt, M. M. (2007). Awareness and regulation of emotion in typical and atypical development. In J. J. Gross (Ed.), *Handbook of emotion regulation* (pp. 269–286). New York: Guilford Press.

Stein, M. B., Walker, J. R., & Forde, D. R. (2000). Gender differences in susceptibility to posttraumatic stress disorder. *Behavior Research and Therapy, 38*, 619–628.

Stevens, A., Dionne, E., & Dwyer, J. (2007). Popular and fad diet programs: Nutritional adequacy, safety, and efficacy. In J. D. Latner & G. T. Wilson (Eds.), *Self-help approaches for obesity and eating disorders: Research and practice* (pp. 21–52). New York: Guilford.

Stice, E., Marti, C., Spoor, S., Presnell, K., & Shaw, H. (2008). Dissonance and healthy weight eating disorder prevention programs: Long-term effects from a randomized efficacy trial. *Journal of Consulting and Clinical Psychology, 76*(2), 329–340.

Stone, M. H., Hurt, S. W., & Stone, D. K. (1987). The PI 500: Long-term follow-up of borderline personality disorder in-patients meeting DSM-III criteria: 1.Global Outcome. *Journal of Personality Disorders, 1*, 291–298.

Strom, L., Pettersson, R., & Andersson, G. (2000). A controlled trial of self-help treatment of recurrent headache conducted via the internet. *Journal of consulting and Clinical Psychology, 68*, 722–727.

Strupp, H. H., & Anderson, T. (1997). On the limitations of therapy manuals. *Clinical Psychology: Science and Practice, 4*, 76–82.

Sutzke, T., Aitken, L., & Stout, C. (1997). Maximizing treatment outcome in managedcare: A useful technological adjunct. *The Independent Practitioner, 17*, 27–29.

Sysko, R., & Walsh, B. T. (2007). Guided self-help for bulimia nervosa. In J. D. Latner & G. T. Wilson (Eds.), *Self-help approaches for obesity and eating disorders: Research and practice* (pp. 92–117). New York: Guilford.

Takala, J. P. (2007). Spontaneous distance from crime. In H. Klingemann & L. C. Sobell (Eds.), *Promoting self-change from addictive behaviors: Practical implications for policy, prevention, and treatment* (pp. 127–137). New York: Springer.

Tavris, C., & Aronson, E. (2007). *Mistakes were made (but not by me): Why we justify foolish beliefs, bad decisions, and hurtful acts*. New York: Harcourt.

Taylor, C. B., & Jones, M. (2007). Internet-based prevention and treatment of obesity and body-dissatisfaction. In J. D. Latner & G. T. Wilson (Eds.), *Self-help approaches for obesity and eating disorders: Research and practice* (pp. 141–165). New York: Guilford.

Thaler, R., & Sunstein, C. R. (2008). *Nudge: Improving decisions about health, wealth, and happiness*. New York: Caravan Books.

Thiels, C., Laireiter, A. R., & Baumann, U. (2002). Diaries in clinical psychology and psychotherapy: A selective review. *Clinical Psychology and Psychotherapy, 9*, 1–37.

Thiels, C., Phil, M., Schmidt, U., Treasure, J., Garthe, R., & Troop, N. (1998). Guided self-change for bulimia nervosa incorporation use of a self-care manual. *American Journal of Psychiatry, 155*, 947–953.

Thiels, C., Schmidt, U., Troop, N., Treasure, J., & Garthe, R. (2000). Binge frequency predicts outcome in guided self-care treatment of bulimia nervosa. *European Eating Disorders Review, 8*, 272–278.

Tillfors, M., Carlbring, P., Furmark, T., Lewenhaupt, S., Spak, M., Eriksson, A., et al. (2008). Treating university students with social phobia and public speaking fears: Internet delivered self-help with or without live group exposure sessions. *Depression and Anxiety, 25*, 708–717.

Titov, N., Gavin, A., & Schwencke, G. (2008). Shyness 2: Treating social phobia over the Internet: Replication and extension. *Australian & New Zealand Journal of Psychiatry, 42,* 595–605.

Titov, N., Gavin, A., Schwencke, G., Probny, J., & Einstein, D. (2008). Shyness 1: Distance treatment of social phobia over the internet. *Australian & New Zealand Journal of Psychiatry, 42,* 585–594.

Tolin, D. F., & Foa, E. B. (2006). Sex differences in trauma and posttraumatic stress disorder: A quantitative review of 25 years of research. *Psychological Bulletin, 132,* 959–992.

Toneatto, T., & Nett, J. C. (2007). Natural recovery from problem gambling. In H. Klingemann & L. C. Sobell (Eds.), *Promoting self-change from addictive behaviors: Practical implications for policy, prevention, and treatment* (pp. 113–118). New York: Springer.

Toro, P. A., Rappaport, J., & Seidman, E. (1987). Social climate comparison of mutual help and psychotherapy groups. *Journal of Consulting and Clinical Psychology, 55,* 430–431.

Townsend, D., Nicholson, R. A., Buenaver, L., Bush, F., & Gramling, S. (2001). Use of a habit reversal treatment for temporomandibular pain in minimal therapist contact format. *Journal of Behavior Therapy and Experimental Psychiatry, 32,* 221–239.

Tsai, A. G., & Wadden, T. A. (2007). Commercial and organized self-help programs for weight management. In J. D. Latner & G. T. Wilson (Eds.), *Self-help approaches for obesity and eating disorders: Research and practice* (pp. 179–204). New York: Guilford.

Tsai, A. G., Thomas, A. W., Womble, L. G., & Byrne, K. J. (2005). Commercial and self-help programs for weight control. *Psychiatric Clinics of North America, 28,* 171–192.

Turpin, G., Downs, M., & Mason, S. (2005). Effectiveness of providing self-help information following acute traumatic injury: Randomized controlled trial. *British Journal of Psychiatry, 187,* 76–82.

Tuschen-Caffier, B., Pook, M., & Frank, M. (2001). Evaluation of manual-based cognitive-behavioral therapy for bulimia nervosa in a service setting. *Behavior Research and Therapy, 39,* 299–308.

Tyrer, P. (2005). Temporal change: The third dimension of personality disorders. *Journal of Personality Disorders, 19,* 573–580

Tyrer, P., Seivewright, N., Ferguson, B., Murphy, S., & Johnson, A. L. (1993). The Nottingham study of neurotic disorder: Effect of personality status on response to drug treatment, cognitive therapy, and self-help over two years. *British Journal of Psychiatry, 162,* 219–226.

Umhau, J. C., & Dauphinais, K. M. (2007). Omega-3 polyunsaturated fatty acids and health. In L. L'Abate (Ed.). *Low-cost approaches to promote physical and mental health: Theory, research, and practice* (pp. 87–101). New York: Springer.

U.S. Department of Commerce (2002). *A nation online: How Americans are expanding their use of the internet.* Washington, DC: Government Printing Office.

US Department of Health and Human Services (1999). *Mental Health: A report of the Surgeon General.* Rockville, MD: Center for Mental Health Services, National Institutes of Mental Health.

van Bastelaar, K. M. P., Pouwer, F., Cuijpers, P., Twisk, J. W. R., & Snoek, F. J. (2008). Web-based cognitive-behavioural therapy (W-CBT) for diabetes patients with co-morbid depression: Design of a randomized controlled trial. *Bio Med Central Psychiatry, 8,* prepublication—page numbers currently unavailable.

van Boeijen, C. A., van Balkom A. J. L. M., van Oppen, P., Blankenstein, N., Cherpanath, A., & van Dyck, R. (2005). Efficacy of self-help manuals for anxiety disorders in primary care: A systematic review. *Family Practice, 22,* 192–196.

Van Den Berg, S., Shapiro, D. A., Bickerstaffe, D., & Cavanagh, K. (2004). Computerized cognitive-behaviour therapy for anxiety and depression: A practical solution to the shortage of trained therapists. *Journal of Psychiatric and Mental Health Nursing, 11,* 508–513.

van Straten, A., Cuijpers, P., & Smits, N. (2008). Effectiveness of a web-based self-help intervention for symptoms of depression, anxiety, and stress: Randomized controlled trial. *Journal of Medical Internet Research, 10,* 1–12.

Vangelisti, A. L. (2009). *Sourcebook of hurt feelings in close relationships*. New York: Cambridge University Press.

Vangelisti, A. L., & Beck, G. (2007). Intimacy and fear of intimacy. In L. L'Abate (Ed.), *Low-cost approaches to promote physical and mental health: Theory, research, and practice* (pp. 395–414). New York: Springer.

Vermilvea, E. G. (2000). *Growing beyond survival: A self-help toolkit for managing traumatic stress*. Baltimore: Sidran Press.

Vincent, N., Walker, J. R., & Katz, A. (2008). Self-administered therapies in primary care. In P. L. Watkins & G. A. Clum (Eds.), *Handbook of self-help therapies* (pp. 387–417). Mahwah, NJ: Erlbaum.

Vingerhoets, A., Nyklicek, I., & Denollet, J. (Eds.). (2008) *Emotional regulation: Conceptual and clinical issues*. New York: Springer.

Vinnars, B., Barbar, J. P., Noren, K, Gallop, R., & Weinryb, R. M. (2005). Manualized supportive-expressive psychotherapy versus nonmanualized community-delivered psychodynamic therapy for patients with personality disorders: Bridging efficacy and effectiveness. *American Journal of Psychiatry, 162*, 1933–1940.

Voluse, A., Korkel, J., & Sobell, L. C. (2007). Self-change toolbox: Tools, tips, websites, and other informational resources for assessing and promoting self-change. In H. Klingemann & L. C. Sobell (Eds.), *Promoting self-change from addictive behaviors: Practical implications for policy, prevention, and treatment* (pp. 239–255). New York: Springer.

Von Korff, M., Moore, J. E., Lorig, K., Cherkin, D. C., Saunders, K., Gonzalez, V. M., et al. (1998). A randomized trial of a layperson-led self-management group intervention for back pain patients in primary care. *Spine, 23*, 2608–2615.

Wade, W. A., Treat, T. A., & Stuart, G. L. (1998). Transporting an empirically supporting treatment for panic disorder to a service clinic setting: A benchmarking strategy. *Journal of Consulting and Clinical Psychology, 66*, 231–239.

Wakefield, P. J., Williams, R. E., Yost, E. B., & Patterson, K. M. (1996). *Couple therapy for alcoholism: A cognitive-behavioral treatment manual*. New York: Guilford Press.

Walsh, R., & Shapiro, S. L. (2006). The meeting of meditative disciplines and western psychology: A mutually enriching dialogue. *American Psychologist, 61*, 227–239.

Watkins, P. L. (2008). Self-help therapies. In P. L. Watkins & G. A. Clum (Eds.), *Handbook of self-help therapies* (pp. 1–24). Mahwah, NJ: Lawrence Erlbaum Associates.

Watkins, P. L., & Clum, & G. A. (Eds.). (2008). *Handbook of self-help therapies*. Mahwah, NJ: Erlbaum.

Webpsych. (2009). *InnerLife*. A proprietary software program.

Weeks, G., & L'Abate, L. (1982). *Paradoxical psychotherapy: Theory and practice with individuals, couples, and families*. New York: Brunner/Mazel.

Weise, C., Heinecke, K., & Rief, W. (2008). Biofeedback-based behavioral treatment for chronic tinnitus: Results of a randomized controlled trial. *Journal of Consulting and Clinical Psychology, 76*, 1046–1057.

Weissman, M., Markowitz, J., & Klerman, G. L. (2000). *Comprehensive guide to interpersonal psychotherapy*. New York: Basic Books.

Weissman, M., Markowitz, J., & Klerman, G. L. (2007). *Clinician's quick guide to interpersonal psychotherapy*. New York: Oxford University Press.

Wells, A., Garvin, V., Dohm, F.-A., & Striegel-Moore, R. (1996). Telephone-based guided self-help for binge eating disorder: A feasibility study. *International Journal of Eating Disorders, 21*, 341–346.

West, D. M., Gore, S. A., & Lueders, N. K. (2007). Behavioral obesity treatment translated. In J. D. Latner & G. T. Wilson (Eds.), *Self-help approaches for obesity and eating disorders: Research and practice* (pp. 243–264). New York: Guilford Press.

Westen, D. (2000). The efficacy of dialectical behavior therapy for borderline personality disorder. *Clinical Psychology: Science and Practice, 7*, 92–94.

Westen, D., Dutra, L., & Schedler, J. (2005). Assessing adolescent personality pathology. *British Journal of Psychiatry, 186*, 227–238.

Westin, D., Novotny, C. M., & Thompson-Brenner, H. (2004). The empirical status of empirically supported psychotherapies: Assumptions, findings, and reporting in controlled clinical trials. *Psychological Bulletin, 130*, 631–663.

White, J. (1995). Stresspac: A controlled trial of a self-help package for the anxiety disorders. *Behavioral Cognitive Psychotherapy, 23*, 89–107.

WHOQoL Group (1998). Development of the World Health Organization WHOQoL-BREF Quality of Life Assessment. *Psychological Medicine, 28*, 551–558.

Widiger, T. A., & Frances, A. J. (1989). Epidemiology, diagnosis, and comorbidity of borderline personality disorder. In A. Tasman, R. E. Hales, & A. J. Frances (Eds.), *American psychiatric press review of psychiatry* (Vol. 8, pp. 8–24). Washington, DC: American Psychiatric Press.

Widiger, T. A., & Weissman, M. M. (1991). Epidemiology of borderline personality disorder. *Hospital and Community Psychiatry, 42*, 1015–1021.

Wiens, S., & Ohman, A. (2007). Probing unconscious emotional processes: On becoming a successful masketeer. In J. A. Coan & J. B. Allen (Eds.), *Handbook of emotion elicitation and assessment* (pp. 65–90). New York: Oxford University Press.

Wiersma, D., De Jong, A., & Ormel, J. (1988). The Groningen Social Disabilities Schedule: Development, Relationship with I.C.I.D.H., and Psychometric Properties. *International Journal of Rehabilitation Research, 11*, 213–224.

Wildman, R. W. (1992). Gambling. In L. L'Abate, J. A. Farrar, & D. A. Serritella (Eds.), *Handbook of differential treatments for addictions* (pp. 211–229). Boston: Allyn & Bacon.

Williams, C. (2003). New technologies in self-help: Another way to get better? *European Eating Disorders Review, 11*, 170–182.

Williams, J. M. G., Teasdale, J. D., Segal, Z. V., & Kabat-Zinn, J. (2007). *The mindful way through depression: Freeing yourself from chronic unhappiness*. New York: Guilford Press.

Wilson, G. T. (1996). Manual-based treatments: The clinical application of research findings. *Behavior Research and Therapy, 34*, 295–314.

Wilson, C. C., & Turner, D. C. (Eds.). (1998). *Companion animals in human health* (pp. 61–90). Thousand Oaks, CA: Sage.

Winder, C. L. (1957). Psychotherapy. *Annual Review of Psychology, 8*, 309–310.

Winett, R. A., Tate, D. E., Anderson, E. S., Wojcik, J. R., & Winett, S. G. (2008). Preventing weight gain with internet programs. In P. L. Watkins & G. A. Clum (Eds.), *Handbook of self-help therapies* (pp. 325–353). Mahwah, NJ: Erlbaum.

Winfield, H. R., & Harvey, E. J. (1993). Determinants of psychological distress in relatives of people with chronic schizophrenia. *Schizophrenia Bulletin, 19*, 619–626.

Winzelberg, A., Luce, K. H., & Taylor, C. B. (2008). Self-help therapies for eating disorders. In P. L. Watkins & G. A. Clum (Eds.), *Handbook of self-help therapies* (pp. 163–185). Mahwah, NJ: Erlbaum.

Wisdom, J. P., & Baker, E. C. (2006). Getting out of depression: Teens' self-help interventions to relieve depressive symptoms. *Child & Family Behavior Therapy, 28*, 1–11.

Wollert, R. W., Knight, B., & Levy, L. H. (1980). Make today count: A collaborative model for professionals and self-help groups. *Professional Psychology, 11*, 130–138.

Woody, S. R., & Sanderson, W. C. (1998). Manuals for empirically supported treatments: 1998 update. *The Clinical Psychologist, 51*, 17–21.

Wright, J., Clum, G. A., Roodman, A., & Febbraro, G. A. M. (2000). A bibliotherapy approach to relapse prevention in individuals with panic attacks. *Journal of Anxiety Disorders, 14*, 483–499.

Yeaton, W. H. (1994). The development and assessment of valid measures of service delivery to enhance inference in out-come based research: Measuring attendance in self-help group meetings. *Journal of Consulting and Clinical Psychology, 62*, 686–694.

Yeung, B. (2008). Succor, succor in the court. *Miller-McCune: Turning Research into Solutions*, August, 61–69.

Young, A. S., Chinman, M., Forquer, S. L., Knight, E. L., Vogel, H., Miller, A., et al. (2005). Use of a consumer-led intervention to improve provider competencies. *Psychiatric Services, 56*, 967–975.

Young, B. H., Ruzek, J. I., Wong, M., Salzer, M. S., & Naturale, A. J. (2006). Disaster mental health training: Guidelines, considerations, and recommendations (54–79). In E. C. Ritchie, P. J. Watson, & M. J. Friedman (Eds.), *Interventions following mass-violence and disasters: Strategies for mental health practice* (54–79). New York: Guilford Press.

Zanarini, M. C., Frankenburg, F. R., Dubo, E. D., Sickel, A. E., Trikha, A., Levin, A., et al. (1998). The Axis I comorbidity of borderline personality disorder. *American Journal of Psychiatry, 155*, 1733–1739.

Zanarini, M. C., Frankenburg, F. R., Hennen, J., & Silk, K. R. (2004). Mental health service utilization by borderline personality disorder patients and Axis II comparison subjects followed prospectively for 6 years. *Journal of Clinical Psychiatry, 65*, 28–36.

Zanarini, M. C., Frankenburg, F. R., Khera, G. S., & Bleichmar, J. (2001). Treatment histories of borderline patients. *Comprehensive Psychiatry, 42*, 144–150.

Zuckerman, E. (2003). Finding, evaluating, and incorporating internet self-help resources into psychotherapy practice. *Journal of Clinical Psychology, 59*, 217–225.

Index